ANNALS OF THE NEW YORK ACADEMY OF SCIENCES

Volume 315

BRAIN DEATH:
INTERRELATED MEDICAL AND SOCIAL ISSUES

Edited by Julius Korein

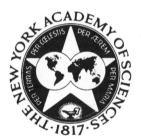

The New York Academy of Sciences
New York, New York
1978

Library of Congress Cataloging in Publication Data

Main entry under title:

Brain death.

(Annals of the New York Academy of Sciences; v. 315)
1. Brain death—Congresses. 2. Coma—Congresses. 3. Death—Proof and cer-
tification—Congresses. I. Korein, Julius. II. Series: New York Academy of Sciences.
Annals; v. 315. [DNLM: 1. Brain death—Congresses. W1 AN626YL v. 315 / W820
B814 1977]
Q11.N5 vol. 315 [RA1063.3] 508'.1s [616.8'04'7]

78–24423

PCP
Printed in the United States of America

ISBN 0–89072–073–8

BRAIN DEATH:
INTERRELATED MEDICAL AND SOCIAL ISSUES

ANNALS OF THE NEW YORK ACADEMY OF SCIENCES

VOLUME 315

November 17, 1978

BRAIN DEATH: INTERRELATED MEDICAL AND SOCIAL ISSUES *

Editor and Conference Chairman
JULIUS KOREIN

Conference Cochairmen
J. FEIN AND K. YOUNGSTEIN

CONTENTS

---

* This series of papers is the result of a conference entitled Brain Death held
on November 16, 17, and 18, 1977 by The New York Academy of Sciences and
cosponsored by the New York Blood Center, Inc.

Financial assistance was received from:

- THE COMMONWEALTH FUND
- HOFFMANN-LA ROCHE, INC.
- THE HENRY J. KAISER FAMILY FOUNDATION
- MERCK SHARP & DOHME POSTGRADUATE PROGRAM
- NICOLET INSTRUMENT CORPORATION
- SANDOZ, INC.
- ANNE WEISENTHAL

PREFACE

Julius Korein

Department of Neurology
New York University Medical Center; and the
EEG Laboratories, Bellevue Hospital Center
New York, New York 10016

The meaning and diversified usage of the term *death* have been a major preoccupation of mankind. In my early training in medicine, I encountered this problem and formed a philosophy which I expressed in a poem that ended with the line, "Death is the closing of an eye of God." Discourse on the *concept* of death has been, in the past, primarily relegated to philosophers, theologians and creative individuals in the fine arts. In contrast, rather than dealing primarily with the concept of death, medical science seeks *criteria* to define and diagnose the death of an individual. The advent of new discoveries and applications of modern medicine has allowed life to be prolonged. Life-support systems have been developed that may temporarily replace many vital functions such as those of the cardiac, respiratory and renal systems. Organ transplantation has become a mode of therapy. Increased knowledge has been derived about the significance of the brain in relation to the functioning of an individual. All these are among the many factors that have led to a recrudescence of interest in the problem of death. Scientific exploration designed to restate the "classical" definition of death by the development of criteria of death to include brain death has had a marked impact on society. Both concepts and criteria are being re-evaluated by all social strata, including the legislative and judicial sectors of different governments. It is not surprising that the extensive changes in our thinking about meaning and usage of the term *death* over the past two decades have led to confusion and disagreement.

There are, therefore, multiple purposes to this volume on brain death and associated problems. It is most important to define, delineate, and present pragmatic criteria which will allow the physician to reliably make the diagnosis of death of an individual when his brain is dead. Implicit in this determination is the relationship of the problem to society in general, the meaning of the concepts of life and death, as well as the ability of medical science to develop criteria in order to differentiate brain death from other diagnostic entities. The confusion that has been evident in the field of medicine itself includes the linguistic limitations of ambiguous terminology that has been often transmitted to and amplified by the legal profession, philosophy, the news media and the public in general.

There are a variety of specific nontrivial biologic and nosological problems that must be dealt with, and these have been compounded on occasion by gross distortion and misunderstanding. It is paramount, therefore, that terminology be used as precisely as possible to clarify these issues. Currently, in 18 states legislation has been passed defining death either in terms of irreversible cessation of spontaneous respiratory and cardiac function (i.e., the "classical" definition of death) or, if these functions are maintained artificially, in terms of irreversible (total) brain destruction. Either of the above definitions are equally acceptable for the pronouncement of death in these states. The necessity for having such

1

general alternate statutes to pronounce death in every state is reflected by the consensus of contributors to this volume.

It should be made unmistakably clear that the alternative definition of brain death does not replace the classical definition of death but only adds another set of criteria that may be used in the pronouncement of death under highly specified conditions. These conditions exist in the intensive care unit (ICU), for example, where the technology and specialized personnel for resuscitation, monitoring, and maintenance of life-support systems are available. Furthermore, the reader must be aware that these laws do *not* represent an intrinsic concept that there are two different kinds of death, in that brain death is actually central to both sets of criteria. If an individual suffers irreversible total circulatory and respiratory failure, death of the brain inevitably follows immediately, certainly within a few minutes if not seconds. It is only with the advent of modern medical advances used in the ICU that we face the relatively infrequent situation in which the brain dies before other systems that are maintained by life-support and resuscitation technology. Therefore, both definitions are actually predicated on an implicit *concept* of brain death. The reader must again note that the *concept* of brain death is different from the *criteria* which the physician uses for the diagnosis of brain death.

Part I of this volume defines and introduces the evolution of the multifaceted problems of human death generally and brain death specifically in the context of medicine and society. Medical problems are primarily dealt with in Part II, which is divided into several subsections. The clinical and laboratory criteria of brain death are presented and discussed as well as aspects relating to brain metabolism. Problems relating to electroencephalography, intracranial blood flow, and studies on survival after anoxia are also examined. The clinical and laboratory criteria discussed are those that have been developed and frequently used by many independent practitioners and investigators to determine the diagnosis of brain death. The presentation by Ingvar *et al.* stresses other forms of irreversible noncognitive states (the apallic syndrome) which clearly do not meet the criteria of brain death. In the papers and discussions in and after Part II, the problems of terminology, criteria and the differentiation of patients who are "brain-dead" are contrasted with those of a complex group of patients who may also be in an irreversible coma.

Posner's admirable attempt to clarify and differentiate the medical diagnosis of brain death from other forms of altered states of consciousness along with the subsequent discussion forms Part III. This presentation on coma and other altered states of consciousness including brain death may be read to obtain an overall orientation of the medical problems. Although there is a continuous attempt to clarify the terminology used throughout this volume, the tabular grouping of definitions is dealt with succinctly in Part III.

The papers in Part IV detail additional ancillary studies that have been used to confirm the diagnosis of brain death as well as the neuropathologic findings that may relate to such diagnoses. These ancillary studies may be of great value in the diagnosis of a specific patient. The presentation by Milhaud relating to a prolonged test for apnea using oxygen serves to accentuate the wide variety of tests for apnea which have proven difficult to standardize. The problems and limitations of tests for apnea are discussed in other parts of this volume. Of major significance is the conclusion that neuropathologic examination of the brain per se does not necessarily correlate with the clinical criteria of brain death; gross and histologic examination of the brain using current techniques of light microscopy will only reveal a characteristic picture of autolysis and destruction of the brain many hours after intracranial circulation has ceased.

In Part V, prognosis and prediction of quality of survival is presented for both children and adults who are in comatose states. This section is clearly not primarily involved with brain death. Rather, it is a discussion of those forms of prolonged altered states of consciousness which include persistent vegetative states, other chronic comas, and noncognitive states. Many of these syndromes represent irreversible situations such as previously described by Ingvar *et al.* in Part II, i.e., the apallic syndrome. They all must be clearly distinguished and separated, by means of appropriate medical criteria, from brain death. Naturally, it is most essential to establish adequate criteria for patients in reversible states where cognition may return. Although there are advocates (such as Veatch in Part VI) who would consider the *concept* of brain death to include *cognitive death*, the public and the medical community are not yet generally prepared to accept the approach that these individuals should be considered dead. The status of these patients in irreversible noncognitive states is similar to that of the viable anencephalic monster and raises associated tangential problems relating to extraordinary care, ethics, morality and the economics of utilization of medical resources. Beyond this, even after one clearly distinguishes these sets of medical problems (i.e., persistent vegetative states) from brain death, still other tangential issues automatically arise that relate to the rights of the individual and the terminally ill patient. Rather than avoid these topics, they are introduced as separate issues and should not be confused with the issues relating to brain death. The conflicting views about these groups of patients are therefore presented primarily by members of the nonmedical fields of law and ethics in subsequent sections. The medical management of these patients, especially those in prolonged coma or other forms of altered states of consciousness, is the secondary major problem with which this volume concerns itself. These patients represent an unresolved, poorly defined group of neurologic disorders which will require further extensive research, social evaluation, and legislative consideration. This is a situation that will become more pressing as time goes on. This tenuous, less well-defined group of patients who cannot be termed brain-dead by existing criteria but who are in a prolonged irreversible noncognitive state accentuates the futility of what may be considered "extraordinary care," including repeated and unwarranted resuscitation and prolonged treatment. Management of such patients is emotionally ungratifying to their physicians, nurses, family and society at large; they also represent an increasing economic burden in application of both medical and fiscal resources. It is this rather distasteful problem that must be explored in even greater detail.

Before proceeding to a discussion of other parts of this volume, it should be noted that a major set of medical criteria of brain death and associated problems has been dealt with and elaborated upon. We can expect that the criteria for brain death will be further refined in relation to clinical problems such as the test for apnea and laboratory verification. The latter includes portable tests for intracranial circulation and electrophysiologic or other forms of testing of brain-stem function. It would appear in the light of current technology that we already have the capability of establishing a set of clinical and laboratory criteria that is essentially fail-safe in allowing the physician to diagnose brain death. There may be a potential error in misdiagnosing a patient as being "alive" who is in fact dead, but this is entirely acceptable. From the wealth of experience of the contributors to this volume, it appears virtually certain that once an adult patient is brain-dead (including meeting the criterion of absent intracranial circulation), the conventional criteria of death (e.g., irreversible cardiac arrest) will be met within a week. Therefore, the diagnosis of brain death and the diagnosis of death without utilization of special criteria may be unequivocally established by using time as the arbiter.

The limitations of any single clinical or laboratory test have been dealt with in detail as have situations such as drug intoxication, which may give misleading information in the use of a specific criterion. However, it is the composite clinical and laboratory picture, including the history of the patient, that allows the physician to make the final and appropriate diagnosis. No single test can be allowed to replace the clinical judgment of the physician who, in the face of uncertainty, may allow further time to pass and repeat his examination until there is no doubt of the diagnosis. Other medical problems associated with the diagnosis of brain death include those of organ transplantation and will be discussed in the final section of this volume.

This Preface will be followed by a list of terms and their definitions as they have been used in the past and are currently being used in this volume. Ambiguities and overlapping meanings will be noted. Editorial comments will be made throughout this volume in an attempt to clarify the authors' use of terminology. The reader should refer to this list of definitions if there are any questions as to the usage of terminology in the text and in my presentation on brain death in Part I. For example, the term *brain death* will be considered to involve irreversible destruction of the contents of the intracranial cavity down to the first cervical spinal cord segment. This therefore includes the cerebral hemispheres, the brain stem, and the cerebellum. Although the terms *brain death* and *cerebral death* have most often been used synonymously in the past and at times in this volume, the need to avoid such overlapping usage with more strictly defined terms will become apparent to the reader. We will attempt to avoid this confusion and consider cerebral death as indicating irreversible destruction of both cerebral hemispheres alone. The term *systemic death* indicates irreversible cardiorespiratory dysfunction. Brain-stem death per se will not be considered as brain death. The problems related to permanent loss of cognition with or without arousal and terms such as persistent vegetative states, apallic syndrome, and other noncognitive states are also more fully discussed in Part V.

Part VI deals with philosophical, ethical, social, and religious factors and stresses the *concept* rather than the *criteria* of brain death. Proponents who wish to consider an individual who is in an irreversible noncognitive state as being dead should attend especially to Veatch's presentation. Although cogent arguments are presented as to why the term brain death should not be used, sufficient pragmatic criteria, if not concepts, have been developed to enable the physician to make this diagnosis. Carse's penetrating insight into the causes underlying the role medicine plays in society is dramatic, interesting, and relevent and I would recommend that every physician read his paper. Finally, Hauerwas, in his own inimitable style, clearly gives a rational approach to the religious concepts of brain death and associated problems. The discussions of these three papers often reflect the confusion between concepts and criteria relating to brain death.

Legislative problems relating to brain death, other irreversible states, and the rights of the individual are presented in Part VII, and the apparent conflicting views relating to law, philosophy, and medicine are in many ways reflected in the attempts to develop appropriate legislative structures. Beresford continues the discussion of cognitive death, while Capron continues elucidation of the legal definition of death (see also his paper in Part I). Horan gives a strict definition of brain death in relation to the classical definition as opposed to any other forms of cognitive death using currently established criteria. He cautions against extension of the concepts to criteria that will allow a patient in an irreversible, noncognitive state to be considered as dead, in contrast to Veatch's position. Finally, Assemblyman Keene describes the success and limitations of the Natural Death Act in California after it has been in effect for one year. The compromises and modifications of the initial version of this Act will give the reader an idea of how difficult it is to enact such a bill into law and implement it so that it becomes effective in terms of the individuals who require its use. This type of law may stand at the center of a controversy. There are situations where legislation is limited but serves a purpose and is to be preferred to none. There are, however, other examples of proposed legislation that are so restricting and limited, in their definition of brain death, for example, that it would be preferable to have no legislation whatsoever if the choice is given. This is illustrated by Rabbi Tendler's proposition in Part VIII for a law on brain death which includes specified criteria. This last section also concludes with clinical problems relating to intensive care units, discussed by Suter, and organ transplantation, discussed by Veith. Part VIII also includes a final discussion by Milhaud with some details on the legal and medical aspects of organ transplantation in France.

It is hoped that this volume will allow the reader to comprehend the enormity of the problem, the potential sources of confusion and ambiguity. This may allow him to select those portions that will clarify both the conceptual and utilitarian aspects of brain death so that they may be used in a meaningful and pragmatic manner. Guides and direction for future research abound in this volume, and it is interesting to contemplate what changes will evolve in the construct of brain death and associated problems over the next decade.

I would like to acknowledge the aid of The New York Academy of Sciences as well as that of the Cochairmen, Dr. J. Fein and Mr. K. Youngstein and those participants who chaired the individual sessions of the Conference on Brain Death: Drs. F. Plum, R. Veatch, R. Beresford, and Mr. A. Capron. In addition, I wish to acknowledge Ms. P. Kronhaus's efforts in assisting me in organizing this volume and the Conference from which it was derived. I also wish to thank the Editorial Staff of The New York Academy of Sciences, and especially Mrs. J. Cullinan, for their skillful editorial assistance.

TERMINOLOGY, DEFINITIONS, AND USAGE

CONSTRUCT

An object, perception or idea that is systematically put together in a orderly manner from components, facts or impressions. Note that a construct may range from highly philosophical concepts such as "truth" or "good" to actual perceptions and observations of material objects such as "chair" or "city." Both concepts and criteria can be considered constructs.

CONCEPT

A concept is an idea or set of thoughts pertaining to a class of objects or processes. The concept of death represents an idea about what death is, such as "the soul leaving the body." Concepts must not be confused with criteria, as defined below. Concepts may be used, but are not necessarily required to develop criteria. (See especially the paper by Veatch.)

CRITERIA

Criteria are a set of standards against which observations are compared to allow the individual to make a judgment. For example, one of the criteria for death is total unresponsiveness. Based on this criterion, the presence of unresponsiveness is determined by observations and tests which will allow a judgment to be made (along with the use of other criteria) as to whether the individual is dead. The use of criteria represents an operational activity in order to come to a decision about a situation. The reader should keep in mind the confusion that exists in parts of this volume, between concept and criteria especially in the discussions.

DEATH

The classical definition of death of a human being is related to the criteria used, i.e., those used by a physician, which identifies this state. Inherent in the definition is that the state is irreversible and there is the implicit assumption that it occurs at a specific moment. Most often, these criteria are defined in terms of cessation of vital functions. These include loss of cardiorespiratory and neural functions. Criteria for determining such loss are the absence of heart beat, blood pressure, breathing, motor activity and total unresponsivity. Other criteria have been suggested to confirm the diagnosis with greater certainty, including the onset of rigor mortis and even putrefaction, but most practitioners of medicine and law would accept the above as adequate for the pronouncement of death. Other terms that may be used synonymously with the definition of death include systemic death and the commonlaw definition of death (see Capron, Part I). Death has also been considered a process (see Korein, Part I). It is the thesis of many of the contributors to this volume that brain death be considered equivalent to death of an individual.

6

0077-8923/78/0315-006 $01.75/0 © 1978, NYAS

BRAIN DEATH

Brain death is defined as irreversible destruction of the neuronal contents of the intracranial cavity. This includes both cerebral hemispheres, including cortex and deep structures, as well as the brain stem and the cerebellum. An equivalent term is *total brain infarction* to the first cervical level of the spinal cord. The criteria for determining brain death will be the subject of many papers in this volume. In order to develop appropriate criteria to diagnose brain death, it is not required that every neuron in the brain be destroyed. Rather, it implies that the extent of destruction and consequent irreversible neuronal dysfunction is so great that regardless of any supportive measures, irreversible cardiac arrest and death of the adult human being is inevitable within one week. Death of the human being (as previously defined) and brain death ultimately mean that all neuronal structures in the brain will die. The two definitions conceptually define death in the same manner, that is, death of the brain. However, the criteria used by a physician to arrive at the diagnosis of death in contrast to brain death differ. These derived diagnoses are equivalent, both representing the death of an individual.

CEREBRAL DEATH

Strictly speaking, cerebral death is defined as irreversible destruction of both cerebral hemispheres exclusive of the brain stem and cerebellum. However, cerebral death has been and is often still being used as a synonym for brain death. In most situations criteria for determining "cerebral death" may include components of brain-stem function, for example, apnea. In such situations the progression from cerebral death to total brain death is often frequent and complete. Rarely, clinical situations arise, however, in which the cerebral hemispheres alone may be involved in the destructive process, but the brain stem is spared. These exceptions may lead to a chronic comatose or noncognitive state which must be considered as another diagnostic category, to be defined below. Therefore the use of "cerebral death" as a synonym for "brain death" is not generally advocated. To avoid confusion an attempt will be made to identify the manner in which the term *cerebral death* is used and whether or not it is being used as a synonym for brain death.

COMA DÉPASSÉ

Coma dépassé is a term originally used by a school of French neurophysiologists in 1959. The term referred to patients who were in unresponsive coma, are apneic, and who have had no electrophysiologic activity in deep or superficial structures of the cerebrum. In 1970 the additional criterion of absence of intracranial blood flow was included to define coma dépassé. Thus, in effect, if *all* these criteria are met the term, which has been translated to mean ultra coma or beyond coma (and on several occasions was unfortunately translated to mean irreversible coma), may be used as equivalent to brain death as defined above.

BRAIN-STEM DEATH

There are several groups of investigators and clinicians who have considered irreversible destruction of brain-stem structures with absent brain-stem function per se as equivalent to death of the human being. Patients in this state, however, may have evidence of electroencephalographic activity and cerebral circulation, and therefore are generally not considered as meeting the criteria for brain death. Such patients may eventually become brain-dead or persist for a prolonged period in a comatose state if given appropriate supportive measures.

NEOCORTICAL DEATH

This term has been used to describe the destruction of cortical neurons bilaterally while deep structures of the cerebral hemispheres such as the thalamus and basal ganglia may be intact along with the brain stem and cerebellum. Other intracranial structures may be involved to a varying degree, however. Such patients infrequently may present a problem in the differential diagnosis of brain death. They most often, however, have a limited to complex repertoire of brain-stem reflexes, which clearly distinguishes them from patients with other conditions. The term apallic syndrome may be considered as essentially similar to neocortical death, although some investigators contest this (see the article by Ingvar *et al.*).

UNRESPONSIVE COMA

The deepest state of coma, where the patient usually has no response to external stimuli and no spontaneous movements. Such patients may, however, have spinal reflex responses such as withdrawal of a leg to painful stimuli and/or deep tendon reflexes in the extremities (see the article by Allen *et al.*).

PERSISTENT VEGETATIVE OR NONCOGNITIVE STATES

These terms are clinical descriptors of a set of irreversible states. The pathologic substrate involving neural structures is not always clearly definable. Attempts at classifying these syndromes neuropathologically are represented by the terms *neocortical death* and *apallic syndrome*. The lack of precision of this terminology is reflected by the multiplicity of neuropathologic lesions found in the brains of patients in persistent noncognitive states. For example, they may have severe bilateral cortical destruction, or bilateral involvement of deep structures of the cerebrum including the thalamus and basal ganglia. Such patients may also have involvement of the ascending reticular formation of the brain stem. Often they have combinations of lesions in many of these and other loci.

The clinical picture reflects the destruction of critical elements of the central nervous system, leaving the patient in an irreversible condition in which there is no evidence that he or she has any sense of awareness. Higher functions of the brain are absent, and there is no purposeful response to external stimuli. Some investigators and clinicians differentiate those patients who have absent awareness but may be *aroused*. Arousability may be either clinical (e.g., eye-opening or other complex reflex activity in response to noxious stimuli) or physiologic (e.g., alteration of EEG pattern in response to external stimuli). Arousability per se does not necessarily imply cognitive function or sense of awareness, but suggests some residual function of the ascending reticular formation. The patient is not a sentient individual.

These patients do have vegetative function which includes a large variety of simple and complex reflex patterns. These may be limited to pupillary reflex to light or spontaneous respirations, but may range to highly complex stereotyped patterned behavior such as decerebration, yawning and other high-level brain-stem reflexes. Other terms that have been used to describe this state are coma vigil and akinetic mutism. The surviving anencephalic monster may be considered in a state analogous to that of these patients. These patients are *not* brain-dead. If appropriate resuscitative procedures are utilized, these patients may be maintained in this state for many years.

Problems with such patients are detailed in the papers by Ingvar *et al.*, Posner, Levy *et al.*, Beresford, and other contributors to this volume. The variation of usage of these terms must be critically evaluated by the reader.

APALLIC SYNDROME

The syndrome resulting from absence or destruction of the pallium, that is, the neocortical structures of the cerebrum. This term has its major usage in attempting to give one localization for the complex clinical picture of persistent noncongitive state. However, in most of these patients, the anatomic state of destruction may include deep structures of the cerebral hemispheres as well as portions of the cerebellum and brain stem. (See also the definitions of neocortical death and persistent vegetative or noncognitive states.)

IRREVERSIBLE COMA

This term is an umbrella which covers a variety of irreversible states, for example, brain death, cerebral death, and persistent noncognitive states. Unfortunately, it has also been used as an exclusive synonym with brain death and cerebral death. This usage is erroneous and leads to confusion. Therefore, it is suggested that this term only be used with qualification.

RESPIRATOR BRAIN

The presumed end point of brain destruction as defined pathologically in a patient who is brain-dead and maintained on a respirator and complete life-support adjuncts. The difficulty in use of this term and its relationship with autolysis of brain structures are discussed more completely in the papers by Pearson *et al.* and Walker. The main difficulty in most definitions is that they do not include the relationship to cessation of intracranial circulation. It appears that the pathologic process may occur up to 20 hours after cessation of intracranial blood flow. Neuropathologic examination of the brain prior to this time may therefore be misleading.

APNEA

Apnea is the inability of an individual to breathe spontaneously. The problem with the criteria arises once the patient is placed on respiratory support. There is a large variety of tests to determine whether the patient can, in fact, regain spontaneous respiration if he does not simply override the respirator. Limitations, problems and difficulties in obtaining a straightforward, simple definition of apnea are discussed in various parts of this volume, such as in the article by Posner. The paper by Milhaud *et al.* especially represents one extreme view of defining apnea.

CEPHALIC REFLEXES

Cephalic reflexes are those requiring intact brain-stem structures. Most significant are those involving pupillary reaction to light and extraocular movements (oculocephalic and vestibular reflexes). This is most clearly explained in the paper by Allen *et al.* These are vegetative phenomena as opposed to cognitive function.

SPINAL REFLEXES

Spinal reflexes are those requiring intact spinal structures. Since brain death may occur with a viable spinal cord present, the presence of spinal reflexes does not militate against the diagnosis of brain death.

—Julius Korein

DEATH: HISTORICAL EVOLUTION AND IMPLICATION OF THE CONCEPT

Benjamin Boshes

Department of Neurology
Northwestern University Medical School
Chicago, Illinois 60611

For primitive man death was a mystery, an absence of life that he looked upon with a mixture of fear, fascination and superstition all the while he sought to alter it by ritual dances and incantations. At first death suggested deep sleep, but finally early man began to regard it as a transition from one life to another, and burial became a rite of passage. He prepared the body, and inhumation, a practice known only to man, became part of the ritual. The paleolithic people not only interred their dead but also provided them with food and other equipment, implying the belief that the dead have needs in the next life.

These early customs would suggest that man refused to accept death as the definitive end of life and insisted that something of the individual continued to survive the dying experience. The concept of a personal extinction through death was unknown until the sixth century B.C., when it appeared in the metaphysical thinking of Indian Buddhism. This did not find expression in the Western world until the time of the Greek philosopher, Epicurus, in the third century B.C.

The mortuary rituals and funeral customs reflected the culture from which they were derived. Some provided tools, ornaments and food; others covered the corpse with red ochre, the color of blood, to revitalize the dead one. The corpse was sometimes placed in the fetal crouch, interpreted by some as evidence of the belief in rebirth. Yet other cultures bound the limbs tightly in this position, implying a fear that the dead might return to do harm. The Greeks and the Romans believed that the dead must cross a barrier dividing the world of the living from that of the dead, the river Styx, across which the boatman, Charon, carried the corpse in whose mouth a coin was placed to pay for the trip. Many groups describe bridges of death, a crossing, and the nineteenth-century poem "Crossing the Bar" by Lord Tennyson continues the idea.

The concept of resurrection of the dead is found in the eschatologies of the various ancient cultures, but nowhere is the preparation more clearly demonstrated than in the practices in ancient Egypt. Here the body was put through an elaborate mortuary ritual which included mummification to preserve the corpse from disintegration. In pursuit of eternity, the pharaohs planned and built tombs within great pyramids and into the chambers came the best furniture, jewelry, tools and pictures of the deceased and his family. Perhaps the greatest Egyptian treasure of all was the tomb of Tutankhamun, built around 1400 B.C. and luxurious in funerary equipment.

The Egyptians were not alone. In Peru and in China tombs were found with life-prolonging substances such as jade placed in the orifices of the corpse, substances alleged to have life-prolonging properties. Crosses or crucifixes were laid on the Christian dead and sometimes in the Middle Ages the consecrated bread of the Eucharist was buried with the body. If the dead were a priest, he

11

0077–8923/78/0315–0011 $01.75/0 © 1978, NYAS

might be buried with a chalice and a paten, the instruments of his office. Death and funerary rites have always commanded sacred consideration because there is the sense that the dead must be prepared for their next experience.

Inhumation or burial was the most general method of disposal throughout the ages. To some it symbolized a return to the womb of Mother Earth; to others it served to remind: "For dust thou art, and unto dust thou shall return." Sometimes the body was laid directly on the earth with or without clothes. The use of coffins dates back to 3000 B.C. in Egypt. Later, in the Christian era, these sculptured containers gave much information about the attitude toward death. The Egyptian pyramids began to appear about 3000 B.C. and through the ages have been followed by such structures as the Taj Mahal in India and the mausoleum for Lenin in Red Square in Moscow. The importance of the tomb as a place of existence for the dead became so great that in some even toilet facilities were added. Because of the belief that the dead were actually living in the structures, some burial sites were converted into shrines where thousands came to seek miracles of healing or to earn religious merit.

The ritual of burial required that the deceased be brought to a place of burial or cremation. The ancient Egyptians carried the embalmed body on a sledge, accompanied by mourners and priests. The Mohammedans ported their corpse on an open bier, followed by women relatives with dishevelled hair and by hired mourners as well. This body was interred with its right side towards Mecca. In Hinduism the funeral procession moves to the place of cremation and it is a great honor to be a carrier. All relatives come to the funeral, and even enemies attend, because death transcends interpersonal animosities during life. To view the dead body is a good omen, for death has dignity. The body is burned to free the soul and the cremation is the ultimate purifying act. Sometimes a hollow tube, a holy straw, is used to guide this soul in its route outward where it may enter into another living being, be it man or animal. The soul remains immortal here, and death anniversaries are a time for celebration, not for grief.

In Bali, Indonesia, the Hindu ceremony of cremation is altered in that the body is carried inside a gilded papier-mâché animal or a tower which is set afire. It is never made clear exactly where the body is placed so as to confuse the evil spirit and ensure the soul freedom as it leaves. In the custom of *satī* (or suttee), still practiced in remote villages of India, the widow crouches by the bier on which she hurls herself to be immolated in the flames consuming the corpse of her husband. This is an old concept of purification by fire of the woman who will thus not be touched by another man, and it prepares her soul for the next life. The Parsi cult in Bombay place the bodies of their dead in "towers of silence," where vultures pick away the flesh. When the bones are clean, they are dropped to the bottom of a well which opens to the sea. This is freeing the soul for transmigration without contaminating the earth or air.

Christian funerary rituals were developed in medieval Catholicism and were closely related to the doctrinal belief concerning purgatory. The entire ceremony was marked by black clothes, unbleached wax candles, solemn tolling of church bells. The coffin was carried to the church, trailed by a sad cortege and accompanied by sounds of mourning and the smells of incense.

In some cultures, the body was dismembered for burial. Thus, the Egyptians removed the viscera, which were preserved in four canopic jars. The Romans buried one finger joint that was disconnected from the hand. In medieval Europe the heart and sometimes the intestines of important persons were

interred in separate places, for example, William the Conqueror, whose body
was buried at St. Étienne at Caen, his heart in Rouen Cathedral, and his intestines in the Church of Chalus.

Post-funerary ceremonies were held in various cultures, not only to mourn
the dead, but also to purify the mourners. These included the wearing of old
or colorless clothes, shaving of the hair, or letting it grow long and unkempt.
Avoidance of amusement, denial of emotional gratification, and other forms of
mortification were common practices. Some of this practice represented respect
for the dead, but it has also been seen as a protective device for the survivors,
who seek to divert the ill humor of the dead spirit away from them while they
are still enjoying the life of this world. Death was regarded as fearful and evil,
and everything about it had to be purified. The Parsis cleansed the room in
which the dead lay, including all articles in contact with the body. In other
cultures, dancing and athletic contests took place, intended to generate vitalizing
forces to benefit the dead. The funeral banquet of the Christians, the "shivah"
of the Jew, the meal on the return of the mourners to the home of the deceased
are all part of these rituals and have as their purpose the encouragement of the
living to go on and to return to the activities of this world.

Following the burial it was customary to place a tombstone or a marker on
the grave with an accompanying inscription. Sometimes a picture or sculpture
of the person buried was included. In early Christian catacomb burials, the
deceased was depicted on the plaster of the walls where the body was laid,
represented in dress appropriate to the office, such as a queen or knight. However, in the later Middle Ages, when there was preoccupation with the horror
and degradation of death, below the effigies of the deceased, as they were known
in life, were placed other effigies of their naked, decaying corpses. These were
the "memento mori" tombs of the period.

In some cultures provisions were made for communication with the dead.
The earliest Romans buried their deceased next to the hearth in their houses,
and when laws prohibited this custom, they interred the body just outside the
city walls. They believed that the dead continued to live in intimacy with
their family and from this concept sprang up a "cult of the dead." It was the
custom to gather periodically near the dead body to tighten the bonds that tied
him to the living. Tombs were constructed with seats in a semicircle to accom-
modate the visitors.

Other customs provided for continued expiation to God in hopes of alleviat-
ing the sufferings of the departed soul. Wealthy Christians facing purgatory
endowed monasteries, and chapels were established by a family where masses
could be said regularly for the repose of the soul of the dead and those of his
relatives. To this day the Jewish believer awaits anxiously the birth of a son
or grandson who will "be" his Kaddish. This paean of benediction written in
Aramaic expresses the highest and noblest aspiration of the Jewish faith and
is used in every religious ceremony, even in daily prayers. It speaks nothing of
grief, but only of the praise of God, and phrases from the Kaddish become
part of the Lord's Prayer. It also became a mourner's prayer and the living
Jew uses it as a means of assuring his future. When the time comes he must
have a loved one, a son or a grandson, to say "Kaddish" for him after he is
gone, he hopes, to his heavenly paradise.

All of the foregoing draws only lightly on the treasury of record, the customs
and practices of human beings, as separate from other animals, as they have
faced the question of death. The mystery of death constituted a fearful problem,

and in order to cope with it man developed an ideology and a ritual to handle its emotional challenge. This was built into his religious life. All religions are concerned with post-death security, the linking of mortal man to an eternal realm, whether it be achieved by ritual magic, divine assistance, or mystic enlightenment.

As human societies become more sophisticated, particularly in recent times, the traditionalistic eschatologies begin to lose their import. Medieval concepts of death and judgment are not as meaningful, and beliefs that inspired some of these images and traditions have been forgotten or abandoned. The elaborate funeral processions are gone, except for a dignitary of state An assassinated President John Kennedy will have a cortege, the riderless black horse, boots turned backward, the coffin drawn on an artillery caisson. The shrines are gone, except in Red Square for Lenin, or Yad-va-Shem in Jerusalem for the recorded names of those who died in the Holocaust. Funerals are streamlined, having only a simple procession sometimes limited to the family. Cemeteries are no longer the elaborate art-filled *campo santi* of Italy. Instead they are landscaped lawns with simple flat markers, no monuments, no mausoleums, no obelisks. Modern society has a longer expectancy of life and a higher standard of living, but the mystery of death and its impact on the emotions has not lessened. Instead man now faces death less equipped and more hopelessly than at any other time in his history. Let us examine what is happening.

Today's man no longer finds a deep resource in religion. His educated mind does not let him accept the mystical philosophies of earlier periods. The priest, the rabbi, or the minister is not seen as endowed with magical powers, and current religious ritual does not fulfill his need. The devout Catholic misses his Latin Mass, the Jew his ritual incantation. With the industrialization of society, generalized education and rapid growth of mass communication, modern man finds himself in a world where he must deal with ecology, civil rights, over-population, violence, international crises and the threat of war. His scientists have conquered infection and improved medical care, but no insight has been provided about the termination of life—death. Furthermore, all about him is a social revolution. The rise of democracy provides egalitarian status for every-one, and each man is free, an individual with rights; he expects equal justice. Therefore, he has the right to resist implied and vested authority and to chal-lenge abuse. Inherent in this is the question of right to decision of life or death by medical authority: "Is the individual subject to the decision of the doctor or does he belong to himself?" Thus is man seeking, even in death, to determine his own destiny. Some are frightened by what is happening about them and are dismayed by the experimentation and accomplishments of the "technological priesthood." Powers once attributed to God, such as massive destruction by earthquakes and floods, can be matched by man. The atomic scientist with his nuclear bomb can readily destroy civilization. Man even has some control over death-producing processes. The modern physician can neutralize the effect of previously fatal bacteria; he can start a heart that has stopped; and he can substitute a machine for a failing lung-heart system to maintain a patient in-definitely. The ethicist queries, "Does the person so managed have a choice as to whether he wishes to be saved?" Do the people about him, his family, those who love him, have a voice in the decision or is this exclusively the prerogative of the physician?

Now come further questions. Is the patient on a heart or lung machine still a person? If the assisted organs were suddenly deprived of the support, they could not go on for more than a few minutes. Therefore, is that individual alive or is he purely a biologic preparation, *anima ex machina?* Does a person who has a known failing heart, and who anticipates that it may stop suddenly only to be resuscitated by modern techniques, have the right to ask not to be helped? Does the man who has suffered a broken neck that has left all four extremities permanently paralyzed have the same privilege? How shall we do it?—not feed him? not treat his infected bladder or decubitus ulcers? In a recent report from Massachusetts General Hospital, massively burned patients who are described as in a state where "survival is unprecedented," are given a choice. These persons have an early significant period when they are calm, clear, not in severe pain and readily communicated with. After a careful study which ends in the conclusion "survival is unprecedented," the patient is told and given the choice of full treatment to sustain life as long as possible, including resuscitative measures, or treatment to control pain and other discomforts but which "let the end come naturally." This is in contrast to the physician-only decision to withhold intensive care in absolutely hopeless cases. The patient's decision, either way, is scrupulously carried out.

A person facing death goes through stages, which have been clearly described by Dr. Elizabeth Kübler-Ross. First he denies the possibility of death. Then he works through further steps of anger, bargaining for time, depression, and finally acceptance. The last step perhaps parallels the mysterious period of the past when an individual was able to turn to his god, to his saints. The traditional rituals gave him a "handle" of support and he did not have to think or to explain. It was part of his faith, his belief. Today we find the person without this handle and usually in a strange hospital or nursing home. He is bitter, unhappy, isolated and complains that he is not being visited. Finally he gives into all of his feelings with, "My time has come, I guess it's all right."

Now, asks the ethicist, may not this person die with dignity? May he not prepare a document, written or by word, expressing his wish? Must he be subjected to a hopeless medical course which is a continuous, albeit futile, process of intravenous needles, nasogastric tubes, repeated sternal thumping the electroshock to the chest for heart standstill, when he knows that all of this may glean him only another day or another week? May he not die in his own way? Massively burned patients are permitted to do so. This is the basis of the Living Will that is being employed in various parts of the country. The concept is not new, but it was a poet who said it earlier. In 1817 William Cullen Bryant in "Thanatopsis" wrote the familiar words:

> So live, that when thy summons comes to join
> The innumerable caravan, which moves
> To that mysterious realm, where each shall take
> His chamber in the silent halls of death,
> Thou go not like the quarry-slave at night,
> Scourged to his dungeon, but, sustained and soothed
> By an unfaltering trust, approach thy grave
> Like one who wraps the drapery of his couch
> About him, and lies down to pleasant dreams.

Was not Bryant asking for death with dignity? In this age dying people at their final moment usually do not invoke God. The only dying words I recall were heard when I was a young intern at the Cook County Hospital in Chicago in 1930. A young Mexican dying of miliary tuberculosis cried repeatedly, "Pobre mama"—"My poor mother."

If the patient does not make the decision to stop or continue resuscitation, who should? Who has the right to order, "Do not resuscitate"? Shall the patient be asked? Should the family make the decision? The latter situation is often distressing for a physician because some of the family members will say, "Do not resuscitate; if we cannot have our mother intact, we do not want her to survive." Others insist: "Please do everything, don't hold back any measures that may help no matter how little it contributes." The pressure on the physician from both sides is enormous. Yet does he have the right to the decision? This matter has become so complex that in some hospitals committees have been set up to help to make the decision. Medical and lay people, including lawyers and clergy, are represented. This group is advisory and works in consultation with the attending physician. The considerations are submitted to the family before orders not to resuscitate are instituted.

These committees, carefully planned, reflecting a broad segment of society and acting only in an advisory capacity, have already been informally called "God committees." From a Harvard Law School professor comes the question, "For whose good are these new statements aimed? Are they aimed at freeing the patient from a tyranny of a technologic (or bureaucratic professional) imperative 'to keep alive at all cost,' a tyranny that many thinking persons fear as a more or less distinct menace to their well-being and liberty in their last days? Or are they aimed at freeing society from the burden and expense of caring for a growing multitude of extravagantly demanding moribund persons?" The critic points up the value of the Living Will for such an instance in which fundamentally the patient makes the decision, but he also admits that both the Living Will and the Critical Care and Optimum Care Committees' concepts will have to be tested for legality. In short, the decision for a final procedure at death in these terminally ill patients, and there are tens of thousands of them always with us, will end in the courts. The handwriting is already on the wall.

Our advancing technology has brought us the question of the meaning of brain death, the problem of active and passive euthanasia. Our socioethical state carries the imperatives of individual rights, of privileges of privacy. We are faced with the dilemma of deciding who may make the decision to terminate treatment for a person who is a minor or a mental defective or for one who is mentally ill or irreversibly unconscious and unresponsive. Is the word of a court the full solution? Even these decisions are subject to appeal and reversal. In the meantime, what about the person, the subject himself, during the often slow sociolegal process?

I have come far from the caveman who was bewildered because his mate or friend did not arouse from what appeared to be a very deep sleep. Now we look at the totally unresponsive body, breathing because a machine forces air and oxygen into the lung, continuing metabolic process because food has been introduced intravenously or through a nasogastric or gastrostomy tube. The body is warm; the heart is beating and we ask, "Is this humanhood?" I stop at this point.

This is why we are all gathered here, persons representing the medical sciences, law, ethics, religion, and sociology. I am reminded of one of the most meaningful moments in my medical career, some 50 years ago. Professor Robert Frederick Zeit, a beloved, erudite pathologist of our faculty, had come out of retirement for a few weeks to give us a special course on cancer. In the final lecture he described the result of a lifetime of effort in research on malignancy. Certainly he had found no solutions, but he summed up eloquently in his soft German-English, "And when you reach the top of the mountain, you are no closer to heaven; only the horizon is more clear."

In this volume we shall attempt to climb a mountain concerned with brain death and death itself. I am not sure that we will end up closer to a heaven of wisdom on the subject, but certainly our horizons will be more clear.

BIBLIOGRAPHY

1. NATIONAL GEOGRAPHIC. 1977. Egypt. The dazzling legacy of an ancient quest. **151**(3): 292–312.
2. EDWARDS, I. E. S. 1975. Tutankhamun: Its Tombs and Its Treasures. The Metropolitan Museum of Art and Alfred A. Knopf. New York, N.Y.
3. VIVEKANANDA, S. Life After Death. : 14. Advaita Ashrama. Calcutta.
4. The New Encyclopedia Britannica Macropedia. Encyclopedia Britannica, Inc., Chicago & London. (Death, **5:** 527–529; death rites and customs, **5:** 533–538; eschatology, **6:** 958–962).
4a. BOSHES, B. 1977. *Ibid.* Death. Medical and Health Annual. : 227–229.
5. KÜBLER-ROSS, E. 1969. On Death and Dying. Macmillan. New York, N.Y.
6. POPE PIUS XII. 1958. The prolongation of life. The Pope Speaks **4:** 393–398.
7. GEELHOLD, G. W. 1977. Life and death: Who decides? Pharos, January 7–12.
8. FRIED, C. 1976. Terminating life supports out of closet. New Eng. J. Med. **295:** 390–391.
9. VEATCH, R. 1976. Death, Dying, and the Biological Revolution: Our Last Quest for Responsibility. Yale University Press. New Haven, Conn.
10. DYCK, A. J. 1973. Ethics and Medicine. Lenacre Quarterly : 182–200.
11. Optimum Care for Hopelessly Ill Patients. 1976. New Eng. J. Med. **295:** 362–364.
12. RASKIN, M. T., J. D. GELLERMAN & N. R. RUE. 1976. Orders not to resuscitate. New Eng. J. Med. **295:** 364–366.
13. BOK, S. 1976. Personal directions for care at the end of life. New Eng. Med. **295:** 367–368.
14. BRONSTEIN, H. 1977. The Meaning of the Kaddish. North Shore Cong. Israel. Glencoe, Ill.
15. GILMER, W., JR. 1976. Living Wills. J. Legal Med. **32:**
16. The right to die. *The New York Times,* July 3, 1973.
17. JENNETT, B. & F. PLUM. 1972. Persistent vegetative state after brain damage. Lancet **1:** 734–737.
18. Refinements in criteria for the determination of death: An appraisal. JAMA **221:** 46–53.
19. 1968. A definition of irreversible coma—Ad Hoc Committee of the Harvard Medical School. JAMA **205:** 337–340.
20. 1968. Black's Law Dictionary, 4th Ed. : 488. West Publishing Co. St. Paul, Minn.
21. KOREIN, J. & M. MACCARIO. 1971. On the diagnosis of cerebral death. Clin. Electroencephalogr. **2:** 178–199.
22. BOSHES, B. 1975. A definition of cerebral death. Ann. Rev. Med. **26:** 465–470.
23. WALKER, A. E. 1975. Cerebral death. *In* The Nervous System. The Clinical Neurosciences. **2:** 75–87. Raven Press. New York, N.Y.
24. 1972. A report by the Task Force on Death and Dying of the Institute of Society, Ethics and Life Sciences. An appraisal. JAMA **221:** 48–53.
25. 1976. The Quinlan case hinged on "privacy." Med. World News : 43–44.
26. KITTRIDGE, F. I., JR. 1976. After Quinlan. J. Legal Med. : 23–31.
27. BERESFORD, H. R. 1977. The Quinlan decision. Problems and legislatives. Ann. Neurol. **2:** 74–81.

28. 1977. An appraisal of the criteria of cerebral death. A collaborative study. JAMA **237:** 982–986.
29. CAPRON, A. M. 1973. Determining death: Do we need a statute? Hastings Center Rep. Vol. **3.**
30. CAPRON, A. M. & L. R. KASS. 1972. A statutory definition of the standards for determining human death. Univ. Pa. Law Rev. **121:** 87–118.
31. FLETCHER, J. 1972. Indicators of humanhood: A tentative profile of man. Hastings Center Rep. Vol. **2.**

THE PROBLEM OF BRAIN DEATH: DEVELOPMENT AND HISTORY *

Julius Korein

Department of Neurology
New York University Medical Center; and the
EEG Laboratories, Bellevue Hospital Center
New York, New York 10016

INTRODUCTION

Brain death is reviewed and analyzed from medical, biological, and historical perspectives. Understanding of the terminology used is imperative prior to undertaking such an endeavor. The meaning of the words *construct, concept* and *criterion* are, therefore, explicitly defined. The usage of the terms *death* and *brain death* are discussed and throughout this paper these are separated from other sets of medical problems and social issues, such as those relating to irreversible noncognitive states, organ transplantation and the "right to die." Death is not considered an event, but rather a process related to the dissolution of a living system. The definition of a living system involves derivations from thermodynamics, information theory, control systems, value theory and the dynamics of irreversible states. The critical component of the living system may then be defined. In the human organism, the brain is the critical component. Brain death then becomes equivalent to death of a person.

Development of criteria that will allow the physician to diagnose brain death, the death of an individual, is then considered within the medical and social milieu. Historically, initiation of the major events in the evolution of these criteria is considered to have begun with the allocution of Pope Pius XII on the prolongation of life in 1957. These events include medical studies, social critiques, and statutes, all of which reflect the initial confusion about the subject. Medical research, however, has gradually increased the specificity of terminology as well as clinical and laboratory criteria to be used, allowing the accurate and reliable diagnosis of brain death. Ancillary laboratory techniques include electroencephalography as well as studies relating to brain circulation and metabolism. No single clinical or laboratory criterion can be used to arrive at a diagnosis of brain death. Rather, it is the composite of these criteria combined with the physician's medical judgment, etiologic and temporal factors, and consideration of the appropriate differential diagnosis that leads to the appropriate judgment and management of any given patient.

FUNDAMENTAL CONSIDERATIONS

Constructs, Concepts and Criteria

To insure appropriate utilization of the terms construct, concept and criteria, we will begin by stating their dictionary definitions. *Construct* (noun) refers to

* Revised manuscript received June 7, 1978.

an object, perception or idea that is systematically put together in an orderly manner from components, facts or impressions. *Concept* (noun) is an abstract notion, idea, thought or opinion which may be generalized. *Criteria* (noun, pl.) refer to standards, tests, rules or measures by which correct or valid judgments can be formed. Both concepts and criteria may be considered to be constructs. Fundamental to our thesis is the concept that death of a human being is the irreversible loss of those functions that we consider the essence of an individual. Such concepts have led to the development of criteria of death in terms of irreversible cessation of vital functions, i.e., cardiovascular, respiratory and central nervous system activity. The premise underlying the concept of brain death is that there is a single critical vital system, the brain, whose irreversible destruction is both a necessary and sufficient condition in considering an individual as dead. This notion is derived from a large mass of clinical and experimental observations indicating that the essence of the human organism, including both internal and external behavior, is subserved by the brain, which is irreplaceable. It should be made unmistakably clear that we are not dealing with a conceptual duality. Brain death is essential to any concept pertaining to death of a person. What we are considering are dual criteria in deriving the diagnosis of death. That is, death may be diagnosed either by the "classical" criteria, which relate to vital functions, or, under highly circumscribed conditions, by the criteria for brain death. Although the concept of brain death would imply the destruction of every neuron in the brain, in utilizing criteria it is sufficient to obtain evidence that the critical mass of neurons is destroyed and the remainder irreversibly dysfunctional, thus reaching a singularity or step-function involving a state of the entire brain from which there is no return. In this sense, there is a virtual identity between destruction and irreversible dysfunction of neurons.

It is the criteria for brain death that are of major concern to the physician who must make the diagnosis of death by using either classical methods or the equivalent diagnosis of brain death. The criteria that the physician uses are primarily based on concepts and observations that relate to living systems generally and to the human organism specifically. In addition, these criteria are being continually refined by clinical and experimental research. Current criteria are based on available technology, knowledge and concepts of brain function. Although there are limitations and difficulties in applying these criteria, sufficient experience has been amassed which allows their practical application to diagnose brain death. Confusion exists because of imprecise terminology, the intrinsic nature of the problem, and the frequent confounding of brain death with other issues that are tangentially related. An attempt will be made to dispel these underlying sources of confusion. Tangential areas, which include problems relating to vegetative states, organ transplantation, the rights of the individual, and decision-making relating to these issues by members of a given society, will be discussed. These different situations first must be distinguished from the problem of brain death per se, and second must be categorized, defined precisely, and differentiated from each other.

Terminology and Definitions

Operational definitions presented are based on medical criteria. The criteria themselves will be subsequently detailed later in this paper and elsewhere in this volume. *Systemic death* or *death* will refer to the diagnosis of death by conventional means. *Brain death* will refer to the diagnosis of death by means of criteria indicating total and irreversible brain dysfunction. This includes dysfunction of all neuronal components in the intracranial cavity, that is, both cerebral hemispheres, brain stem and cerebellum. *Cerebral death,* which has often been used synonymously with brain death, will, in the context of this paper, refer only to destruction of the cerebral hemispheres excluding the brain stem and cerebellum. *Brain-stem death* will be considered to have occurred if irreversible stem dysfunction is demonstrated in the presence of cerebral activity. We should note at this juncture that brain death and systemic death are considered equivalent. In contrast, neither cerebral nor brain-stem death alone, as defined, are the same as brain death or death. Often, however, cerebral or brain-stem death may be rapidly followed by irreversible dysfunction of the remainder of the brain, thus resulting in "total" brain death.

The term *irreversible coma* will be used as an umbrella that includes brain death and other non-brain-dead states. These include, for example, cerebral or brain-stem death, as defined above. This category also refers to other groups of poorly defined irreversible states. Terminology used to describe these situations includes irreversible noncognitive state, persistent vegetative state, neocortical death, and the apallic syndrome, among others. The essential criterion used in defining these disease states is evidence of irreversible lack of cognition, often in the presence of vegetative function. Brain function can be dichotomized into cognitive and vegetative behavior. It is necessary to have intact structures in both the cerebral hemispheres and the brain stem for cognition to occur. By cognition, we include elements of alert awareness, perception, mentation, reasoning, problem-solving, memory, and decision-making. Cognition includes purposeful behavior in response to internal and external stimuli which relate to the inherited and learned goals of the organism. The neural circuitry underlying these functions has a relatively high degree of modifiability. In contrast to cognitive behavior, vegetative functions include complex stereotyped, repetitive patterns that do not require awareness. These functions are, at the highest level, complex reflex patterns related to relatively fixed neuronal circuitry and may occur in the absence of the cerebral hemispheres. Other examples of vegetative behavior are decerebrate posturing, breathing, and oculocephalic reflexes.

Structural lesions of the brain which are known to cause irreversible noncognitive states are those that involve the entire cerebral cortex bilaterally, or the deep structures of the cerebrum (thalamus and basal ganglia) bilaterally, or the reticular formation at the core of the brain stem. Combinations of these lesions may result in similar states. Thus, we may differentiate between patients who meet the criteria of brain death and those who are in an irreversible altered state of consciousness but are unequivocally not brain-dead.

These definitions are stressed because of the controversial issue in considering cerebral death, brain-stem death, and irreversible noncognitive states as representing death of the individual and, therefore, being equivalent to brain death and death. This problem is not trivial and will be further elaborated elsewhere in this volume. Furthermore, these conditions should be considered in the differential diagnosis of irreversible coma and should be distinguished from conditions such as the de-efferented (locked-in) syndrome and reversible coma by using appropriate criteria.

Prior to presenting further details on the development of terminology and criteria pertaining to brain death, we will explicitly state a set of basic constructs in attempting to understand the living system and then differentiating the varied states of the human organism.

CONCEPTS AND CRITERIA OF LIFE AND DEATH

Process versus Event

The definition of death, while often made in a straightforward and simplistic manner, is in fact a highly complex construct which has many intricate facets and ramifications. Because of the limitations of knowledge surrounding the problem of death, the concepts and criteria that developed were applied in a relatively direct and pragmatic manner by man in various societies. Death has been considered with reference to the state of the organism in an all-or-none manner, that is, that an individual organism is either dead or alive. This notion is both simplistic and naive since death is not an *event*, but a *process*. The controversy over the nature of this process was discussed in 1971 by Morison[1] and Kass.[2] The process of death occurs over a finite period. Since the process may be brief, the duration and means of evaluating the state of the organism are often limited. Practical requirements over the past several thousand years demanded a *yes* or *no* answer to the question of whether or not an individual was dead. Therefore, it was both reasonable and convenient to consider death as an event. Actually it is now known that death involves a complex series of changes which, if they occur rapidly enough, asymptotically approach the commonly used concept of an event. Prior to the advent of applications of modern science and technology to biology, the development of deeper understanding of the physiology of living systems, the utilization of intensive care units (ICU), and the therapeutic use of organ transplantation, the distinction between death as a process and death as an event had limited significance. However, as the utilization of resuscitation and life-support systems increased, the necessity of defining the process of death has become essential. Although a statement of the *moment* of death is required by many agencies in our society, this "moment" may, in fact, be a period of long duration that cannot be precisely stated. The presumed end state of a multicellular organism, when all of its cells are dead, is not the moment of death, nor is the time of pronouncement of death necessarily the moment of death, since many cellular components of the organism may still be alive. We must, therefore, consider the dynamic, organizational, and cellular aspects of the deteriorating human organism in order to redefine the process of death.[3, 4] Perhaps then we may obtain utilitarian criteria to define the moment of death.

Definition of Death in Relation to Life

Implicit within the concept of death is the concept of life; therefore, some operational criteria of life and irreversibility must be included in the definition of death. Further, it must be kept in mind that there are other states in nature to which these constructs, *life* and *death,* are not directly applicable. For example, a stone, a crystal or an amino-acid molecule cannot be considered either living or dead, although the latter may have been a component of a living system. The transition from complex molecules that are not alive to those that are alive or have the potential for life involves a series of step-functions, including interaction with their environment. These complex structures may then achieve a state that fulfills the criteria of a living system. Additional criteria are required to define the system as human organism or a person. A virus may be a highly complex molecule which in its crystalline state is not alive, but potentially may become alive if its environment changes. This occurs when the virus infects a host cell. A goldfish instantaneously frozen after being dropped into liquid nitrogen is similarly not alive but neither is it dead, despite the fact that its metabolic activity is zero. It has the potential of becoming alive by placing it in water. These states that potentially may lead to life have been referred to as a form of suspended animation and clearly involve the function of the system at a given time, the nature of its environment and reversibility of transition from a static to a dynamic state.

The classical concept of death of the human organism is couched in terms relating to the "cessation of life," life being defined in terms of criteria dealing with *vital* functions.[5, 6] These vital functions included those of circulation, respiration, and responsivity to external and internal stimuli, i.e., sentience and purposeful movement. When all these functions are absent and there is no possibility of their return, the individual is considered to be in a state described as dead. A major consideration in these classical constructs of death is irreversibility of the state. As previously noted we shall refer to this classical definition of death as systemic death. More specific elements of the definition of death, and therefore implicit in the definition of living systems, have been developed to include metabolic activity, energy utilization, information processing, and the nature, structure and direction of changes in the organism. Therefore we will attempt to conceptualize the problem of defining a living system based on current scientific advances and then consider how they relate to the problem of death. Such constructs have been presented in Wilson's text on physiology[7] and elsewhere.[8] An approach to develop an experimental model based on brain energetics to differentiate between reversible loss of function and irreversible loss of viability is exemplified in the paper by Fein.[9] These definitions consider the living organism in terms of the thermodynamics of open systems, information theory, control systems (e.g., negative feedback systems), and game or value theory.[10-16] The complexity and direction in which the system moves through an environment can be considered in terms of the energy expended to increase negentropy (or the organization of the system) at the expense of the environment.[17-19]

Open Systems, Thermodynamics, and Information Theory

All living organisms are members of a class of open systems. Open systems exchange both energy and matter with the environment. These systems generally tend towards a steady state, i.e., stationary, nonequilibrium state, by keeping entropy production to a minimum. Entropy may be defined as a measure of *disorganization*. These systems have a variety of internal mechanisms that operate on the energy and matter entering and leaving the system. Their internal irreversible processes always operate to lower the amount of entropy production. As Prigogine has stated: "This result has an immediate bearing on the stability of stationary states. When a system is in the state of minimum entropy production . . . it cannot leave the state by a spontaneous irreversible change. If, as a result of some fluctuation, it deviates slightly from the state, internal changes will take place and bring the system back to its initial state." [17] This may result in a decrease of the total entropy of the system with compensatory increase of environmental entropy. That is, the internal mechanisms may operate on the energy and matter entering and leaving the system such that the system becomes more organized while the environment becomes disorganized. From the thermodynamic point of view, there is no violation of the Second Law of Thermodynamics, which states that the entropy in any real process increases. The degradation of environmental energy and matter more than compensates for the increase of organization in the system. The living organism, then, is an example of this class of open systems. Such a system functions as an interacting composite of irreversible real processes and originates or evolves in a spontaneous manner given the appropriate interacting components of the system's internal and external environments and the boundary conditions. Since the living organism consists of innumerable dependent variables which are linked one to the other, it is actually never in a steady state but is metastable. As one variable changes to a *steady* position, it may be coupled to another which has shifted away from its *stable* state. Therefore, the total system *tends* toward a steady state, which is the most stable solution of all critical variables. It is this general trend and progression of states as time passes that is of major interest in considering reversibility and irreversibility in the living organism.

Information, in the engineering sense, can be defined as a measurable physical quantity which is related to and transmitted by means of patterns of energy and matter. Thermodynamic entropy at the atomic-molecular level is identical with negative entropy (negentropy). Therefore, information or negentropy can be considered as a measure of *organization*. The state of organization of a living organism may be quantifiable in terms of negentropy. This informational measure represents the number of equiprobable states of a system at a given moment in time. Thus, the use of thermodynamics, statistical mechanics, and information theory allows a quantitative representation of a living organism in terms of its organization or its number of equiprobable states. Greater organization results in a decrease in the number of equiprobable states of a system.

Control Systems and Value Theory

All living organisms have a variety of mechanisms that obtain, select, process, compare, store and utilize information from their environment and their own internal state to produce a goal-oriented output in the form of biological behavior. Thus, the organism contains within it simulations of itself, the environment, and potential future states of both. The portion of the organism's organizational structure utilized for information-processing leading to simulating the state of the system itself and the environment at any given moment also participates in controlling its goal-directed behavior, i.e., future states of the system. These aspects of the system will be referred to as control systems. In simple organisms, such as a virus, virtually the entire system is the control system. In more complex multicellular organisms, specific structures may develop to form a master control system which supersedes all other subsidiary systems. In man, the brain is the critical control system. The DNA molecules in a single cell reflect the past experience of the species with environments over an evolutionary time scale. These molecules are the genetic blueprint and major determinants of the structure of a given living organism. The neuronal and synaptic structures in the human brain not only reflect their evolutionary development, but their interactions also reflect the relatively short-term experience of the individual person over his lifetime. The neuron itself does not reproduce, but it alters its connections with other neurons by either being destroyed or by means of growth of its dendritic tree, thus increasing the number of synapses and/or by increasing production of neuro-transmitter agents at the synapse.

The organism contains a variety of intra- and intercellular mechanisms which serve as control systems. Depending on their boundary conditions (e.g., membrane structure), they may act as a multicellular organ. These control systems range from enzymes to immunologic and hormonal systems, but reached their culmination in the development of the central nervous system (CNS). These multilevel systems operate on the organism and the environment to keep entropy production at a minimum and to increase the organization of the individual or group. They are comprised of a variety of servo-decision mechanisms programmed by evolution and experience, directed towards the goal of the living system, i.e., to select outputs in response to a given input from the available future simulated states which have the smallest increment in entropy production. The central nervous system output is primarily in the form of feed forward and feedback neural loops.

Information or negentropy only quantifies the organization of the system but gives no indication as to its *value* at a given moment. Value of information depends on the degree to which a given system can utilize that information to tend towards the steady state by keeping entropy production to a minimum, i.e., maintain the goals of the system as changes occur. It is a measure of the fit or adaptibility of living systems with the given environment at a given time as well as an indication of how successfully this adaptation is maintained as time passes. Value, then, or meaning of information, clearly differs from the quantity of information. It is a relative measure that depends upon the system one is dealing with and the effectiveness of its goal-oriented behavior. We may consider a quantity of information that is identical in form being received by several different living systems which will have totally different values relative to the system receiving it. For example, a bacterium with no visual receptors and limited control-system capacity may be compared to an earthworm, which has more complex sensory transducers and control systems, and these may be further contrasted to a man with highly developed visual receptors and an extensive control system. The spoken words, "Stop, there is a cliff," may have no value to the first system, be of possible minimal value (as a vibration) to the second system, but be of enormous value to the last system, resulting in behavior that will prevent a possible sudden future increase in entropy. The quantity of the information itself is identical in all three circumstances. In considering the value of the organization of a total organism at a given time, we must relate it to changes in the system and to the state of the environment. It is conceivable that both a fish and a nonaquatic bird may have the same quantity of information in terms of its total molecular structure, but the value of that organization is highest for the fish in water and for the bird in air, while the value of their structure approaches zero if their environments are reversed. The measure of value is dynamic and changes as the structure of the system and the environment change. A well-known example of this is sickle-cell anemia.

Patients with the disease and the trait in a cool, northern environment, where malaria is not endemic, may be considered to suffer from an illness that has negative value in terms of the individual's life and progeny. However, if individuals with the same disease are in a tropical zone, where malaria is rampant, their "illness" protects them from malarial infestation and thus, in *that* environment, has a significant degree of positive value for the individual and his progeny.

Irreversibility, Brain Death, and The Critical System of the Human Organism

The significance of the theoretical concepts previously described may be used as a foundation for discussing transitions of living systems into a variety of states that may or may not be irreversible. The terminology we will adopt includes energy utilization of the organism, the complexity of organization of the system, information-processing by the system, the direction in which these parameters change and its reversibility in a given environment. The value of both the information relating to the structure of the organism and that which is received and processed to form an output by the organism allows the physician to develop criteria in order to make a determination of irreversibility and brain death. It is the interaction of the physician with the patient by means of information transfer related to history, physical examination, and laboratory tests to obtain a diagnosis that not only defines the situation but also predicts the outcome. Essentially, all disease states are evaluated in this manner. The situation involving brain death is one highly specific representation of this informational evaluation and transaction between a patient and physician.

In approaching the problem of brain death, we must define death of cells, organ systems, components of the organism, and the organism itself. It is our thesis that death of the human organism may be equated with irreversible destruction of the critical system of that organism. The critical system is that system which is irreplaceable by an artefice, be it biological, chemical, or electromechanical. Further, the critical system subserves the essential behavioral characteristics of the individual. Virtually all organ systems are replaceable in man, with one exception, and that is the brain. The heart can be replaced by a pump, the kidneys by an appropriate dialysis unit, endocrine glands by hormonal replacement therapy, and so on. A limb may be artificial, but when it comes to the neuronal cells that comprise the central nervous system, an individual is born with a fixed number that do not reproduce. A neuron may grow by increasing its dendritic tree and interconnections, and the soma may support growth of a crushed axon, but if the soma is destroyed, this is an irreversible process. The brain depends on the neurons for its function, and the organism depends on the brain. If the brain is irreversibly destroyed, the critical system is destroyed, and despite all other systems being maintained by any manner whatsoever, the organism as an individual functioning entity no longer exists. If the critical system, i.e., the brain, in a man is destroyed, the human organism is no longer in a state of minimal entropy production; its state will progressively become more disorganized by spontaneous irreversible fluctuations. Therefore it will never return to its initial state as a sentient human being. The time course may be prolonged by artificial means, depending on the adequacy of functioning subsidiary control mechanisms, but the outcome of dissolution of the system is just as certain as that resulting from irreversible cardiac arrest. Elsewhere in this volume data will be presented indicating that when brain death (that is, death of the cerebral hemispheres, brain stem and cerebellum) occurs, irreversible cardiac arrest will inevitably follow regardless of the maintenance of all resusatative procedures. No investigator contributing to this volume has presented evidence that irreversible cardiac arrest may be postponed more than a week (exclusive of that in infants and children), and most often these final irreversible changes occur prior to 48 and even 24 hours after brain death. This is clearly not the situation in which there may be an irreversible noncognitive state with persistence of brain-stem structures, and although the argument may be raised that in such states the personality of the individual is destroyed, their vegetative functions, including spontaneous cardiorespiratory activity, may persist for years with appropriate life-support measures. There are several reasons that are presented for not considering patients in irreversible noncognitive or vegetative states as being brain-dead. The determination of such irreversibility is still undergoing investigation, and prognostication is not always sharply defined. Furthermore, it is occasionally difficult to differentiate a patient in a purely noncognitive state from one who still has some semblance of cognition. Since communication is the key in making this determination (e.g., by means of eye movements in a patient with a locked-in syndrome), the possibility exists of situations in which the brain may respond to external stimuli in a manner that only can be observed by changes of electroencephalographic or cerebral blood flow activity. This may occur in a patient in whom the brain stem and cerebrum have been separated by a hemorrhage in the intracollicular region. Such a patient may have significant cerebral hemispheric function and brain-stem function, but be in an irreversible noncommunicative state. In the majority of patients, appropriate clinical and laboratory evaluation allows the reliable diagnosis of persistent vegetative or noncognitive state, such as in the case of Karen Ann Quinlan. Management of these patients is analogous to that of patients in other forms of irreversible chronic coma and anencephalic monsters who survive for prolonged periods. It is not unreasonable that many contributors to this volume would consider extending the definition of death of a person to such patients. However, this must await guidelines based on more precise clinical research to prevent potential abuse and misdiagnosis. Currently, there is no significant degree of social acceptance of such a concept. It is for these reasons that we do not wish to confuse patients in this group with those who are brain-dead, as defined by means of criteria which will be elaborated upon both in this paper and elsewhere in this volume.

We reiterate that there are not two different concepts of death; we maintain, rather, that two different sets of criteria may be used to diagnose death. The conventional definition of death includes irreversible cessation of cardiorespiratory function which is rapidly followed by brain death within minutes if not seconds. Brain death, in contrast, is a situation arising as an outgrowth of resuscitative and life-support technology; it applies to the infrequent situation in which the brain dies while other systems are maintained artificially or are still viable. Both the "classical" definition of death and that of brain death are based on irreversible cessation of brain function. There is no inherent dichotomy of logic in this construct. Therefore, brain death is the functional equivalent of systemic death of an individual. This may be further illustrated both experimentally and clinically. If a dog's head is experimentally severed from the body and kept alive by an appropriate life-support system and the same is done to a dog's body, the essence of the animal's "personality" is in the head, not the corpus. The head in such an experiment will eat, salivate, blink, sleep and respond to stimuli to which it has previously been conditioned, such as its name being called. If a human is quadriplegic because of a cervical spinal cord transection, but has a normal brain, he may be kept alive by a life-support system; unquestionably he is a person who is aware and responds appropriately to external stimuli. However, if a person's cerebral hemispheres were destroyed by a shotgun blast, with subsequent deterioration of the brain stem, the temporary maintenance of his body by modern scientific methods does not mean that a human life is being maintained. To press the analogy to an extreme, we may culture skin cells from a person and keep them growing in artificial media for months. If we stop growing these cultured cells, however, this does not constitute the killing of a person, although we are destroying DNA molecules and tissues related to that person.

For the reasons stated above, the brain will be accepted as the critical system of the human organism and brain death as irreversible destruction of that system. We will not accept any other terminology or condition (other than death) as being equivalent to brain death. Previous use of terminology that considers brain death and cerebral death as synonymous will be ignored.[20] Chronic irreversible comas and noncognitive states where significant components of the brain are destroyed will not be considered as equivalent to brain death. The problem of defining the critical system of the critical system and of practically applying such subdivision clinically is of more than passing importance. This topic requires further research and will be discussed in detail elsewhere in this volume (see especially the paper by Ingvar[21]). Therefore, in order to distinguish brain death, we will now briefly review the establishment of criteria that may be used to make this diagnosis.

HISTORICAL REVIEW AND DEVELOPMENT OF CRITERIA

The Proclamation of Pope Pius XII

The distinction between death of an organism and death of components of the organism was considered as a practical problem by a group of anesthesiologists who maintained patients on life-support systems although there was no evidence of brain viability. These patients had irreparable destruction of the brain. The question arose in the application of technical advances whether it was appropriate to keep the corpus or body "alive" in the absence of a brain, and the problem was presented in 1957 to Pope Pius XII. This resulted in a papal allocution which was published in the following year, entitled "The Prolongation of Life."[22] Among the many significant statements contained in this document, two will be stressed. The first was that the pronouncement of death was not the province of the church but the responsibility of the physician: "It remains for the doctor . . . to give a clear and precise definition of 'death' and the 'moment of death' of a patient who passes away in a state of unconsciousness." The second point was that there came a time in the course of a patient's disease where the situation was *hopeless* and death should not be opposed by *extraordinary* means. The definitions of the words "hopeless" and "extraordinary" were not precisely stated in medical terminology, but it was clear that in hopeless cases resuscitative measures could be discontinued and death be unopposed. It was at this time that brain death and associated problems become the subject of increasing general interest. Historically, this proclamation initiated the surge in concept development, research, application and controversy in use of the construct "brain death." Using the papal allocution as a point of departure, the history of the problem of brain death will be reviewed.

Neurologic Studies and Coma Dépassé

During 1959 several groups of French neurophysiologists were involved with salient research in patients who were in extremely deep coma. They coined the term "coma dépassé," which was literally translated as "beyond coma" or "ultra-coma," and by some authors, unfortunately, as "irreversible coma." The results of these studies were published by Fischgold and Mathis,[23] Jouvet,[24] and Mollaret and Goulon [25] in 1959. The patients they studied were in deep states of unresponsive coma, in which the absence of spontaneous respiration necessitated the use of a respirator. These patients, in addition, were areflexic. Studies performed included electroencephalography (EEG) as well as multiple electrophysiologic recordings from the surface of the cortex and deep structures of the cerebrum such as the thalamus. The finding of absent electrophysiologic activity was considered by these investigators as confirmation of irreversible dysfunction of the brain. Some of these authors also described the neuropathologic findings on postmortem examinations. These findings, if a sufficient period of time had elapsed between the cessation of brain function (more precisely, cessation of brain circulation) and the cessation of cardiac function (i.e., systemic circulation), revealed a pathologic picture indicating massive necrosis and autolysis of the brain, later described by Walker et al.[26] and Lindenberg [27] as a "respirator brain." Earlier descriptions of the neuropathologic findings were presented by Bertrand et al.[28] in 1959, Mollaret et al.[29] in 1959, and Kramer in 1963 [30] and 1966.[31] Both Walker [26] and Pearson [32] have discussed the problem of neuropathologic findings in brain death and will detail these in subsequent presentations in this volume.[33, 34] It should be noted that only later the additional criterion relating to absent cerebral circulation was also included as part of the constellation of coma dépassé, as stated by Fischgold in 1970.[35]

In 1968, with the increased use of organ transplants as a therapeutic modality, there was further intensification of research and interest in the problem of brain death. This resurgence was manifested by studies in clinical neurology, EEG, cerebral blood flow, cerebral metabolism and neuropathology as well as in many nonmedical disciplines relating to the medicolegal, ethical, and other aspects of brain death. Attempts were made to define the criteria more precisely, and although terminology was often vague and diagnostic criteria were in a state of flux, as information became available, the construct labeled brain death did in fact begin to achieve a level of precision and reliability that allowed pragmatic use of the term. Partial limitations of the concept did not invalidate appropriate application. Although currently there is confusion in terminology and explicit criteria for brain death are not yet entirely uniform, refinements allow a reasonable approach to the dynamic problem of accurately diagnosing brain death. One of the purposes of this volume, in fact, is to present the current state of the research and applications aimed at solving this problem.

The Harvard Criteria and the Declaration of Sydney

Most often quoted are the Harvard criteria,[36] developed in 1968, which define cerebral death as irreversible coma (brain death) in terms of the following characteristics:

1. Absence of cerebral responsiveness
2. Absence of induced or spontaneous movement
3. Absence of spontaneous respirations (requiring the use of a respirator)
4. Absence of cephalic and deep-tendon reflexes
5. Absence of drug intoxication or hypothermia
6. Presence of a *flat* EEG
7. Persistence of these conditions for 24 hours

Although the Harvard criteria may be and have been used effectively, they have within them a set of limitations that requires close scrutiny. The 24-hour period is essentially arbitrary. The definition of a flat EEG required more precise standardization. With respect to drug intoxication, (1) its detection was not always possible; (2) many patients would be on drugs for therapy and still be brain-dead from other causes; and (3) there was no discussion of the interaction of drugs with other factors causing the coma. The amount of information available on this problem is limited.[37, 38] Other limitations of clinical criteria should be noted. It is the absence of cephalic reflexes, especially fixed dilated pupils, which is more germane to the diagnosis of brain death; deep-tendon reflexes are often present and are of limited significance. The evaluation of absence of spontaneous respiration is a relatively complex procedure. One only tests the mechanism that initiates respiration by increase of arterial pCO_2; one never tests the mechanism whereby breathing is initiated by decreased arterial pO_2 since that test may constitute a situation that would increase brain damage.[39] Finally, induced movements, such as stereotyped patterned leg withdrawal, may be related to an intact spinal reflex arc in patients with brain death.

The terminology used also left much to be desired. The term *irreversible coma* could be used to describe patients who are not brain-dead, but who are in a variety of chronic comas or in persistent vegetative states, as previously noted. The common practice of considering *brain death* and *cerebral death* as equivalent terms may lead to confusion. This is most evident when one considers the status of the brain stem; for example, the cerebrum may be destroyed and the brain stem remain intact, or the reverse may occur. Rarely, the cerebrum and brain stem may be completely separated from each other.[40] These subjects relating to a critique of the Harvard criteria have been discussed and will be further expanded upon in other papers presented in this volume by Molinari[41] and Allen *et al.*,[42] who will discuss in detail the clinical criteria of brain death.

In 1968, the Declaration of Sydney was made, which added two important statements to the problem of the diagnosis of brain death in relation to organ transplantation. The first was a reaffirmation that death is a process, and that in a multicellular organism a large mass of cells might be alive but that this did not indicate that the organism as a whole was alive. Second, it declared that in situations related to organ transplantation, the pronouncement of death should involve two physicians unrelated to the transplant procedure itself.[43] The medical aspects of this topic will be discussed by Veatch[44] and other ramifications of the problem of transplantation will be noted elsewhere in this volume.

Significance of the EEG

In 1969 a series of papers by Silverman *et al.* relating to a retrospective study sponsored by the American Electroencephalographic Society more precisely defined and discussed the significance of the flat or isoelectric EEG, and the term *electrocerebral silence* was subsequently advocated.[45-47] Problems in attempting to standardize the EEG techniques including the use of maximal amplification, maximal intraelectrode distances and duration of recording were most recently specified by the American EEG Society in 1976.[48] Further prospective studies sponsored by the National Institutes of Health included evaluation of the use and limitations of the EEG as an adjunct in the diagnosis of brain death.[37, 49] The problems of utilization of electroencephalography will be detailed in this volume by Bennett,[50] Hughes,[51] and Goldensohn.[52]

Revised and Ancillary Criteria

Additional research, primarily by European investigators,[53-65] on cerebral blood flow (CBF) and cerebral metabolic rate of oxygen consumption considered the problem of diagnosis of brain death in relation to intracranial circulation and oxidative metabolism. The addition of absent intracranial circulation must be considered as a most important ancillary criterion in the establishment of brain death, especially if any uncertainty exists in utilizing other criteria. The value of four-vessel angiography is undisputed although a simpler technique that will allow bedside evaluation of CBF is being sought. In this volume, Fein will discuss brain energetics, while Hass and Hawkins will cover other aspects of the cerebral metabolism related to intracranial lesions. Subsequently, Braunstein,[66] Kricheff,[67] and their coworkers will detail applications of cerebral blood flow studies related to radioisotope techniques, including validation by femoral carotid angiography that may be used clinically as an adjunct in the diagnosis of brain death. The radioisotopic bolus method, as described by these investigators in collaboration with Korein,[68-73] may prove to be a practical, simple, innocuous bedside evaluation of the critical deficit in cerebral circulation which will aid the clinician in the diagnosis of brain death. Other ancillary techniques that may be of aid in establishing the diagnosis of brain death will also be presented in this volume. (See especially the remarks of Goodman in the discussion sections of this volume.) Some of these ancillary criteria have been previously reviewed by Smith and Walker.[74]

APPLICATIONS OF CRITERIA IN THE DIAGNOSIS OF BRAIN DEATH

Medical Judgment, Current Criteria, and Differential Diagnosis

If we accept the thesis that the brain is the critical system of the human organism and that death of the brain does, in fact, represent death of the organism as a whole, then we face the nontrivial problem of applying appropriate criteria in unequivocally diagnosing brain death. The diagnosis allows an error to be made only in diagnosing a dead brain as alive. It is never, under any circumstances, permissible to diagnose a living brain as dead. Therefore, the criteria utilized must be skewed to insure no misdiagnosis of the second kind. Depending on the circumstances, we may use all clinical and laboratory tests that are locally available and relevant. We must always use clinical judgment to temper the choices of tests and their interpretations in making the diagnosis of brain death. One cannot understate the primacy of using medical judgment in establishing a diagnosis of brain death. Such judgment dictates several preliminary contingencies. First, no single clinical or laboratory criterion is adequate to make the diagnosis of brain death since the potential for error, although at times is exceedingly small, exists nevertheless. Second, if doubt in the diagnosis exists, the factor of time may always be extended until this doubt is erased by repeated clinical or laboratory evaluations. Third, it is almost always desirable to have an etiologic basis for the diagnosis. Although there are exceptions, it is obvious that limited clinical and laboratory tests will confirm the diagnosis of brain death in a patient with massive destruction of the brain due to a gunshot wound. In contrast, in diagnosing brain death in a patient in coma of unknown etiology, caution must be used to determine that the situation is not reversible. Under these circumstances, confirmatory tests often must be performed and even repeated that will allow the diagnosis to be made without equivocation. Finally, the circumstances that surround the patient are crucial, especially in infants and children, in whom the resistance of the brain to anoxia and decreased cerebral blood flow is demonstrably greater than in the adult. Research in applying criteria in this situation has been presented by Ashwal et al.,[75] and aspects of this problem are discussed in this volume by Pampiglione.[76]

Current suggested criteria following the NINDS Study [37] appear to be a reliable approach to the problem in adults and these are presented in TABLE 1. These criteria, as well as others, will be discussed in detail in this volume.

The differential diagnosis of states that may mimic brain death includes any reversible situation. This is mostly commonly related to drug intoxication. However, reversibility has been reported in patients with hypothermia, encephalitis and cerebral insult in acute stages. Infrequently, clinical and EEG criteria of brain death are seen in patients who are apneic and comatose and who may be in a reversible state; studies revealing the absence of cerebral circulation may be of aid in confirming the diagnosis of cerebral death, but other confirma-

TABLE 1

Prerequisite:	All appropriate diagnostic and therapeutic procedures have been performed (diagnosis established).
Criteria (to be present for 30 minutes at least six hours after the onset of coma and apnea):	Coma with cerebral unresponsivity Apnea Dilated, fixed pupils Absent cephalic reflexes Electrocerebral silence
Confirmatory test:	Absence of cerebral circulation

tory tests indicating absent brain-stem function are required to diagnose brain death. Other conditions that may be irreversible, such as persistent brain-stem involvement, must also be excluded. The differential diagnosis of brain death is discussed in detail by Posner; the relevent problems, prognosis and quality of survival after severe cerebral anoxia in adults and children are presented in the papers by Ingvar *et al.* and by Pampiglione *et al.;* and the general prognosis of persistent vegetative states will be detailed in the report by Levy *et al.*

Technology, "Extraordinary" Care, and Transplantation

The diagnosis of brain death is not meant to replace the conventional diagnosis of death. The use of criteria of "brain death" is highly restricted. These restrictions are directly related to a specific, appropriately equipped hospital environment where the technology and personnel for resuscitation and maintenance of life-support systems are available. Thus, one does not apply the criteria of brain death outside of the ICU or an equivalent facility associated with the operating room or emergency ward. Only in such environments is it reasonable to use the diagnosis of brain death as equivalent to systemic death. Under most circumstances, death is still and will be diagnosed by conventional means, although the occurrence of brain death is more common now because of advanced technology. Most individuals die systemically and the death of the brain follows rapidly. Brain death may be viewed as an artefact of modern medical advances. The necessity for developing the criteria to diagnose brain death, as previously mentioned, was initially based on termination of "extraordinary" efforts to maintain an individual's body when there was no hope of recovery of brain function. To continue such efforts not only represents a study in futility, but also siphons off highly technical limited medical resources and available personnel from patients who can be helped. To maintain the function of the body of a brain-dead patient only because the technical means exist is a moral and economic atrocity that has evolved through a perversion of modern science. There are circumstances, however, in which maintaining life-support systems in a brain-dead individual is both medically and morally sound. These circumstances are related to organ transplantation. If the patient prior to his condition has agreed to donate his organs, or if the relatives later agree that his organs may be used for transplantation, it is incumbent on the physician to maintain those organs in the best possible state to allow a successful transplantation. The management of these problems in the ICU generally, and how they relate to transplantation, are the topics of Suter [77] and Veith [78] in this volume.

Other Medical and Social Ramifications of the Construct of Brain Death

The ramifications of introducing the construct of brain death are multiple and complex.[79] These include ethical, religious, legislative and judicial factors as well as a set of medical problems pertaining to the role of the physician in relation to the patient and society. Since other contributors to this volume will cover many of these issues, these final comments will be restricted to ramifications that are more directly related to medicine.

The role of the physician in a problem such as brain death is, as it should be, explicit. It is the physician who must make the diagnosis and pronouncement of brain death. The judgment relating brain death to systemic death is the physician's responsibility. If there is an unambiguous legal precedent or a law in a given state defining death in terms of brain death, the physician will utilize that precedent or law. If there is no legal precedent or law, the confines of medical practice followed by the physician's colleagues within his professional environment must be utilized. (See, for example, Reports of the American Neurological Association.[80]) Since it is the physician's responsibility to evaluate the patient in order to establish a diagnosis of brain death, there is no reason to consider that this pronouncement requires a consensus of opinion or a committee. One does not diagnose a medical condition by a committee, although appropriate consultation may be required. In situations related to organ transplantation it may be prudent or advisable to adhere to the stipulation set down in the Declaration of Sydney that two physicians who are not involved with the transplant procedure concur in the diagnosis.

This situation, i.e., diagnosis of brain death, must be carefully distinguished from other types of problems related to the management of patients who are in persistent vegetative states [81] or are terminally ill or in other extreme situations that do not involve brain death. This set of problems, which excludes brain death, may range from that of withholding resuscitation from patients with terminal carcinoma, discontinuing life-support procedures in patients who are in a variety of irreversible states, or deciding which patient should be placed on dialysis in relatively acute situations when resources are limited. These problems may involve the decision of a physician or a combined decision of the physician and the family or even a committee. This is not to suggest that a committee be utilized for every aspect of these difficult medical problems but only to indicate that situations exist in which the physician's interaction with the patient and society might be more formalized and appropriate protocols developed for decision-making management of patients in these extreme circumstances.[82] The unfortunate use of the terms "active" and "passive" euthanasia may be considered as an example. Although one may argue with the terminology on a variety of grounds, there are unequivocal pragmatic differences among the following illustrations. Injection of a toxic substance for the purpose of killing a patient is not the same as removal of life-supporting systems from a patient who is in irreversible coma (but not brain-dead), and these are both different from refraining to resuscitate a patient with terminal carcinoma and multiple metastases who has gone into cardiac arrest. Although in the past physicians have taken on this painful responsibility, it would appear that in the future such decisions may be planned and formed in conjunction with the patient, the family, the hospital facility, and the social matrix one is dealing with. Appropriate regional policy decisions on many levels must be made if this path is to be followed.

CONCLUSION

The diagnosis of brain death is highly specific and is based on the assumption that the brain is the critical system in the human organism. It may be considered equivalent to systemic death under circumstances in which life-support technology is applied in the appropriately equipped ICU. There is no single clinical or laboratory criterion that can be used to make the diagnosis.

Multiple criteria tempered by clinical judgment are mandatory to make the diagnosis and to insure irreversibility of brain destruction. It is the physician's responsibility to determine the diagnosis by the means he has available. Since brain death is a process, the choice of duration of criteria to determine the *moment* of death may be developed by the physician. It would facilitate the physician's task if specific laws equating brain death with systemic death were available. The problem of brain death should be clearly distinguished from other diagnostic entities relating to use of life-support systems and from other irreversible medical situations.

REFERENCES

1. MORISON, R. S. 1971. Death: Process or event? Science **173:** 694–698.
2. KASS, L. R. 1971. Death as an event: A commentary on Robert Morison. Science **173:** 698–702.
3. KOREIN, J. & M. MACCARIO. 1970. On the diagnosis of cerebral death—a prospective study. (Presented at the 7th International Congress of Electroencephalography and Clinical Neurophysiology, Sept. 13–19, 1969). J. EEG Clin. Neurophysiol. **27:** 700 (abstract No. 130).
4. KOREIN, J. & M. MACCARIO. 1971. On the diagnosis of cerebral death: A prospective study on 55 patients to define irreversible coma. Clin. EEG **2:** 178–199.
5. WINTER, A. 1969. The Moment of Death. : 84. Charles C Thomas. Springfield, Ill.
6. BERGEN, R. P. 1969. Law and medicine: Death, definition and diagnosis. JAMA **208:** 759–160.
7. WILSON, J. A. 1972. Principles of Animal Physiology. : 10–29, 91–156, 213–218. Macmillan. New York, N.Y.
8. KOREIN, J. 1966. Towards a general theory of living systems. *In* 3rd International Conference of Cybernetic Medicine. A. Masturzo, Ed. : 232–248. Francesco Giannino and Figli. Naples.
9. FEIN, J. This volume.
10. JOHNSTONE, J. L. 1921. The Mechanism of Life. Edwards Arnold & Co. London.
11. ROTHSTEIN, J. 1952. Information and Thermodynamics. Phys. Rev. **85:** 1.
12. WIENER, N. 1948. Cybernetics. John Wiley & Sons. New York, N.Y.
13. SZILARD, L. 1964. On the decrease of entropy in a thermodynamic system by intervention of intelligent beings. Behav. Sci. **9:** 301–310, 1964. (Translated by A. Rapoport and M. Knoller. From: Z. Phys. **53:** 840–856, 1929.)
14. VON NEUMANN, J. & O. MORGENSTERN. 1953. Theory of Games and Economic Behavior. Princeton University Press. Princeton, N.J.
15. MARSCHAK, J. 1956. Cost of decision making. Behav. Sci. **1:** 67–78.
16. KHARKEVICH, A. 1960. On the value of information in problems of cybernetics. : 53–57. Moscow. *In* Computing Reviews. By E. M. Fels. **4:** 190, 1963.
17. PRIGOGINE, I. 1955. Thermodynamics of Irreversible Processes. Charles C Thomas. Springfield, Ill.
18. VON BERTALANFFY, L. 1969. General Systems Theory. George Braziller. New York, N.Y.
19. SCHRÖDINGER, E. 1947. What is Life? Cambridge University Press. New York, N.Y.
20. REMOND, A., ED. 1975. Handbook of Electroencephalography and Clinical Neurophysiology. Clinical EEG, II. Vol. 12. Elsevier. Amsterdam.
21. INGVAR, D. This volume.
22. PIUS XII: The Prolongation of Life (An address of Pope Pius XII to an International Congress of Anesthesiologists, Nov. 24, 1957). *In* The Pope Speaks. : 393–398, Nov. 4, 1958.

23. FISCHGOLD, H. & P. MATHIS. 1959. Obnubilations, comas et stupeurs. Electroenceph. Clin. Neurophysiol. **11:** Suppl. Masson. Paris.
24. JOUVET, M. 1959. Diagnostic électro-sous-cortico-graphie de la mort du système nerveux central au cours de certains comas. Electroenceph. Clin. Neurophysiol. **11:** 805–808.
25. MOLLARET, P. & M. GOULON. 1959. Le coma dépassé. Rev. Neurol. **101:** 3–15.
26. WALKER, A. E., E. L. DIAMOND & J. MOSELEY. 1975. The neuropathological findings in irreversible coma. J. Neuropath. Exp. Neurol. **34:** 295–323.
27. LINDENBERG, R. 1971. Systemic oxygen deficiencies: The respirator brain. *In* Pathology of the Nervous System. J. Minckler, Ed. : 1583–1617. McGraw-Hill. New York, N.Y.
28. BERTRAND, I., F. LHERMITTE, B. ANTOINE & H. DUCROT. 1959. Necroses massives de système nerveux central dans une survie artificielle. Rev. Neurol. **101:** 101–115.
29. MOLLARET, P., I. BERTRAND & H. MOLLARET. 1959. Coma dépassé et necroses nerveuses contrales massives. Rev. Neurol. **101:** 116–139.
30. KRAMER, W. 1963. From reanimation to deanimation. Acta Neurol. Scand. **39:** 139–153.
31. KRAMER, W. 1966. Extensive necrosis of the brain development during reanimation. Proc. 5th Intern. Congr. Neuropath. Excerpta Medica Internet. Congr. Series No. **100:** 33–45.
32. PEARSON, J., J. KOREIN, J. HARRIS, M. WICHTER & P. BRAUNSTEIN. 1977. Brain death. II. Neuropathological correlation with the radioisotopic bolus technique for evaluation of critical deficit of cerebral blood flow. Ann. Neurol. **2:** 206–210.
33. WALKER, A. This volume.
34. PEARSON, J. *et al.* This volume.
35. FISCHGOLD, H 1970. Electroencephalography and organ transplantation. Electroenceph. Clin. Neurophysiol. **29:** 209.
36. 1968. A definition of irreversible coma. Report of the Ad Hoc Committee of the Harvard Medical School to Examine the Definition of Brain Death. JAMA **205:** 85–88.
37. 1977. An Appraisal of the Criteria of Cerebral Death. A Summary Statement. A Collaborative Study. Sponsored by the National Institute of Neurological Diseases and Stroke (Contract NO1–NS–1–2316). JAMA **237:** 982–986.
38. POWNER, D. 1976. Drug-associated isoelectric EEGs—A hazard in brain death certification. JAMA **236:** 1123.
39. PLUM, F. & J. B. POSNER. 1972. The Diagnosis of Stupor and Coma, 2nd Ed. F. A. Davis. Philadelphia, Pa.
40. KOREIN, J. 1975. Neurology and cerebral death—Definitions and differential diagnosis. Trans. Am. Neurol. Assoc. **100:** 61–63.
41. MOLINARI, G. This volume.
42. ALLEN, N. *et al.* This volume.
43. GILDER, S. S. B. 1968. Twenty-second World Medical Assembly [Sydney, Australia]: Death and the W.M.A. Brit. Med. J. **3:** 493–494.
44. VEATCH, R. This volume.
45. SILVERMAN, D., M. G. SAUNDERS, & R. S. SCHWAB, ET AL. 1969. Cerebral death and electroencephalogram: Report of Ad Hoc Committee of American Electroencephalographic Society on EEG Criteria for Determination of Cerebral Death. JAMA **209:** 1505–1510.
46. SILVERMAN, D., R. I. MASLAND & M. G. SAUNDERS, ET AL. 1970. Irreversible coma associated with electrical silence. Neurology **20:** 525–533.
47. GRASS, E. R. 1969. Technological aspects of electroencephalography in the determination of death. Am. J. EEG Technol. **9:** 77–90.
48. 1976. Guidelines in EEG. : 21–28. American Electroencephalographic Society.
49. BENNETT, D., J. HUGHES, J. KOREIN, J. MERLIS & C. SUTER. 1976. An Atlas of EEG in Coma and Cerebral Death. Raven Press. New York, N.Y.

50. BENNETT, D. This volume.
51. HUGHES, J. This volume.
52. GOLDENSOHN, E. This volume.
53. INGVAR, D. H. 1969. Cerebral blood flow and EEG in coma, apallic syndromes and akinetic mutism. Presented at IX Symposium Neuroradiologicum. Göteborg, Sweden.
54. INGVAR, D. H. 1971. EEG and cerebral circulation in the apallic syndrome and akinetic mutism. Electroenceph. Clin. Neurophysiol. 30: 272–273.
55. INGVAR, D. H. & L. WIDEN. 1972. Hjarndod. Lakartidningen 69: 3804–3814.
56. BROCK, M., C. FIESCHI, D. H. INGVAR, N. A. LASSEN & K. SCHURMANN, EDS. 1969. Cerebral Blood Flow. Springer Verlag. Berlin.
57. BROCK, M., K. SCHURMANN & A. HADJIDIMOS. 1969. Cerebral blood flow and cerebral death. Preliminary report. Acta Neurochir. 20: 195.
58. GOODMAN, J. M., F. S. MISHKIN & M. DYKEN. 1969. Determination of brain death by isotope angiography. JAMA 209: 1869–1872.
59. VLAHOVITCH, B., P. FREREBEAU, A. KUHNER, B. STOPAK & C. GROS. 1969. L'arrêt circulatoire intra cranien dans las mort du cerveau—Étude des angiographies avec injection sous pression. Presented at IX Symposium Neuroradiologicum, Göteborg, Sweden.
60. VLAHOVITCH, B., P. FREREBEAU, A. KUHNER, B. STOPAK, B. ALLAIS & C. GROS. 1972. Arrêt circulatoire intracranien dans la mort du cerveau: Angiographie avec injection sous pression. Acta Radiol. 13: 334–349.
61. BES, A., L. ARBUS & Y. LAZORTHES, ET AL. 1969. Hemodynamic and metabolic studies in "coma dépassé": A search for a biological test of death of the brain. M. Brock, C. Fieschi, D. H. Ingvar, et al., Eds. : 213–215. Springer Verlag. Berlin.
62. GROS, C., B. VLAHOVITCH, P. FREREBEAU, A. KUHNER, M. BILLET, G. SAHUT & G. GAVAND. 1969. Critères arteriographiques des comas dépassés en neurochirurgia. Neurochirurgie 15: 477–486.
63. HASS, W. K., J. RANSOHOFF, D. H. WOOD & A. WALD. 1970. Continuous in vivo monitoring by mass spectrometry of human blood gasses and cerebral blood flow. Trans. Am. Neurol. Assoc. 95: 255.
64. BUECHELER, E., C. KAEUFER & A. DUEX. 1970. Zerebrale Angiographie zur Bestimmung des Hirntodes. Fortschr. Roentgenstr. 113: 278–296.
65. SHALIT, M. N., A. J. BELLER, M. FEINSOD, A. J. DRAPKING & S. COTEY. 1970. The blood flow and oxygen consumption of the dying brain. Neurology 20: 740–748.
66. BRAUNSTEIN, P. et al. This volume.
67. KRICHEFF, I. et al. This volume.
68. KRICHEFF, I. I., P. BRAUNSTEIN, J. KOREIN & K. COREY. 1972. A simple bedside evaluation of cerebral blood flow in the study of cerebral death (abstract). Neuroradiology 4: 129.
69. BRAUNSTEIN, P., J. KOREIN & I. I. KRICHEFF. 1972. Bedside assessment on cerebral circulation. Lancet : 1291, June 10.
70. BRAUNSTEIN, P., I. I. KRICHEFF, J. KOREIN & K. COREY. 1973. Cerebral death: A rapid and reliable diagnostic adjunct using radioisotopes. Nucl. Med. 14: 122–124.
71. KOREIN, J. 1973. On cerebral, brain and systemic death. Current concepts of cerebrovascular disease. Stroke 8: 9–14.
72. KOREIN, J., P. BRAUNSTEIN, I. I. KRICHEFF, A. LIEBERMAN & N. CHASE. 1975. Radioisotopic bolus technique as a test to detect circulatory deficit associated with cerebral death. 142 Studies on 80 patients demonstrating the bedside use of an innocuous IVF procedure as an adjunct in the diagnosis of cerebral death. Circulation 51: 924–205.
73. KOREIN, J., P. BRAUNSTEIN, A. GEORGE, M. WICHTER, I. I. KRICHEFF, A. LIEBERMAN & J. PEARSON. 1977. Brain death. I. Angiographic correlation with the

radioisotope bolus technique for evaluation of critical deficit of cerebral blood flow. Ann. Neurol. **2:** 195–205.

74. SMITH, A. J. & A. E. WALKER. 1973. Cerebral blood flow and brain metabolism as indicators of cerebral death. Johns Hopikns Med. J. **133:** 107–109.

75. ASHWAL, S., A. J. SMITH, F. TORRES, M. LOKEN & S. CHOU. Radionuclide bolus angiography: A technique for verification of brain death in infants and children. J. Pediat. In press.

76. PAMPIGLION, G. This volume.

77. SUTER, C. This volume.

78. VEITH, F. This volume.

79. WALKER, A. E. 1977. Cerebral Death. Professional Information Library. Dallas, Texas.

80. JENNETT, W. B. & F. PLUM. 1972. The persistent vegetative state: A syndrome in search of a name. Lancet **1:** 734–737.

81. 1977. Report of the Committee on Irreversible Coma and Brain Death. (Revised Statement Regarding Methods for Determining that the Brain is Dead.) Trans. Am. Neurol. Assoc. **102:** 191–193.

82. HUGHES, C. J.: Supreme Court Decision of New Jersey. A-116, September term, 1975. In the matter of Karen Quinlan, an alleged incompetent. Decided March 31, 1976.

SOME PRELIMINARY REMARKS ON BRAIN DEATH

Richard Roelofs

Department of Social Medicine
Montefiore Hospital and Medical Center
Bronx, New York 10467

Dr. Korein has summarized the developments leading to the present recognition of brain death and cerebral death as relatively well defined and distinguishable clinical entities. Many topics of medical and scientific interest remain to be explored, e.g., the reliability of various diagnostic procedures and the precise nature of the relevant structural features and functional mechanisms of the brain. These and much more will be discussed in the papers to follow. But medical recognition of brain death has given rise also to new questions of ethics and social policy, as well as to philosophical puzzles and disputes about the definition of human life and death. Should we say that a patient with a ruined brain is dead? If not, can we agree that a patient with a ruined brain may justifiably be allowed to die? What if only the cerebral cortex is ruined: is such a person dead? May active therapy be withdrawn from such a patient? These questions are also on the agenda of this conference, and are to be addressed in detail later on. My purpose here is only to direct attention to them, and to sketch some possible replies.

I shall begin, then, with the question: should we say that a patient with a ruined brain is dead? It seems to me that there are at least three different sorts of questions which might be formulated in these words, and it is important to distinguish them at the outset.

First, there is the question about the logical or conceptual connection between having a ruined brain and being dead; that is, we may be asking whether brain death is a kind of death in the way that a square is a kind of rectangle. When physicians undertake to answer this question they are playing the philosopher's game on the latter's home turf. What is needed to answer the question is an analysis of our concept of death.

Second, there is the question about the epistemic connection between having a ruined brain and being dead; that is, we may be asking whether the fact that a patient has a ruined brain is a good and sufficient reason for saying that the patient is dead. Notice that we might very well agree to employ brain death in this way, as a criterion of death, even if we did not agree that brain death is a kind of death. Philosophers might want to say something about the conditions under which it would be reasonable to do this, but in the end the adequacy of brain death as a criterion of death would be a matter for medical experience to decide.

Finally there is the question as to whether there should be some connection between having a ruined brain and being legally dead; that is, we may be asking whether employment of brain death as a criterion of death should be embodied in statute (perhaps for the protection of physicians or for the benefit of viable patients who must compete for scarce resources). We might think this unwise even if we agreed that brain death is an adequate criterion of death in medical or biological terms. But I shall say nothing more about this third

0077–8923/78/0315–0039 $01.75/0 © 1978, NYAS

version of our question; here I gladly defer to Professor Capron. I would like to say just a bit more about the first and second versions. Is brain death a kind of death? Is brain death a useful criterion of death? We can, of course, ask exactly analogous questions about cerebral death, and in what follows I shall suggest that the answers may well be different. But the conceptual issue has first to be settled somehow.

I wish that I could shed more light on the concept of death. There is little help to be gotten from the literature. In all that has been written about death and dying in recent years, almost no attention has been paid to the analysis of the concept, and most of us would be embarrassed if we were asked to spell out in different words what it is that we are saying about a patient when we say that this patient is dead. But I think it may be possible to identify one element that must be included in any plausible analysis of the concept of death, and to use this in turn to answer the question whether brain death (or cerebral death) is a kind of death.

This much, I think, is clear: our concept of death involves the concept of an irretrievable loss. If a patient recovers after having been pronounced dead, we don't say that he was dead and is alive again; we say that (contrary to all appearances) he wasn't dead after all. It may be thought that this can happen only when physicians and coroners are careless. But to rest content with this is to overlook a most interesting feature of our concept of death, namely, that it is not merely false but logically absurd to suppose that anyone survives death or recovers from it, ever.* Hence, to say that a patient is dead commits us to a prediction concerning the indefinite future. But from this it follows that no description of the patient's present condition can be equivalent to the statement that the patient is dead. Now, brain death and cerebral death are presented in the scientific literature as conditions that can be found to obtain (or not to obtain) in the case of particular patients at some particular time (or over some finite interval of time). The conclusion to be drawn is that brain death and cerebral death cannot be kinds of death. They are not new concepts or definitions of death; indeed, they are not even candidates for such roles.† But although it is impossible to suppose that brain death and cerebral death can function as kinds or alternative concepts of death, it is at least initially plausible that they might function as criteria of death. A criterion of death is a state of affairs, typically some bodily condition of the patient, which suffices to justify the judgment that the patient is dead. What counts as a good and sufficient reason here, and how we come by it, would be a long and complicated story. Events at the surface of the body, or information displayed by medical devices, serve as criteria of the well-defined bodily conditions which are in turn taken as criteria of death. The traditional criteria, absence of pulse and of respiration, fill the bill quite nicely: a relatively brief lapse of these functions is correlated, both inductively and by means of theory, with the immediate onset of long-term degenerative changes, the reversal of which is beyond all rational expectation. Much the same can be said in favor of brain death as a criterion of death, with this important difference: that the diagnosis of brain death, at least, is supposed to support the judgment that the patient is dead even when degenerative change is being held at bay by mechanical perfusion and ventilation. Cerebral death,

---

* By definition, death is an irreversible state in medicine and biology.—*J.K.*

† This volume is replete with disagreement with this statement, but the reader must separate *concept* of death and *criteria* for death.—*J.K.*

however, is not in the same way correlated with the onset of systemic autolysis. If it is to be accepted as a criterion of death some altogether different argument will have to be offered in its behalf.

I want to turn now to some of the ethical questions that seem to be involved in acceptance of the brain death or cerebral death criteria. It is sometimes suggested that to adopt brain death or cerebral death as a criterion of death would be wrong because, in some circumstances at least, to do so would result in violations of individual rights. The vision evoked here is of a helpless patient being denied expensive therapy or robbed of his kidneys on the pretext that he is dead when he is (really) still alive. Is there anything to this suggestion? I think not. Of course a proposed criterion of death might be unreliable in the sense that it could be satisfied by a good many patients who are not dead at all. But this, if true, would be a direct argument against adopting it as a criterion; we would not need to invoke any moral arguments in order to reject it. Again, even a reliable criterion might be mistakenly applied, that is, we might think that it is satisfied in some particular instance, when in fact it is not satisfied. If such mistakes are *likely* to be made, due to difficulty of application, that would clearly count against the proposed criterion. But the mere fact that mistakes *can* be made does not count against it.

If a criterion of death is both reliable and relatively easy to apply, and is found to be satisfied by a particular patient, then in that case we can have no reason to think that this patient is (really) still alive. It seems very natural to conclude from this that we may employ any criterion of death whatever, so long as it is adequate in the ways just mentioned, without infringing anyone's rights. The living and the dead will have just the rights that they had before. The only consequence of employing a different criterion is that we may be able to tell more precisely who is alive and who is dead. Of course if our new criterion is more adequate than the old, that is, if it does indeed help us make fewer mistakes about who is alive and who is dead, then we will now treat some persons as dead who would formerly have been treated as living. But this doesn't at all mean that the new criteria result in the infringement of any patient's rights; the correct account of this situation is that previously (because of the inadequacies of diagnostic tools or the fear of legal liability) we were treating dead people as though they were alive, and so perhaps according them treatment to which they had no rightful claim.

This is all true as far as it goes. Yet I think it would be a mistake to conclude that shifts in criteria of death would leave everything ethically and legally just as it was before. If there are scientific and therapeutic motives for shifting the criteria (for example, to provide more material for research, or more and better organs for transplantation), then it must be the case that under new criteria the person who is dead will be more useful than before. It may be possible to sustain some of his organs for a longer period, perhaps indefinitely, and hence he may be subjected to certain kinds of treatment that were never previously contemplated. You will recall that a few years ago Professor Hans Jonas attacked the so-called "Harvard criteria" in an essay entitled "Against the Stream." He did not allege that these criteria would legitimize the removal of life support from patients before they were truly dead. His objection was that these criteria would create a new class of dead persons in whom certain vital functions might be sustained or simulated indefinitely for research and therapeutic purposes. It is interesting to note that Jonas did not bother to argue that it would be wrong to treat dead persons in this fashion. He seemed to take that moral judgment as indisputably obvious, and proceeded to argue that, since the criteria proposed by the Harvard Ad Hoc Committee would be liable to this abuse, they ought not to be adopted. The prospect of exploiting an artificially animated cadaver for the benefit of the living was, in his view, simply intolerable. This view may be mistaken, but it is hardly odd or unheard of. Organ donation is not yet widely popular, and consent for autopsy is notoriously difficult to obtain. It appears that there is still considerable social resistance to treating the dead as a kind of renewable resource. Of course, the fact that many people share Professor Jonas's repugnance does not show that there is something objectively wicked about maintaining platoons of warm pink corpses as blood banks, experimental subjects, and the like. I shall not attempt to argue this question here. I only want to point out that it is a serious question, an interesting question, a question for which our customary modes of thought and action concerning the dead may provide no ready answer. If it is true that shifting criteria of death create new categories of dead persons, it may turn out that our moral obligations with respect to persons in these new categories may not be just the same as those which we have acknowledged heretofore in dealing with the dead.

I have tried to suggest some of the ways in which persons skilled in logical analysis or moral philosophy might make a contribution to the discussion of brain death and cerebral death. I should like to say just a few words now about the possible relevance of theology and religious tradition. Of course it is not to be expected that the theologian, any more than the philosopher, would be so bold as to propose an independent criterion of death sharply at odds with those accepted by physicians. As for the concept of death, I have already remarked that in my view scarcely anyone has said anything helpful on that score. At considerable risk of oversimplification I shall venture to assert that the job of religion is to provide an extended metaphor for the world rather than a logical or causal account of it. Hence the theologian's task is to find just the right words to say, in obedience to the ruling metaphor, what death is *like;* he is less concerned, or not concerned at all, with the definition of death or with specifying the conditions under which death may be expected to occur. Moreover the metaphors provided by theology are intended to edify, that is, to influence practice. Hence, again, the theologian's interest lies in how one faces death or cares for the dying, not in any speculative determination of the boundary between life and death. But his concern for the proper metaphor or picture may very well bring the theologian into the discussion in a different way, as a critic of certain arguments offered on behalf of neurologic criteria of death.

Someone might, for example, argue as follows: "What a person *is,* is his brain. But once this is admitted, it is obvious that brain death is a reliable criterion of death. For if what a person *is,* is his brain, then any good and sufficient reason we have for saying that his brain is dead, will also be a good and sufficient reason for saying that this person is dead." Now it seems to me that even if they were inclined to accept the conclusion of this argument, Christian and Jewish theologians might well find the initial premise objectionable. Some might say that this premise conflicts with the metaphor that ought properly to govern our talk about persons and their bodies. Others might say that this premise itself suggests a wholly misleading metaphor. In both cases, however, the objection is that it is inappropriate to identify a person with some particular organ or organ function. Let's consider these objections in turn.

Religious believers of a dualistic persuasion will see the body as a vehicle, a tool, a house for the soul; from this point of view, no part of the body is any more closely identified with the person than any other, for the person and his body are conceived as belonging to totally different orders of reality. Believers of this persuasion will of course concede that certain parts of the body are critically important, in the sense that if these parts are severely damaged the person will cease to animate that body. But this leaves open all the possibilities that are adumbrated in the metaphor: that we may exchange one vehicle (or tool, or house) for another that is as good or better than the original, or that we may get along more simply without such encumbrances. To say that a person *is* his brain is to dismiss this metaphor out of hand, and thereby to undermine the religious form of life that is informed by it.

There is another line of religious tradition which, while refusing to make this sort of distinction between a person and his body, might nevertheless decline the invitation to agree that what a person is, is his brain. From the standpoint of this tradition all talk of the body as merely a vehicle, tool, or house for the soul is profoundly suspect. It looks, indeed, very much like an alien deposit of pagan philosophy, undermining biblical faith by suggesting that the body is of secondary importance, that this world is not our home and its problems are of no concern to us. Perhaps in reaction to this, the nondualistic religious tradition exalts life in human community, life that involves family nurture, productive work, and political action; and it recognizes the body as essential to that life. Moreover a nondualistic religion, whether Jewish or Christian, frankly celebrates bodily delights and is expressed by bodily actions: eating and drinking, dancing and kneeling, playing, singing, hearing, speaking, embracing, and making love, are as important to it as any processing of information. The person for whom such a religion is the form of life is a fully embodied person. He will not concede that he *is* his brain, or his cerebrum, because to do so would be to suggest, now, that persons are related to bodies as programmable components are related to the executive components of a computer, that is, as distinguishable parts of one complex material system. A theologian speaking from within this religious tradition would say that this is misleading; no *part* of the body is any more closely identified with the person than any other, because a person simply *is* a body behaving in appropriate ways over time.

But it does not follow from what has been said that there must inevitably be religious objections to the adoption of brain death or cerebral death as criteria of death. For these criteria need not be stated or defended in ways which identify the individual person with any part or function of the central nervous system. Nor is it necessary for partisans of these criteria to claim that permanent loss of consciousness or purposive function is equivalent to death. To make the case for brain death or cerebral death as criteria of death it only needs to be shown that such criteria enable earlier or more reliable identification of individuals who fall under our common concept of death.

This brings us back to the questions with which we began, clearly construed now as questions about the adequacy of certain criteria. Should we say that a patient with a ruined brain is dead? And what if only the cerebral cortex is ruined? Do either of these provide us with good and sufficient reason for saying that the patient is dead? I shall here only state my own conviction, without argument, that a case can be made for brain death as a supplemental criterion of death in cases where heart and lung action are being artificially sustained. It seems to me much more doubtful that cerebral death should be accepted as such a criterion. No one seriously doubts that a decerebrated frog survives his loss of brain tissue, and it is difficult to see, in the absence of special assumptions that have not yet been made clear, why the human case should be treated differently. A decerebrated human being is indeed a pitiful spectacle, and we may well feel that to be in such a condition is a fate worse than death. But this is not an argument for adopting a new criterion of death. It is perhaps an argument for a rational euthanasia policy.

BIBLIOGRAPHY

1. FLEW, A. 1964. Body, Mind, and Death. Macmillan. New York, N.Y.
2. JONAS, H. 1974. Philosophical Essays. Prentice-Hall. Englewood Cliffs, N. J.
3. KOREIN, J. 1973. On cerebral, brain, and systemic death. Stroke 8: 9–14.
4. STENDAHL, K. 1965. Immortality and Resurrection. Death in the Western World: Two Conflicting Currents of Thought. Macmillan. New York, N.Y.

THE DEVELOPMENT OF LAW ON HUMAN DEATH

Alexander Morgan Capron

University of Pennsylvania Law School
Philadelphia, Pennsylvania 19104

INTRODUCTION

The preceding presentations have developed the historical and contemporary meanings of death and have emphasized that physicians' present capacity to extend human life (or what may merely be bodily functions independent of human life) creates not only medical difficulties but ethical and religious ones as well. The task of this paper is to relate those medical and moral difficulties to the problems faced by society in attempting to respond through its official institutions to the medical reality. The issues that are introduced here will be developed more fully throughout this volume.

The law has always been concerned in some fashion with human death. "In this world, nothing is certain but death and taxes," as Franklin reminded us— and upon the fact of death, or its presumed occurrence, societies have seen fit to have many decisions made concerning property and family, civil rights and criminal punishment, and so forth. But in recent years the questions of when death does (or should) occur, and what may follow after it, have become more complex for the law.

Within the confines of this presentation, I address three legal developments concerning human death which manifest varying degrees of success: first, statutes on the transplantation of cadaver organs, an area marked by rapid adoption and uniformity but in which the basic issues treated in this volume were not resolved; second, the creation of new standards for determining that death has occurred, a field in which, without speed or complete agreement, a sensible consensus seems to be emerging; and third, statutes on the termination of care for irreversibly ill patients, where after several years of legislative consideration a spate of bills—poorly drafted and premature—has been adopted within the past 14 months. After a brief discussion of the first topic and an introduction to the second, which I discuss at greater length subsequently in this volume, the bulk of my attention is devoted to the problems in the leading treatment-termination statutes.

ORGAN TRANSPLANTATION

The transplantation of organs and tissue from one human being to another has a considerable history. Some efforts at grafting go back many years, and the procedure of greatest concern for our purposes, kidney transplantation, was first performed in this country thirty years ago.[1] The early transplants were performed using live donors, but with the availability and growing sophistication of immunosuppressive drugs during the late 1950s and 1960s, physicians came increasingly to rely on organs from dead bodies. (Today cadavers account for nearly 70 percent of all transplanted kidneys and the success rates for this group are improving.[2])

0077–8923/78/0315–0045 $01.75/0 © 1978, NYAS

Physicians working in this field found, however, that their progress was being impeded by the law.[3] To maximize the probability of success, organs should be removed from a donor as soon as possible after death is declared. The confusion existing in the law at the time over the authority to order removal of the kidneys greatly complicated doctors' efforts. Disputes arose among relatives, each of whom claimed priority, and between the views of relatives and the wishes expressed by the potential donor prior to death.[4] The law spoke in terms like "quasi-property"[5] that indicated a marked unsureness about the proper disposition of these contentions. These problems reflected both the law's prior inattention to the factual situations confronting transplanters and legislative actions taken more than a century earlier in response to a related but different medical phenomenon—grave robbing.

Rights over Corpses

The law that had grown up concerning the disposition of dead bodies did not reflect society's careful consideration of the relative interests of transplanters, patients and family members in the context of this new medical procedure, but rather was concerned with the disputes that sometimes arise within families about who ought to dispose of a relative's earthly remains and in what manner it ought to be done. It is hardly surprising that the rules, which can be traced back centuries to before the dawn of scientific medicine, did not adequately speak to the issues of transplantation in the 1960s. The resulting uncertainties left many people concerned for potential liability if they were later found to have acted improperly; this raised a need for prior judicial permission, which plainly ran afoul of the need for prompt action. Until the law on the relative authority of a decedent and of various family members was clarified, a serious roadblock existed to widespread reliance on cadaver organs, particularly in the treatment of renal failure.

Grave-Robbing Statutes

The second obstacle to progress in this field originated in the early nineteenth century. At that time society was faced with the understandable but excessive entrepreneurial zeal of individuals who seized upon the coincident need of medical schools for human cadavers for the training of students and the availability of such specimens in graveyards. Society's response was to adopt statutes making tampering with human bodies, including their use or sale, a crime under very broad provisions.[6] Although the purpose of these grave-robbing statutes would seem not to reach to kidney transplantation in the mid-twentieth century, the existence of the statutes exposed transplanters to at least potential criminal prosecution.[7]

The Uniform Anatomical Gift Act

In response to the obvious need for updating the law, a few legislatures acted in the mid-1960s,[8] and in 1965 the National Conference of Commissioners on Uniform State Laws, a body composed of law professors, lawyers and judges representing every state, impaneled a special committee to draft a model statute on organ donation. After several years of meetings and consultation with medical and scientific groups, including the Committee on Tissue Transplantation of the Division of Medical Sciences at the National Research Council, the Committee's proposed statute, entitled the Uniform Anatomical Gift Act (UAGA), was approved by the National Conference on July 30, 1968. Even prior to the adoption of this final version, several state legislatures had enacted prior drafts of the Uniform Act. Within a few years, every American jurisdiction had enacted this statute, a record unparalleled in the history of the National Conference.

Remaining Problems of Supply

Despite the ready success with which the statute met in the states, it did not lay to rest all of the problems in this field.[9] First, the number of people in the prime age groups for kidney donors who have taken advantage of the act's provision to make known their desire to have their organs donated to medicine upon their death is very, very small. Second, despite the supposedly binding nature of such determinations, physicians are still reluctant to act upon the deceased's indicated wishes if the family strongly objects, particularly if their objection is framed in terms of the deceased allegedly having changed his or her mind and revoked the apparent donation upon which the physician proposes to act. Third, the necessary cooperation between the neurosurgeons and neurologists (who are most likely to be in charge of patients who might be donors) and the transplant surgeons (who have need for organs for their renal patients) has been difficult to foster. Unless and until organ donation becomes a routine and well-accepted part of death, the formal change in the law is not sufficient to assure that anywhere near all the suitable organs will actually be made available. The burden of requesting a grieving family's permission for the donation falls upon doctors who have little self-interest in assuming it. Although greater success seems to accompany programs that employ persons other than the attending physician to seek permission, there is sharp disagreement on the subject. Moreover, despite the development of several networks of hospitals which share available organs so that they may be employed in patients most closely matched to the donor's tissue type, many problems continue to exist because the general shortage makes available organs a very dear commodity to be shared only reluctantly.[9]

All of these concerns point to the conclusion that the Uniform Act is not generating enough organs, and thus it has been suggested that further changes are needed in the statute.[10] It is beyond the scope of this paper to address such changes other than to note that substantial constitutional issues would be raised if the law were to go much beyond the next possible step, that is, providing that organs are to be taken unless the deceased or perhaps his relatives indicate otherwise.[11]

The Absence of a Definition of Death

Another problem with the Uniform Anatomical Gift Act that is of even greater importance for our topic is that it does not give a substantive definition of the point at which death may be determined. Section 7(b) of the Act merely states that "the time of death shall be determined by a physician who attends the donor at his death or, if none, the physician who certifies the death. This physician shall not participate in the procedures for removing or transplanting a part." This provision of the statute might, on the one hand, be seen as authorizing a physician or hospital to adopt any standard that he, she, or it wishes for determining that death has occurred. Such a view would certainly be conducive to successful transplantation, since the point at which death is declared could be set very early in the dying process, long before any deterioration had occurred in the organ to be transplanted. On the other hand, the very open-ended nature of this provision, and its potential for abuse, led most commentators to conclude that the statute had to be read in the context of existing definitions of death in the law of the state in which the physician operated. Thus, although the Uniform Act was the first contemporary response to the problems addressed in this volume, it was ultimately inadequate in addressing the problem of brain death.

DEFINITION OF DEATH

We come then to the second area in which the law has responded explicitly to the question of human death in recent years. When speaking of law in this context it is important to note at the outset that one is not speaking alone of legislation. In our society there are three major sources of "the law." First are the pronouncements of the people themselves, which take the form of the fundamental charters or constitutions by which society is to be governed and of occasional referenda on election ballots. Second are the statutes enacted by legislative bodies, and the regulations issued by administrators pursuant to those statutes. Third—and perhaps less visible to the lay public but of great significance to society—are the decisions of courts, which sit not only to interpret legislation and constitutions but also to create law on subjects not yet addressed by other lawmakers.

Common-Law Conflict with Medical Developments

On the question of defining when death occurs, the law has traditionally been of the third sort described here, that is, the common law established by the courts. The common-law definition of death, which still prevails in thirty-three American jurisdictions, requires the total cessation of all vital functions. This definition, which grew out of cases involving the disposition of estates and criminal prosecutions, goes back many years, but has been reasserted by courts within the past decade [12] despite medical evidence of the type developed in Dr. Korein's preceding article. Considering the many reasons favoring consistency in the law, the continued adherence by the courts to what may appear a badly outdated rule is not surprising, but it does have some disturbing effects.

These effects became particularly pronounced in 1968, the year in which the Uniform Anatomical Gift Act was put forward for official adoption. At that time the proponents of the Act argued that there was no need for specific legislation on the definition of death.[13] That same year, however, a prestigous ad hoc committee of the Harvard Medical School issued a report defining the

medical state of "irreversible coma," which the committee proposed as establishing a neurologic definition of death.[14] The contrast between the Harvard
criteria, which quickly gained acceptance within the medical community, and
the common-law definition took on particular importance because of the advent
of cardiac transplantation. The drama of a dead man's heart beating in a
living man's chest drew public as well as professional attention. But the underlying problem was a much broader one than that of transplantation alone, and
concern was soon manifest that the law be changed or clarified to allow physicians and lay people to know where they stood on the question of acceptable
standards for declaring death.

The Interests Harmed by the Conflict

Obviously the uncertainty generated by an outdated definition weighs most
heavily as a daily matter on physicians, who, on the one hand, face the risk
of needlessly treating patients who are dead, of wasting otherwise salvagable
organs, and of imposing unnecessary burdens on patient's families if they
continue treatment after death has, in their judgment, occurred, or who on the
other hand, risk civil or perhaps even criminal prosecution for terminating
treatment of a patient who is legally still alive.

But other than physicians' interests are involved. For family members and
for patients aware that the end might be near, there is the uncertainty of
knowing when it is proper to cease treatment without engaging in euthanasia,
and perhaps in some cases there is fear that a physician may alter the proper
standards for death in order to serve medical interests in transplantation. (Back
in the 1960s, this gave rise to many nervous jokes, such as the one about the
patient who hung a sign at the edge of his bed saying "Just sleeping, not dead.")
Moreover, the social interests involved are not only those of patients and family
members, but extend also to the entire society, for the question of death often
affects the disposition of important issues, such as the ownership of property,
tax liability, and the criminal responsibility of persons who cause injuries, which
are matters of basic public policy and not merely ones for private adjudication.
Governmental interests in predictable legal outcomes were endangered by the
incongruence of medical reality and legal rule, and the more fundamental
societal interests in having matters of such moment decided by public mechanisms would not be laid to rest if courts were to defer to medical opinion in a
piecemeal fashion.

Judicial Modification of the Law

It was hardly surprising therefore that the stop-gap solution contained in
the Uniform Anatomical Gift Act proved unsatisfactory. But how, then, ought
the law to be changed? It was suggested by some that the preferable route
would be for the courts to update the common law as cases arose. This has the
advantage of permitting the governmental branch that made the original rule to
modify it and to do so with medical guidance as circumstances dictate.[15] The
advantages of case-by-case adjudication are also its disadvantages, however. For
the rule must await the case and is not announced prospectively, so that uncertainty persists, hardly a benefit when matters of life and death are at stake.

Furthermore, the facts of the case may be said to limit the applicability of the holding. For example, many of the cases that have arisen since 1968 on the subject have concerned situations in which organs were transplanted,[16-19] which might suggest that there is a special kind of death that occurs in organ donors that has no application to the rest of us. Finally, the judicial mode of decision-making is dependent upon the parties for the development of the expert evidence needed to inform the law of the contours of the problem involved, casts that evidence in adversary terms, and does not permit direct public involvement in the framing of the result; moreover, it is much less likely that the results of opinions in such cases will quickly fall into a uniform pattern of decision.

Nevertheless, despite the drawbacks of common-law revision, the recent court decisions have all legally accepted a neurologic definition of death. Indeed, several murder convictions have been sustained on appeal in the face of the defendants' claims that physicians' discontinuation of treatment was the "intervening cause" of death in the victims, who were argued to be still "alive" so long as treatment maintained their respiration and circulation.[20-22] Only in Massachusetts, however, has a state's highest court clearly accepted total and irreversible cessation of brain functions as a legal "definition of death," and even then, "only as it affects [criminal] conviction"[20] without reaching other branches of the law.

A second approach, of which there is one example, would be a judicial interpretation of the Anatomical Gift Act that would establish that the physician's authority under Section 7(b) does indeed extend to neurologic criteria, despite preexisting common law to the contrary. In the *Sulsona* case in New York in 1975[19] the trial court granted a declaratory judgment on petition of the City's Health and Hospitals Corporation to declare that the neurologic criteria of brain death were acceptable under the UAGA provision on death. The judge recognized, nevertheless, that her action was limited to patients who came within the terms of the Anatomical Gift Act and to cases coming before that court and urged the state legislature to provide a state-wide remedy for this problem.

If court cases do not provide a very satisfactory means of redefining death, they may at least increase public awareness of the need for a statutory definition of death. As one recent article observes, "in all but one instance in which litigation has arisen, legislation that recognizes the validity of brain death as a legally accepted standard for determining death has been enacted shortly thereafter. The single exception is New York, where proposals are currently pending before the state legislature."[23] Although these same authors cite the current public distrust of medicine as the impediment to quick adoption of statutory definitions, the major result of litigation seems to have been to convince the leaders of the medical profession in the states in which it arose to abandon their opposition to a statutory definition. While the American Medical Association has repeatedly gone on record against any legislation, physicians more closely involved with the subject have concluded that the expressed medical concern over a premature freezing of current knowledge or an undue interference of the state with medical practice can be overcome by a properly drafted definition.

Statutory Definitions

The first statutory replacement for the common law was adopted in 1970 in Kansas, before the medical cases mentioned above had received judicial decision.[24] With small modifications the Kansas statute was adopted in 1972 and 1973 in three additional states,[25-27] and Oregon in 1975 adopted a statute that proceeds along somewhat similar lines but in much abbreviated terms.[28] All of these enactments have the basic disadvantage that they set forth two alternative standards for determining that death has occurred, those based upon heart and lung functions and those based upon brain functions, and by failing to relate these separate standards not only open the way for potential abuse or misunderstanding but also perpetuate the misconception that there are two different and unrelated types of death. The genesis of the Kansas statute only made matters worse. It originated with the concern of physicians at the University Medical Center that they were in legal jeopardy in performing organ transplantation because the Kansas Supreme Court had adopted the common-law definition of death.[29] Thus, the statute not only presents the idea that there are two different kinds of death, but also gives the impression that the change in the definition of death was sought primarily to let doctors snatch organs from people who otherwise would still be considered alive.

Criticism of the Kansas statute [15] resulted in states' adopting laws since 1974 following one of two alternative approaches. The first was proposed by Dr. Leon Kass and myself in 1972,[30] and legislation along such lines has since been adopted in five states, with modifications in some instances.[31-35] Our model statute provides that death is to be pronounced when a person has experienced irreversible cessation of spontaneous respiratory and circulatory functions, and that in the event that artificial means of support precluded determination that these functions had ceased, a person will be considered dead if in the announced opinion of his or her physician (basing judgment on ordinary standards of medical practice) he or she has experienced irreversible cessation of total brain functioning.

The second model statute, proposed by the American Bar Association (ABA) in 1975,[36] has formed the basis of five state laws (or six, if one counts the somewhat different Oklahoma statute [37]) adopted during the past two years; [38-42] the ABA bill resembles the California statute adopted in 1974.[43] The ABA proposal has the advantage of simplicity since it employs only the second part of the Capron-Kass bill and it speaks only in terms of irreversible cessation of total brain functioning according to usual and customary standards of the medical profession and omits any mention of other acceptable standards for determining death or of how they might be related to brain-functioning standards. This omission is no trivial matter and clearly concerns legislators— properly so since the overwhelming majority of people will still be diagnosed as having died based upon the more traditional cardiopulmonary functions. In response to this problem, California,[43] Georgia,[38] and Idaho,[39] in adopting their statutes, separately provided that the explicit brain-function-based definition does not prohibit a physician from using other usual and customary procedures as the exclusive basis for pronouncing a person dead. Unfortunately, this resurrects the problem of two separate and unrelated standards that flawed the Kansas law.

Despite the differences among the statutes and the opposition or indifference that efforts to adopt statutes have met, it now seems likely that some form of change in the common law will take place in all jurisdictions in the foreseeable future. A special committee of the National Conference of Commissioners on Uniform State Laws has been studying this subject for several years but has as yet been unable to persuade the Conference of the wisdom of its proposals.[44]

Even without a "uniform act," the model statutes now existing may provide the basis for action in the remaining states as indicated by their adoption in numerous states and by the absence of lawsuits they have provoked—suits that remain a threat with the common-law definition or with a poorly drafted statute, such as the one adopted earlier this year by North Carolina,[45] the only state thus far to have departed from one of the model bills. Regrettably, the statute resulting from its innovation seems to be a virtual invitation to litigation so many are the problems and ambiguities it creates.

We leave this topic now, which is explored in greater depth later in this volume, to turn to the third major development of the law on human death, the enactment of statutes concerning the termination of treatment for terminally ill patients.

TERMINATION OF TREATMENT

The question of when treatment should be terminated is the most explosive of the three treated here. It is explosive in the sense that after many years of legislative attempts,[46, 47] in the past year since the adoption of the first statute in California,[48] four other states have enacted similar laws [49–52] and Arkansas,[53] New Mexico,[54] and North Carolina [55] have adopted laws differing substantially in language but similar in intent; a bill patterned after the California act was vetoed by the governor in New Hampshire; and dozens of other states are considering measures along the same lines.[56] (The variations avoid some of the problems of the California statute, discussed below, but add others; the Arkansas and New Mexico laws, in particular, are questionable in extending to involuntary euthanasia since they permit relatives to execute "directives" for incompetent and minor patients.) Furthermore, the subject, which is basically passive euthanasia, is highly charged and understandably excites great public and professional concern. The subject is germane to the topic of brain death because it springs from the same medical technology and because in actual cases people so frequently confuse the question "Is this person dead?" with "Should this person be allowed to die?" The Karen Quinlan case in 1975 and 1976 in New Jersey [57] and the recent Deborah Mari case in Massachusetts [58] are illustrative.

Two Facets of the Problem

Clearly the legislatures are addressing themselves to a very important problem. Two major facets to this problem combine to give it its magnitude and urgency, but are analytically distinct. First, under the present circumstances, patients who are seriously ill, and particularly those who are also mentally incompetent, receive too much treatment. Death for many patients is held off at great cost to their dignity, at great expense to their pocketbooks, at great psychic and emotional burden to their relatives, and perhaps through the imposition of great physical pain and suffering. Second, the decision-making about the extent of treatment is largely in the hands of physicians. Not only are the wishes of family members often overridden, but also, more importantly, a person's own wishes are not capable of being legally effected. This gives rise in all of us, but particularly in those already suffering with a serious and perhaps fatal illness, to the terrible sense that we have lost control over our lives either now or later, once we are no longer physically competent to participate in decisions about our care. This too is a great loss in human dignity.

Were the cause of this problem simply that physicians were intentionally depriving their patients of their rights, the solution would not be far. Indeed, in the area of the treatment of competent patients, there has already occurred a marked shift in medical attitudes and behavior resulting from the increased emphasis on informed consent and patient rights. Most physicians are by now aware that their patients have the right to decide about their own medical care and that the law recognizes a patient's right to decline even life-saving treatment provided that he or she is competent and that the refusal of treatment does not immediately pose a physical risk to another human being or a child in the process of being born.[59, 60] But, of course, the problem of decision-making in incompetent dying patients is not so simple, nor can it be resolved merely by reiteration of the patient's right to make choices about his own care.

Present Confusion in the Law

What role then does the law play in contributing to the present state of affairs? To Shakespeare's line in *Cymbeline* (Act V, Scene 1) that "by med'cine life may be prolong'd, yet death/Will seize the doctor too," one is tempted to further observe that "law will seize the doctor too." Physicians fear that they open themselves to criminal and civil liability if they cease treatment when there is any possibility of saving life. It is not entirely clear whether this is a misperception of current law. It probably is. But the law is unclear about the extent of physicians' obligations to treat. It is probably for physicians themselves to suggest whether or not a particular treatment will be useful in maintaining and restoring a patient's life. Yet the judgment involved is obviously not solely one of medical probabilities but is also one about which reasonable people placing different values on life and on suffering would reach different conclusions. When the patient is competent to decide, it is clearly up to him or her, and not the physician, to apply personal values and make the final decision. But the law is unsettled whether the next-of-kin of an incompetent patient can step into the patient's shoes and make certain decisions about treatment, particularly the judgment to cease treatment. Moreover, physicians are further confused by the debate in the philosophic literature [61, 62] (which spills over into legal cases) about the difference, if any, between a cessation of treatment that leads to death and an active step intentionally bringing about death.

Confusion in the law is not necessarily a bad thing. Confusion may even be desirable if it promotes caution and conservatism in the making of choices that are as weighty and irreversible as those involved in the case of dying patients; society's attachment to the sanctity of life is better protected by conservative choices than it might be by a clarification of the law that was much more permissive.[63] In any event, it is my thesis that the confusion on this subject is not capable of being entirely alleviated by legislative action at this time in our society, and that we do better to live with confusion for a short while than to struggle with bad laws for a long while.

The Patient's Choice as the Underlying Objective

It is, nevertheless, somewhat unseemly for a law professor to argue in favor of confusion. Moreover, there is still great value in attempting to discover the roots of the current problem and in analyzing the legislative responses to this problem. I just suggested that there were two distinct but interrelated facets to the problem. Their analytical relationship arises because the first problem, that of excessive treatment, is dependent upon the judgment of someone as to what is excessive, and this in turn depends upon the judgment of the individual being treated, interference with whose choice is the second facet of the problem before us. Thus it would seem that the underlying objective in this entire area is the preservation of the patient's choice about care and its limits even in the context of terminal illness. If there were agreement on the basic principle of the patient's autonomy even in the fact of terminal illness, then it would not be difficult to adopt legislation providing for means of effecting that autonomy after incompetence occurred. Two major alternatives present themselves— either provision could be made for the appointment of surrogates who would make a person's decisions after he or she became unable to do so or a patient's instructions about the limits of acceptable medical care could be made legally binding on physicians. The former approach has been adopted, although not explicitly in the present context.[64, 65] A statute of the latter type, on which we shall focus, should (1) describe the minimal requisites of binding directions to a physician, (2) provide for a means of assuring the parties involved that the directive accurately represents the patient's wishes (i.e., that the patient was not incompetent when the directive was written and has not revoked it), (3) supply a means of resolving any disagreements that arise about the interpretation of the document and of deciding what to do when circumstances not explicitly covered in the document occur, and (4) punish intentional misstatements of, or deviations from, a patient's wishes.

The California Natural Death Act of 1976

Unfortunately, the leading statute, the Natural Death Act, signed into law on September 30, 1976 in California,[48] does not meet these objectives but rather adds great confusion to the law.[66] It is thus doubly unfortunate that other states have rushed to follow in California's footsteps, although some of them have attempted to avoid its worst missteps.

The California law was inspired by situations like that of Karen Quinlan, whose case was often cited in the legislative debates. Ironically, the California statute is so narrowly drafted that even had Miss Quinlan prepared a directive in the words used by the statute she would not have qualified to have had her directions followed. This curious result and other difficulties quickly emerge from an examination of the California Act.

On its face the Act appears to be straightforward. It states that a "qualified patient" can execute a "directive to physicians" instructing that "life-sustaining procedures" be withheld or withdrawn after he or she becomes incompetent. The statute was intended to lay to rest doubts about the legal efficacy of what are called "living wills." It precludes civil and criminal liability for those carrying out a patient's directive, and makes failure to follow a directive unprofessional conduct which could result in suspension or revocation of a professional's license to practice. Health-insurance policies cannot be made contingent on the execution of such a directive, nor can life-insurance coverage be limited because a directive is executed (i.e., it does not constitute suicide to cease treatment under the Act).

Internal Statutory Problems

Although legitimate questions can be raised about the need to have all patients follow exactly the same directive as set forth in the statute rather than one tailored to a person's own needs, such questions turn out on examination to be least of the problems of a statute that is very complex despite apparent directness and that indeed creates nonsensical results.

Rather than being a term of ordinary usage, the phrase "qualified patient" is given a technical definition by the statute [§7187(e)]. Such a patient is one who is diagnosed and certified by two physicians (who have personally examined the patient and one of whom shall be the attending physician) to be afflicted with a "terminal condition." "Terminal condition" is itself a term defined by the statute [§7187(f)] as an incurable condition caused by injury, illness or disease which will, according to reasonable medical judgment, cause death regardless of the "life-sustaining procedures" employed on the patient. Life-sustaining procedures are defined [§7187(c)] as the medical use of "mechanical or other artificial means," and it is interesting to note that in this morass of definitions the limits of "artificial means" are not set forth by the statute. One is left to wonder whether all of medicine is not by definition artificial and if so what the limits are of "life-sustaining procedures." Second, the procedures must be ones that sustain, restore or supplant a vital function. Third, the procedures must only serve artificially to prolong the moment of death and not be deemed necessary to alleviate pain. Finally, the medical judgment must be that death is "imminent" * whether or not the procedure is used. The result is that the only patients covered by this statute are those who are on the edge of death *despite the doctors' efforts.* The very people for whom the greatest concern is expressed about a prolonged and undignified dying process are unaffected by the statute because their deaths are not imminent.

Moreover, the statute's further provision [§7191(b)] that fourteen days pass between diagnosis of imminent death and signing of a directive renders the category of "qualified patients" a vanishingly small one—only if a miracle occurs will the patient live long enough to sign a directive that will be binding. At the time of signing he or she must, of course, still be fully competent and in possession of sound mental faculties, not overwhelmed by disease or the pain accompanying it or its treatment.

For people outside this category (that is, for the majority of people executing such directives while still healthy but anticipating the infirmities of old age, the burdens of their present physical condition or illness, or simply the chance of being suddenly rendered incompetent to make their own choices) the directive is not binding. The Act [§7191(c)] permits the attending physician to give as

---

* "Imminent" is not defined in the statute, but its accepted meaning is of something that will occur directly, immediately or in a very short time period, without any other intervening event.

much or as little weight "to the directive as evidence of the patient's directions regarding the withholding or withdrawal of life-sustaining procedures" as the physician chooses, and he or she "may consider other factors, such as information from the affected family or the nature of the patient's illness, injury, or disease in determining whether the totality of the circumstances known to the attending physician justify effectuating the directive."

The foolishness generated by the statute does not stop here, however. Another provision of the statute [§7188.5] states that directives executed by patients in skilled nursing homes are without force unless one of the two witnesses required for the directive (who must be someone other than an employee of the nursing home) is a patient-advocate or ombudsman designated by the State Department of Aging. It is precisely the plight of patients in nursing homes that excited great interest in the need for a statute. Yet, ironically, they are not helped by the statute because the companion legislation, which was before the California legislature at the same time as the Natural Death Act, to provide for the creation of patient-advocates was defeated (doubtless because it, unlike the Natural Death Act, would have required the state of California to expend some funds). Thus, there were no people who could act as the necessary witnesses for patients in nursing homes, and such patients were left outside the scope of the statute.

Of course, the problems with the statute may not stand in the way of its application if people choose simply to ignore what it provides and proceed on the basis of what they would like a sensible law to provide. A recent newspaper article about the statute begins with the heart-rending story of a 72-year-old man named Ernie Dias who suffered from diabetes and failing eyesight and had a pacemaker to keep his heart going. After having a stroke he was placed in a convalescent home for mental patients, since court psychiatrists had labeled him mentally deficient. The article reports that he had decided that "enough was enough." He refused to eat or take any medication and spoke of only wanting to die. "But every time he drifted into unconsciousness, nurses would rush him to the hospital to save his life with intravenous feeding." [67] The article then went on to report with obvious approval that hope finally emerged for him when "a counselor who had taken an interest in him discovered California's Natural Death Law. With Dias's signature and those of two witnesses, the nurses were free to stop calling the ambulance." It is hard, of course, to give a legal opinion on such skimpy facts. But it seems highly doubtful that this case actually fell within the scope of the statute, although it would be a good candidate for a properly drawn statute. Consider the following problems: First, if the facility in which he was held was a nursing home, the document would be invalid unless one of the witnesses was official. Second, it is doubtful that Dias was considered of "sound mind," given the basis of the court commitment to a mental-health facility. Finally, and most importantly, at the time the nurses chose to act, Dias was not undergoing a life-sustaining procedure, and the treatment withheld from him, intravenous feeding, is one that could hold off his death indefinitely, so that it cannot be said that death was not "imminent whether or not such procedures are withheld." The journalist describes Dias as "one of surprisingly few Californians to have taken advantage of" the statute. Arguably, it is surprising that anyone qualifies to "take advantage of" this poorly drafted statute.

Broader Problems of Implication

Stepping back from the statute, one perceives that its unfortunate effects are more far-ranging. The principle which the Act puts on the statute books—that there is no obligation to continue treatment when death is about to occur despite the treatment—is now generally accepted.[59, 62] Yet in speaking solely of those patients who have executed a directive using specified language under specific conditions, the Act implies that there is no basis for ceasing treatment of other patients who do not meet all the statutory requirements. Indeed, physicians can be expected to be very reluctant to follow the instructions of anyone (other than a judge, perhaps) to cease treatments not covered directly by the statute. For example, should a family member claim that a patient would not wish treatment to continue, the physicians might counter by saying that "if the patient had wanted that, he would have filled out one of these directives." Moreover, the authority of the family member to speak for the patient in the absence of a directive or in those situations not covered by the directive—in the overwhelming majority of situations when death is not imminent but the dying process is greatly prolonged—is not clarified by the statute, but rather is potentially undermined by it.[68]

Think also of the potential for confusion, agony and even litigation that the statute creates. In any particular case, the actual effects and limitations of the statute will probably not emerge until the patient is already comatose, at which point the family will be operating under a different set of assumptions from those of the physicians and lawyers, because the family will have believed the description given of the statute when it was passed, a description of a statute protective of patient-rights and promising death with dignity.

Worse yet is the potential for mischief in the statute's effect on the rights of noncomatose patients. The Act opens with the bold legislative "finding" (§7186) that ". . . adult persons have the fundamental right to control the decisions relating to the rendering of their own medical care, including the decision to have life-sustaining procedures withheld or withdrawn in instances of a terminal condition."

But just how broad would that right appear to a physician or hospital administrator who looked at this statute? Not very, when one recalls that "life-sustaining procedures" for "terminal conditions" turn out to be those that are utterly superfluous since death is "imminent" even if they are used. Hence, when a competent patient asks that his treatment be ceased, the cautious physician may conclude—erroneously but understandably—that the patient does not have a right to cease treatment unless death is imminent. After all, isn't that what the statute says in plain English? The patient is not covered by the statute and without the statute the right does not exist, for had it existed, the legislature would not have needed to pass the statute. The statement in §7193 that the statute is "cumulative" of "any legal right or responsibility which any person may have to effect the withholding or withdrawal" of treatment merely clouds the question further, especially in light of the declaration in §7186 that "there exists considerable uncertainty" about the legality of termination of treatment even in patients acting "voluntarily and in sound mind."

Some of the bad effects of the statute—for instance, the suggestion just made that the statute may cause physicians to go ahead with treatment in cases where they would previously have been willing to cease it because now either an incompetent patient has failed to fill out a proper directive or a competent one is not on the brink of death—are susceptible to empirical verification or refutation. Many problems may never materialize, although I doubt it. But other of the objections go to the heart of the statute itself, which is so poorly drafted as to be almost worthless. It is thus not surprising that, according to a recent statement by an official of the California Medical Association,[67] while it is estimated that more than 100,000 directives are already in the hands of doctors and patients in California, there have been very few cases in which it has been used.

The Underlying Division of Opinion and Belief

The terrible mess of this legislation is instructive. It cannot be traced to any problem of competence on the part of the legislative committee responsible for the statute. The first draft of the much simpler bill put forward by the Act's chief proponent, Assemblyman Barry Keene, whose defense of the statute can be found elsewhere in this volume, was free of most of these difficulties.[69] Rather, the problems with the statute appear to have resulted from the political compromises (it was amended nine times during the 1976 legislative debates) that the proponents felt pressed to make. Such compromises cannot be brushed aside as the inevitable consequences of competing interests when the results are as disastrous as those of the California Act. Our society does not seem to be in basic agreement on the premises governing medical care for the terminally ill. This subject will, unfortunately, grow more complicated in the years ahead as national health insurance comes about, because the introduction of the public fisc into every medical decision is sure to raise the specter of conflicting interests on the part of governmental decision-makers. In some ways, it would thus be good to resolve this issue in a satisfactory fashion before this additional complicating factor enters the debate. But the rift in views between those favoring patient autonomy and those opposing anything resembling euthanasia is very deep. Until society makes a choice of one over the other, the strictures each would place in the other's bills seem likely to result in a hopeless muddle.

CONCLUSION

The three legal developments about death treated here are interconnected but distinct. The cases that arise in the real world tend to blur those distinctions, but confusion really exists because the law has failed to set to rest all the troublesome questions provoked by medicine's ever more startling ability to preserve life or some of its signs in cases that until recently would have come to a rapid conclusion.

New medical capabilities sometimes present great hope, as in the case of organ transplantation from cadavers. Here society has moved decisively, and the remaining questions are not legal conundrums or problems of unclarity but ones of policy—how much further should we go in procuring organs if present arrangements fail to produce enough?

On the second issue, which is integral to transplantation but much broader, similar uniformity and decisiveness is wanting. But no basic disagreements have emerged, and the difficulties are ones of form (how best to state an agreed-upon conception?) and politics (how to make the issue sufficiently important so as to command the attention of legislators and sufficiently clear to receive the support of organized medicine?).

The major danger for "definition of death" bills is that they will be indiscriminately lumped together with "allowing to die" measures, which understandably excite strong opposition. The questions raised by the opponents about the latter bills (also denominated "death with dignity" or, more lately, "natural death" legislation) reflect fundamental doubts on the advisability of ever giving effect to a patient's choice to terminate life-preserving treatment. Thus, the objections cannot be met by tinkering with the legislation—to satisfy the opponents is to undermine the proponents' intent. Perhaps, until society is ready to resolve this tension in a more direct and conscious fashion, we must content ourselves with the notion that legislation like California's, and cases like Karen Quinlan's, at least have an educational impact on the public.

REFERENCES

1. MOORE, F. D. 1972. Transplant. Simon and Schuster. New York, N.Y.
2. ADVISORY COMMITTEE TO THE RENAL TRANSPLANT REGISTRY. 1973. 11th Report of the human renal transplant registry. JAMA 226(10): 1197–1210.
3. SADLER, A. M. & B. L. SADLER. 1968. Transplantation and the law: The need for organized sensitivity. Georgetown Law J. 57(1): 5–54.
4. Holland v. Metalious, 105 N.H. 290, 198 A.2d 654 (1964).
5. In re Henderson's Estate, 13 Cal. App.2d 499, 51 P.2d 212 (1936).
6. Construction and application of graverobbing statutes. 1973. American Law Reports. 3rd ed. Vol. 52. : 701–727. Lawyers Co-operative Publishing Co. Rochester, N.Y.
7. Cf. Commonwealth v. Berman, Nos. 81821–81822 (Super. Co. Suffolk Co., indictment filed April 11, 1974).
8. SADLER, A. M., B. L. SADLER & E. B. STASON. 1968. Uniform anatomical gift act: A model for reform. JAMA 206(11): 2501–2506.
9. KATZ, J. & A. M. CAPRON. 1975. Catastrophic Diseases: Who Decides What? Russell Sage Foundation. New York, N.Y.
10. SANDERS, D. & J. DUKEMINIER. 1968. Medical advance and legal lag: Hemodialysis and kidney transplantation. U.C.L.A. Law Rev. 15: 357.
11. NOTE. 1968. Compulsory removal of cadaver organs. Columbia Law Rev. 69: 693–705.
12. In re Estate of Schmidt, 261 Cal. App.2d 262, 67 Cal. Rptr. 847 (1968).
13. NATIONAL CONFERENCE OF COMMISSIONERS ON UNIFORM STATE LAWS. 1968. Handbook and Proceedings of the Annual Conference. National Conference, Headquarters Office, Chicago, Ill.
14. AD HOC COMMITTEE OF THE HARVARD MEDICAL SCHOOL TO EXAMINE THE DEFINITION OF BRAIN DEATH. 1968. A Definition of Irreversible Coma. JAMA 205(6): 337–340.
15. KENNEDY, I. M. 1971. The Kansas statute on death: An appraisal. New Eng. J. Med. 285(17): 946–950.
16. Tucker v. Lower, No. 2381 (Richmond, Va. L & Eq. Ct. May 23, 1972).
17. People v. Lyons, 15 Crim. Law Rptr. 2240 (Cal Super. Alameda Co. 1974).
18. People v. Flores, No. 7246-c (Cal. Super. Sonoma Co. Jan. 15, 1974).
19. New York City Health & Hospitals Corp. v. Sulsona, 81 Misc.2d 1002 (N.Y. Sup. Ct. 1975).
20. Commonwealth v. Golston, 366 N.E.2d 744 (Mass. 1977).
21. People v. Saldana, 47 Cal. App.3d 954, 121 Cal. Rptr. 243 (1975).
22. State v. Brown, 8 Ore. App. 72 (1971).

23. VEITH, F. J., J. M. FEIN, M. D. TENDLER, R. M. VEATCH, M. A. KLEIMAN & G. KALKINES. 1977. Brain death: II: A status report of legal considerations. JAMA 238(16): 1744–1748.
24. Kan. Stat. Ann. §77–202 (Supp. 1974).
25. Md. Code Ann. Art. 43, §54F (Cum. Supp 1976) (limits application of brain standard to "known disease or condition").
26. N.M. Stat. Ann. §1–2–2.2 (Supp. 1975) (same as Maryland).
27. Va. Code §32–364.3:1 (Cum. Supp. 1977) (requires concurring opinion of neurologist, neurosurgeon or electroencephographist; adopted March 13, 1973).
28. 1975 Ore. Laws, ch. 565 (adopted July 2, 1975).
29. TAYLOR, L. 1971. A statutory definition of death in Kansas. JAMA 215(2): 296.
30. CAPRON, A. M. & L. R. KASS. 1972. A statutory definition of the standards for determining human death: An appraisal and a proposal. U. Pa. Law Rev. 121(1): 87–118.
31. Alaska Stat. §09.65.120 (Supp. 1977).
32. Iowa Code Ann. ch. 1, §208 (Special Pamphlet, Crim. Laws 1977) (requires second opinion; adopted June 28, 1976).
33. La. Rev. Stat. Ann. §9:111 (West Cum. Supp. 1977) (in case of organ donor, second opinion required; adopted July 27, 1976).
34. Mich. Comp. Laws Ann. §326.8b (Cum. Supp. 1977) (adopted July 14, 1975).
35. W. Va. Code §16–19–1(c) (Cum. Supp. 1977) (adopted March 9, 1975).
36. AMERICAN BAR ASSOCIATION. 1978. Annual Report, February 1975 Midyear Meeting. Vol. 100. American Bar Association, Chicago, Ill.
37. Okla. Stat. Ann. ch. 63, §1–301(g) (West Supp. 1977) (adopted April 28, 1975).
38. Ga. Code Ann. §88–1715.1 (Cum. Supp. 1977) (requires second opinion; adopted April 28, 1975).
39. 1977 Idaho Sess. Laws, ch. 130, §1 (requires second opinion; adopted March 22, 1977).
40. Il. Ann. Stat. ch. 3, §552(b) (Smith-Hurd Cum. Supp. 1977) (part of Uniform Anatomical Gift Act; adopted Sept. 11, 1975).
41. Mont. Rev. Code Ann. §69–7201 (Cum. Supp. 1977) (adopted April 4, 1977).
42. Tenn. Code Ann. §53–459 (1977) (adopted March 18, 1976).
43. Cal. Health & Safety Code §7180 (West Ann. Cum. Supp. 1977) (requires confirmation by second physician; adopted Sept. 27, 1974).
44. NATIONAL CONFERENCE OF COMMISSIONERS ON UNIFORM STATE LAWS. 1977. Handbook and Proceedings of the Annual Conference. National Conference, Headquarters Office, Chicago, Ill.
45. 1977 N.C. Adv. Legis. Serv. ch. 815, §90–320 (part of Natural Death Act; ratified June 29, 1977).
46. BRILL, H. W. 1970. Death with dignity: A recommendation for statutory change. U. of Fla. Law Rev. 22(3): 368–383.
47. SACKETT, W. 1975. Euthanasia: Why no legislation? Baylor Law Rev. 27(1): 3–5.
48. Calif. Health & Safety Code §§7185–7195 (West Cum. Supp. 1977).
49. 1977 Idaho Sess. Laws, ch. 106 (eliminates 14-day waiting period; no penalties for noncompliance with directive).
50. 1977 Nev. Stat., ch. 393 (eliminates 14-day waiting period and requirement of imminence of death despite life-sustaining procedures).
51. 1977 Ore. Laws, S. 438.
52. 1977 Texas Gen. Laws, S. 148.
53. 1977 Ark. Acts 879 (permits others to execute directive for incompetent patient; no penalties for noncompliance).
54. 1977 N.M. Laws, ch. 287 (third party may execute directive for terminally ill minor).
55. 1977 N.C. Adv. Legis. Serv. Ch. 815, §90–322.

56. ZUCKER, K. W. 1977. Legislatures provide for death with dignity. J. Legal Medicine 5(8): 21–24.
57. *In re Quinlan,* 70 N.J. 10, 355 A.2d 647 (1976).
58. *See* HUDSON, R. 1977. Deborah buried; not the debate. *Boston Sunday Globe.* May 15, 1977, p. 1, col. 5.
59. CAPRON, A. M. 1978. Right to refuse medical care. *In* Encyclopedia of Bioethics. W. T. Reich, Ed. Free Press. New York, N.Y.
60. CANTOR, N. L. 1973. A patient's decision to decline life-saving medical treatment: Bodily integrity versus the preservation of life. Rutgers Law Rev. 26(2): 228–264.
61. RACHELS, J. 1975. Active and passive euthanasia. New Eng. J. Med. 292(2): 78–80.
62. RAMSEY, P. 1970. The Patient as Person. Yale University Press. New Haven, Conn.
63. BURT, R. A. 1976. Authorizing death for anomalous newborns. *In* Genetics and the Law. A. Milunsky & G. Annas, Eds. : 435–450. Plenum Press. New York, N.Y.
64. 20 Pa. Cons. Stat. Ann. §5601 (Purdon 1975) (when power of attorney not affected by disability).
65. N.Y. Mental Hygiene Law §78.05 (McKinney 1976) (designation of person to act as committee in case of future incompetence).
66. COMMITTEE ON MEDICINE AND LAW. 1977. Death with dignity. Record of the Association of Bar of the City of N.Y. 32(3): 119–123.
67. MANN, F. 1977. A state that permits you to die. *Philadelphia Inquirer,* Nov. 3, 1977, at 5–A, col. 1.
68. LEBACQZ, K. 1977. On "natural death." Hastings Center Rep. 7(2): 14.
69. GARLAND, M. 1977. Politics, legislation, and natural death. Hastings Center Rep. 6(5): 5–6.

REVIEW OF CLINICAL CRITERIA OF BRAIN DEATH

Gaetano F. Molinari

Department of Neurology
George Washington University Medical Center
Washington, D.C. 20037

INTRODUCTION

Black's Law Dictionary defines death as "the cessation of life; the ceasing to exist; defined by *physicians* as a total stoppage of the circulation of the blood, and a cessation of the animal and vital functions consequent thereon, such as respiration, pulsation, etc." [1]

The first two phrases define death in philosophical and legal terms, but the definition provided by physicians is purely descriptive.

Biomedical technology has long since antiquated this descriptive definition from two perspectives. It has become possible to maintain "circulation of the blood and . . . vital functions consequent thereon . . ." in patients whose brains no longer drive or control movements of the chest and lungs nor regulate intrinsic cardiac muscular contraction, by use of artificial respirators, pacemakers, and certain cardiotropic drugs. Conversely, during open heart surgery, it is common practice to temporarily terminate both intrinsic cardiac pulsation and spontaneous respiratory movements, while the brain and other organs are perfused with oxygen and other vital metabolic substrates by cardiopulmonary bypass machines.

In the latter case, the individual is alive, although the traditional cardio-respiratory signs of life are suspended because precautions have been taken to ensure the viability of the brain; in the case of the brain-damaged patient, artificial respirators and cardiocirculatory support measures may disguise the fact that death may have already occurred. Hence, under these special circumstances, spontaneous cardiopulmonary function has become dissociated from organ viability including that of the brain, and thereby unreliable as the principal indicator of life.

Initially, allocation of limited health-care resources and humanitarian concerns for the families of dying patients prompted physicians to question the prognosis for survival of individuals requiring prolonged use of resusciatative equipment. Ethical questions arose regarding the withdrawal of life-support measures after days or weeks of effort indicated no chance for improvement and a certainly fatal outcome. It was the technical feasibility of organ transplantation, however, and the need for fresh viable cadaver organs for use in living patients that produced the need for a definition of death that could be applied in the shortest possible time and in the presence of persistent vegetative functions including circulation.

From such considerations, the concept of brain death evolved; various alternative descriptive definitions of death were formulated; and the present state of medical, legal and public confusion was generated.

The purpose of this paper is to review the more prevalent descriptions of brain death and to analyze proposed criteria for validity of their implicit bio-

62

0077-8923/78/0315-0062 $01.75/0 © 1978, NYAS

logical principles, and to test their accuracy, scope of applicability, and practicality using a prospectively acquired data base from 503 comatose apneic patients.

Between 1970 and 1972, five hundred and three (503) comatose patients were prospectively followed from time of onset of apnea to final outcome using standardized clinical examinations, reflex testing, and electroencephalograms and, in fatal cases, autopsy protocols.*

Comprehensive evaluations were performed at prescribed time intervals after the accession criteria, coma and apnea, were met. Various specific aspects [2-5] and general conclusions [6-8] of that study have been published, but one of the major and most disturbing findings was that detailed autopsy studies of the brain did not always show signs of autolysis and other features of death of the brain preceding the actual terminal events.[2] In the effort to identify all cases of drug intoxication, many more cases in which drugs may have played a contributive role to the overall picture were found than had been clinically suspected by responsible physicians.[5]

In that study, it was also found that if all cases of drug-induced coma were eliminated, no patient recovered who had had an electroencephalogram showing a 30-minute isoelectric record.[6, 7]

In the light of the salient features of the NINDS Collaborative Study, we will review the various proposed criteria for brain death.

THE HARVARD CRITERIA

In its 1968 report, the Ad Hoc Committee of the Harvard Medical School to examine the definition of brain death [9] described the clinical and electroencephalographic (EEG) characteristics of the nonfunctioning brain.

In the absence of hypothermia and drug intoxication, the Committee suggested that concomitant unresponsive coma, apnea, absence of cephalic and spinal reflexes, and an isoelectric EEG were characteristic of patients with a nonfunctioning brain. Persistence of all of these features for 24 hours was thought adequate grounds to consider the nonfunctional state permanent. The Harvard group defined irreversible coma as the permanent nonfunctioning state of the brain and implied parity between irreversible coma and brain death.

Since collaborative study data indicate that if drugs can be eliminated as a primary or contributing factor by blood-sample analysis, no patient survived who had had a single flat EEG for 30 minutes,[6, 7] then the requirement for persistence for 24 hours may be too conservative, jeopardizing the potential utility of organs. While always accurate in predicting death, but using the criterion of pathologic changes of autolysis, only 8 of 14 brains showed "respirator brain;"[3] very few patients (4 percent) in the collaborative study actually met the Harvard criteria before spontaneous cardiac arrest or termination of support.

---

* Actually, 844 patients were studied in this project. However, many were deferred for a variety of reasons, most commonly due to their late entry into the study.—*J. K.*

CRITERIA BASED ON CLINICAL SIGNS AND DIAGNOSIS

In a clinical and pathologic study of brain death, Mohandas and Chou [10] reported that in patients with brain damage whose nature is known to the physician and which by its nature is known to be irreparable, and who show no spontaneous movement, apnea, and absent cephalic (brain-stem) reflexes, all persistent for *12 hours,* the outcome is invariably fatal. These criteria imply that the prediction of death or a fatal prognosis is tantamount to brain death.

While 67 percent of the patients in the collaborative study would have met these criteria, seventeen (17) had biological activity in the EEG at the time they met them.[8] These criteria permit a margin of error that is unacceptable. This point is of particular interest since a recent report from England suggests that the EEG is not necessary but an optional confirmatory criterion in pronouncing brain death.[11]

CARDIOVASCULAR COLLAPSE

From data derived from a Japanese study of brain death, Ueki and associates [12] reported that a diagnosed gross primary brain lesion, deep coma, bilateral dilated pupils with absent pupillary and corneal reflexes, and an isoelectric EEG predict brain death. In such patients, a fall in blood pressure of 40 mm of mercury persistent for six hours signals that death is imminent.

While these criteria define the proximity of death and may be interpreted as evidence of a dying brain stem,[6] in the collaborative study only 4 percent of the patients would have met these standards.[8] When organ donation is contemplated, hypotension is treated vigorously to maintain organ perfusion. Reversal of the hypotension may in fact restore electroencephalographic activity.

FAILURE OF CEREBRAL CIRCULATION

In a symposium on brain death, reported by Ingvar and Widen in 1973,[13] the criteria recommended for use in Scandinavia in patients with known primary or secondary brain lesions were unresponsive coma, apnea, absence of all cerebral functions including brain stem reflexes, a single isoelectric EEG, confirmed by aortocranial angiography [14] showing no circulation to the brain on two injections of contrast medium 25 minutes apart.

These criteria reduce the temporal delay to an absolute minimum (25 minutes), the circulatory criterion would not be influenced by the presence of drugs that depress cerebral function, and since, collectively, clinical signs, EEG, and cerebral circulation are determined independently of one another, they are cross confirmatory. While they imply that total cerebral infaction is the definition of brain death, variations in the rate at which the circulation to the brain collapses would probably permit a variety of pathologic states to be observed at autopsy.

While the likelihood of 100 percent accuracy is high, in the American collaborative study only seventeen (17) angiograms were taken [6-8] for diagnostic purposes. The use of invasive aortocranial angiography seems impractical in this country.

COLLABORATIVE STUDY CRITERIA

Despite the reticence of American physicians to subject moribund patients to potentially hazardous diagnostic studies, the advantages of a cerebral circulatory criterion to confirm a flat EEG and other clinical indicators of brain death caused the collaborative investigators to adopt a pragmatic approach.

Ancillary to the core investigations, radionuclide bolus transit curves were developed at one center as an indirect, noninvasive method for assessment of cerebral circulation.[15-17]

In a small group of patients, an ultrasonic technique was tried for detection of cerebral pulsation as evidence of persistent cerebral circulation and perfusion.[18]

The investigators recommended therefore that as a prerequisite for considering the diagnosis of brain death, all appropriate diagnostic and therapeutic procedures have been performed.

Since an average of seven hours was required to perform such procedures,[6] and since transient apnea and/or electrocerebral silence that occur initially after a severe head injury, stroke or cardiac arrest will usually recede in a few minutes to hours, criteria should be applied at least six hours after the onset of coma and apnea.

They recommended that the criteria to be met for a period of thirty minutes (30 minutes), six hours after onset, include: coma with cerebral unresponsivity, apnea, dilated pupils, absent cephalic reflexes and electrocerebral silence (isoelectric EEG). Once met, these criteria should be confirmed by some assessment of cerebral circulation indicating absence of "cerebral blood flow." [6]

Since these criteria were derived pragmatically from the analysis of findings and problems encountered in the survey of 503 cases, they have not been validated in a subsequent prospective study.[8] Since pathologic findings did not always confirm brain death, even in patients meeting the more stringent Harvard criteria,[2, 8] the end-point or proof of validity of these criteria remains ill-defined. Prediction of a fatal outcome is not a valid criterion for accuracy of standards designed to determine that death has already occurred.

Nonetheless, when pronouncement of death is necessary in the shortest possible time, the coincidence of independent variables such as clinical signs, EEG activity and cerebral circulation affords the highest degree of security of the diagnosis of brain death.

Some physicians and scholars have resisted the idea of using even more technology at the bedside, specifically, measures for assessment of cerebral circulation, when not even the EEG is available to all physicians called upon to pronounce death.

Alternate criteria have been offered that are more time-consuming but nonetheless may be accurate. Using the same prerequisite, namely, all diagnostic and therapeutic procedures having been performed, cerebral unresponsivity, apnea, absent cephalic reflexes including pupillary, corneal, audioocular and oculocephalic, an EEG showing electrocerebral silence during a 30-minute recording period, all suggest brain death but should be reexamined and confirmed six hours later (total time = 12 hours). In any instance where drugs may contribute to the clinical picture, or diagnosis remains uncertain, brain death may be verified by persistence of all criteria for a period exceeding 48 hours.†

---

† Some of the above criteria are summarized in TABLE 1, which has been modified from Walker,[7] and explicitly listed in TABLE 2, which has been compiled by the editor.

TABLE 1
CRITERIA OF CEREBRAL DEATH *

Parameter	Criteria				
	Harvard [9]	Minnesota [10]	Japan [12]	Sweden [13]	Cerebral Survival [7, 10]
Prerequisites					
Normothermia	Yes [†]	No [‡]	No	No	No
No drug intoxication	Yes	Yes	Yes	Yes	Yes [§]
Diagnostically verified brain lesion	No	Yes	Yes	Yes	Yes
Criteria					
Basic					
Unresponsive coma and apnea	Yes	Yes	Yes	Yes	Yes
Accessory					
Absent cephalic reflexes	Yes	Yes	Yes	Yes	Yes
Dilated, fixed pupils	Yes	Yes	Yes	Yes	Yes
Absent spinal reflexes	Yes	No	No	No	No
Arterial hypotension	No	No	Yes	No	No
EEG with electrocerebral silence	Yes (Confirmatory)	No	Yes	Yes	Yes
Confirmatory					
Absent cerebral circulation	No	No	No	Yes	Yes
Duration of criteria	24 hr	12 hr	6 hr	30 min	30 min to 1 hr but 6 hr after onset of coma and apnea [||]

* Modified from Walker [7] by the editor.
† Yes=required.
‡ No=not required.
§ But not required if absent cerebral circulation is demonstrated.
|| This duration is valid if confirmatory tests show absent circulation; if cerebral circulation studies are not performed, a repeat evaluation of criteria has been suggested by the author.—J. K.

TABLE 2 *

SUMMARY OF SETS OF CRITERIA USED BY DIFFERENT INVESTIGATORS
AND CLINICIANS

Harvard criteria [9]	1. Unresponsive coma
	2. Apnea
	3. Absence of cephalic reflexes
	4. Absence of spinal reflexes
	5. Isoelectric EEG
	6. Persistence of conditions for at least 24 hours
	7. Absence of drug intoxication or hypothermia
Minnesota criteria [10]	1. Basic prerequisite—diagnosis of irreparable cerebral lesion
	2. No spontaneous movements
	3. No spontaneous respiration
	4. Absence of brain-stem reflexes
	5. Persistence of condition unchanged for 12 hours
Japanese criteria [12]	1. Basic prerequisite—diagnosis of primary cerebral lesion
	2. Deep coma
	3. Respiratory arrest
	4. Bilateral dilated pupils and absent pupillary and corneal reflexes
	5. Flat EEG
	6. Abrupt fall in blood pressure of 40 mm Hg with hypotension
	7. Persistence of condition for at least 6 hours
Swedish criteria [13]	1. Unresponsive coma
	2. Apnea
	3. Absent brain-stem reflexes
	4. Isoelectric EEG
	5. Nonfilling of cerebral vessels on two aortocranial injections of contrast media 25 minutes apart
Cerebral survival criteria [7, 19]	1. Basic prerequisite—completion of all appropriate diagnostic and therapeutic procedures
	2. Unresponsive coma
	3. Apnea
	4. Absent cephalic reflexes with dilated, fixed pupils †
	5. Isoelectric EEG
	6. Persistence of the above for 30 minutes to 1 hour, and 6 hours after onset of coma and apnea
	7. Confirmatory test indicating absence of cerebral circulation

* Compiled by the editor.
† See the next paper by Allen et al. on the problem of pupillary dilatation.

SUMMARY

A spectrum of descriptive definitions of death has been formulated based on a variety of observations using currently available clinical methods. These definitions vary widely in objectivity and some fail to distinguish the inevitability of death or irreversible coma from the fact of death. A hopeless prognosis may be an adequate criterion for termination of artificial resuscitation, but the bioethical issue involved is one of "passive" euthanasia and not brain death. A hopeless prognosis without a pronouncement of death itself would seem inadequate grounds to remove viable organs for transplantation.

When organ donation is contemplated, the declaration of death as a past event must be based on cerebral rather than on cardiovascular criteria. At this point in the history of the art and science of medicine, the highest degree of assurance that the brain is dead may be achieved in the shortest possible time, only by using multiple independently measured variables including clinical criteria, electrophysiologic criteria (the EEG), and assessment of cerebral circulation determined either directly or indirectly. As science and technology improve, the degree of objectivity and facility in obtaining objective criteria will also improve.

REFERENCES

1. Black's Law Dictionary, 4th ed. : 488. West Publishing Co. St. Paul, Minn.
2. WALKER, A. E., E. L. DIAMOND & J. I. MOSLEY. 1975. The neuropathology findings in irreversible coma: A critique of the "respirator brain." J. Neuropath. Exp. Neurol. **34:** 295–323.
3. MOSELEY, J. L., G. F. MOLINARI & A. E. WALKER. 1976. Respirator brain: Report of a survey and review of current concepts. Arch. Path. Lab. Med. **100:** 61–64.
4. BENNETT, D. R., J. R. HUGHES & J. KOREIN et al. 1976. Atlas of Electroencephalography in Coma and Cerebral Death. Raven Press. New York, N.Y.
5. WALKER A. E. & G. F. MOLINARI. 1977. Sedative drug surveys in coma. How reliable are they? Postgrad. Med. **61:** 105–109.
6. ANONYMOUS. 1977. An appraisal of the criteria of cerebral death—a summary statement: A collaborative study. JAMA **237:** 982–986.
7. WALKER, A. E. 1975. Cerebral death. In The Nervous System, Vol. **2:** 75–87. Donald B. Tower, Ed. The Clinical Neurosciences. Thomas N. Chase, Ed. Raven Press. New York, N.Y.
8. WALKER, A. E. & G. F. MOLINARI. 1975. Criteria of cerebral death. Trans. Am. Neurol. Assoc. **100:** 29–35.
9. 1968. A Definition of Irreversible Coma. Report of the Ad Hoc Committee of the Harvard Medical School to Examine the Definition of Brain Death. JAMA **205:** 337–340.
10. MOHANDAS, A. & S. N. CHOU. 1971. Brain death: A clinical and pathological study. J. Neurosurg. **35:** 211–218.
11. 1976. Conference of Royal Colleges and Faculties of the United Kingdom: Diagnosis of Brain Death. Lancet **2:** 1069–1070.
12. UEKI K., K. TAKEUCHI & K. KATSURADA. 1973. Clinical study of brain death. Read before the Fifth International Congress of Neurological Surgery. Tokyo, Japan.
13. INGVAR, D. H. & L. WIDEN. 1972. Brain death: Summary of a symposium. Lakartidningen **69:** 3804–3814.

14. GREITZ, T., E. GORDON, G. KOLMODIN & L. WIDEN. 1973. Aortocranial and carotid angiography in determination of brain death. Neuroradiol. **5:** 13–19.
15. KOREIN, J., P. BRAUNSTEIN & I. KRICHEFF, *et al.* 1975. Radioisotopic bolus technique as a test to detect circulatory deficit associated with cerebral death. Circulation **51:** 924–937.
16. KOREIN, J., P. BRAUNSTEIN & A. GEORGE, *et al.* 1977. Brain death: I. Angiographic correlation with the radioisotopic bolus technique for evaluation of critical deficit of cerebral blood flow. Ann. Neurol. **2:** 195–205.
17. PEARSON, J., J. KOREIN & J. H. HARRIS, *et al.* 1977. Brain death: II. Neuropathological correlation with the radioisotopic bolus technique for evaluation of critical deficit of cerebral blood flow. Ann. Neurol. **2:** 206–210.
18. UEMATSU, S. & A. E. WALKER. 1974. Pulsatile cerebral midline echo and brain death. Johns Hopkins Med. J. **135:** 383–390.
19. 1977. An appraisal of The Criteria of Cerebral Death: A summary statement. A Collaborative study. JAMA **238:** 982–986.

CLINICAL CRITERIA OF BRAIN DEATH *

Norman Allen and James Burkholder

Division of Neurology
College of Medicine
The Ohio State University
Columbus, Ohio 43210

John Comiscioni †

Department of Medical Education
College of Medicine
The Ohio State University
Columbus, Ohio 43210

When the concept of brain death was being developed, emphasis was placed upon the loss of function of the central nervous system as reflected in clinical examination. In the studies of Mollaret and associates,[1,2] identification of the state of coma dépassé was stipulated on the basis of isoelectric electroencephalography (EEG) as well as profound coma, absence of spontaneous respirations, dilated pupils, loss of multiple cephalic reflexes, muscle hypotonia, loss of tendon reflexes, loss of medullary automatisms, and hypothermia or hyperthermia and cardiovascular collapse in the absence of supportive measures. The definition of brain death of the Ad Hoc Committee of the Harvard Medical School[3] included the criteria of coma, absence of spontaneous respirations, lack of spontaneous movements, dilated pupils, loss of cephalic reflexes, loss of tendon reflexes "as a rule" and absence of postural responses, with isoelectric EEG as confirmatory evidence.

Since the appearance of these publications, questions have been raised concerning the validity of many of the proposed criteria. In the United States, it has been generally agreed that both EEG examinations, under strict technical conditions, and clinical examinations are required for the diagnosis of brain death.[4,5] On the other hand The Conference of Royal Colleges and Faculties of The United Kingdom[6] has recently taken the position that electroencephalography is not necessary in diagnosis of brain death and that primary reliance is to be placed upon the clinical observation of coma, apnea and absent brainstem reflexes. A similar view was adopted by Mohandas and Chou.[7] With regard to the clinical tests required, it has been noted that spinal reflexes need not be lost in the condition of cerebral death.[8,9] The necessity of dilatation of the pupil has been questioned.[9,10] It has been observed that persistence of complex movements, processed at a spinal level, can occur with complete brain destruction.[11] Recently, the original requirement of vascular collapse has been affirmed by one group[12] but has been considered not essential by another.[9]

In developing clinical criteria for the diagnosis of brain death, the objective should be the formulation of a series of multiple tests which can assess the

* This study was supported by Contract NO1–NS–1–2316 awarded by the National Institute of Neurological and Communicative Diseases and Stroke.
† Deceased.

70

function of the cerebral hemispheres as well as the brain-stem structures. If transitory interruptions of these functions by drug intoxication, hypothermia, anoxia, or vascular shock is excluded, then loss of such functions for a specified time period should indicate a state of diffuse cell death in the brain. The ideal requirement for any one test would be the absence of a response in all cases of brain death and the preservation of the response in all patients who survive or have only partial brain injury without brain death. Unfortunately, such ideal results cannot be expected with many of the individual reflexes and clinical tests usually employed. A given reflex subserved by a particular cranial nerve may be permanently abolished due to local disease while the rest of the brain may be left intact. On the other hand, certain reflexes, such as those mediated by the spinal cord, could be present in cases of brain death and have no meaning with respect to the detection of this condition.

A recent Collaborative Study of Cerebral Survival provided a valuable opportunity for the analysis of validity and utility of clinical signs previously proposed.[13, 14] The study included standardized serial observations on 503 cases screened for possible brain death, supported by electroencephalographic,[15] toxicologic,[16] and pathologic[17] observations. The large body of data accumulated in the study permitted relationships to be examined between presence or absence of clinical signs and such variables as time after onset of coma, EEG activity, and eventual outcome. Outcomes were designated in terms of survival, brain death or cardiac death, with brain death usually being determined on the basis of attending physician evaluation. In analyzing the value of clinical signs, however, it is imperative that correlations be made with precisely defined conditions, such as electrocerebral silence with coma and apnea for a specified time period or pathologic diagnosis of brain death (respirator brain). In order to accomplish such analyses, subsets were derived composed of 102 cases from The Ohio State University Center (Center 6) and 44 survivors from the entire group. Individual and collective data from these two groups were compared with each other and examined for correlation with various operational criteria or specific etiologic entities. The plan for analysis dealt first with the relationship of clinical results to a set of increasingly rigorous definitions of brain death, next with a comparison of the time course of findings in presumptive brain death versus survival, and finally with evaluation of discriminative power of clinical tests based upon phi coefficients.

MATERIALS AND METHODS

The analyses from the Collaborative Study of Cerebral Survival were based upon 503 patients having coma and apnea for 15 minutes as a condition of admission to study. The details of the study and protocol have been described previously.[14, 15, 17] The clinical signs examined included: state of cerebral responsiveness, apnea as determined by the need for artificial respiration and failure of overriding or spontaneous ventilatory efforts, blood pressure by cuff manometer, heart rate, rectal temperature, pupillary reflex, corneal reflex, oculocephalic reflex (doll's-eye response), vestibular reflex (caloric response), audio-ocular reflex (auditory blink reflex), snout reflex (perioral facial reflex), cough reflex, pharyngeal reflex (gag reflex), swallowing reflex, jaw jerk, stretch or tendon reflexes (biceps, triceps, radial, knee and ankle), muscle tone, abdominal reflexes, plantar responses, spontaneous or involuntary movements and their nature, invoked reflex responses and their pattern, and fundoscopy. The initial examination was performed as soon after notification of coma and apnea as possible with subsequent examinations at 6, 12, 24 hours and daily until death or recovery. EEGs were timed to coincide with clinical examinations.

The subset of 102 cases of Center 6 of the study was composed of adults and children over the age of one year examined at Ohio State University Hospitals. The characteristics of this populations were examined by the chi-square method for possible differences from the total population. The following subset differences were significant but were considered favorable for the analysis: higher proportion of patients under age 19, higher proportion of examinations by a senior neurologist, higher number of EEGs completed, higher proportion of cases with electrocerebral silence (ECS) on initial record, longer time interval for death, and higher proportion of autopsy diagnosis of respirator brain. The following conditions were significantly different but were considered irrelevant: more Caucasians, higher number of cerebral trauma diagnoses, and less cases with drug intoxication. Impedances on EEGs were significantly higher; however, this average was only slightly above the median for all centers and was not considered a serious difference. A subset of 44 survivors from the entire study included drug intoxication as well as non-drug-intoxicated cases with multiple diagnoses. Data from this group were extracted so as to permit detailed analysis with outcome and diagnosis. For comparison of presence or absence of clinical signs, cases were identified as presumptive brain death on the basis of electroencephalographic data with ECS, coma and apnea for 24 hours or more. The same group was also used for a study of the time course of clinical findings in comparison with drug-intoxicated and other survivors. For discrimination power of clinical signs, groups of presumptive brain death (coma, apnea and ECS for 24, 12 and 6 hours) were compared with all cases surviving or dying without ever developing ECS. Phi coefficients were computed for each test either individually or in combinations, and the significance of the coefficients was evaluated by the chi-square technique. From the above subsets, groups of cases were selected with cardiac arrest as the primary diagnosis in order to compare findings with those of patients with presumptive brain death and patients without brain death. Another group of primary brainstem disorders was analyzed for clinical signs in comparison with EEG findings.

Since the incidence of certain of the proposed cephalic reflexes in the normal population has not been established in the literature, a survey of 76 normal subjects and 41 hospitalized patients was carried out at Center 6.

RESULTS

Selected Findings in the 503 Cases of the Collaborative Study

Data from the entire study group proved of considerable value in assessing vital signs and incidence of certain reflexes. Body temperature showed no characteristic pattern with regard to outcome. None of the patients subsequently identified by attending physicians as having brain death had initial temperatures greater than 105° F. There was a slight tendency toward moderate hypothermia in these cases, but only 16.7 percent had temperatures below 95° F and only 2 of 114 had a temperature below 90° F. Extreme hypothermia was, in part, avoided by the necessity of warming patients above 90° F for EEG recording.

Comparison of body temperatures of the "cerebral death" cases with other nonsurvivors showed no difference, nor was any discriminative value noted in relation to presence or absence of pathologic diagnosis of respirator brain. There was no major trend toward falling blood pressure. Less than one-fourth of all patients received vasopressor agents. Systolic pressures below 70 mm Hg were found in only 16 percent of the series on initial examination and in less than 25 percent on final examination. Heart rate was also of little value in reflecting outcome and only about 5 percent had severe bradycardia on final examination.

Fundoscopic findings also proved to be of quite limited predictive value. The most common abnormalities were papilledema and other retinal lesions including hemorrhage. Sludging or segmentation of vessels was seen only in cases with fatal outcome from any cause; however, these findings were only identified in 6.5 percent of cases and did not discriminate between cases diagnosed as brain death versus other nonsurvivors.

Of considerable importance in clinical criteria are high completion rates of individual examinations. In some cases examinations may be impossible due to injured or missing body parts or interference from intubation. Reflexes with highest completion rates on initial examination included the following: pupillary, 99.6 percent; corneal, 99.6 percent; oculocephalic, 98.4 percent; audio-ocular, 97.6 percent; snout, 97 percent; arm-tendon reflexes, 99.6 percent; and leg-tendon reflexes 99.2 percent. Vestibular responses were complete in 91.2 percent; whereas pharyngeal, swallow and cough reflexes could be obtained in from 83 to 85 percent.

Correlations of Cephalic Reflexes, Spinal Reflexes, and Motor Findings with Electrocerebral Silence at any Time Period (289 Cases)

In this and the following section, a series of increasingly rigorous operational and presumptive definitions of brain death is described, against which reflex results were compared. The first test was the least stringent one and included all cases from the total population of 503 individuals having the condition of coma, apnea and ECS for any given time duration in the study (TABLE 1). There were 289 such cases. Some of these had subsequent return of biological activities (drug intoxication), hence the group was not a pure sample of presumptive brain death. The incidences of reflex findings were tabulated for examinations conducted at 0 hours (initial examination after entry into study), 12 hours, and the final examination. The latter could have occurred at any time from 0 hour to one week, but in many cases occurred after 0 or 6 hours. The 12-hour group was smaller than the others due to deaths and missed examinations.

On the initial examination, each of the cephalic reflexes was present at least once out of the total number of complete examinations, which ranged from 247 to 282. In the cases of corneal and snout reflexes, these responses were present six times, while the jaw jerk was present seven times. At 12 hours, none was present except for the snout reflex (three times) and the jaw jerk (two times).

These findings contrast sharply with the spinal stretch reflexes. One or more of these reflexes was present in 41 percent (115) out of 283 cases at 0 hours, in 51 percent at 12 hours, and in 43 percent on the final examination. Reflexes in the upper extremities were more often present than were those of the lower.

TABLE 1

FINDINGS DERIVED FROM 289 CASES WITH ECS FOR ANY TIME PERIOD

	0 Hour (247–283 examinations completed)	12 Hours (120–132 completed) examinations
Cephalic reflexes		
Light	5	0
Corneal	6	0
Oculocephalic	3	0
Vestibular	2	0
Audio-ocular	1	0
Snout	6	3
Pharyngeal	3	0
Swallow	3	0
Cough	3	0
Jaw	7	2
Spinal reflexes		
Any reflex	115	67
Arm	104	60
Leg	51	35
Spontaneous movement	36	14
Induced movement	46	23

Spontaneous movements were present at the three periods in 11–13 percent, while induced movements persisted in 15–18 percent.

Thus, cephalic reflexes were present rarely, spontaneous and induced movements occurred more frequently, and spinal reflexes were present in about one-half of cases.

Incidence of Cephalic Reflexes, Spinal Reflexes, and Motor Findings in Presumptive Brain Death Cases Studied at Center 6

From the 102 cases of Center 6, it was possible to select 63 that fulfilled the more rigorous criteria of brain death, namely, coma, apnea and ECS present for 24 hours or longer. None of these patients survived or had a diagnosis of drug intoxication.

All cephalic reflexes were absent from the time of onset of the three criteria in 56 cases (TABLE 2). One or more cephalic reflexes were present in 7 cases throughout the 24-hour period. Among individual reflexes, it was found that the snout reflex and the jaw jerk were most often persistent. The corneal, vestibular, and swallowing reflexes were present on either one or two occasions. In no instance was the light, oculocephalic, audio-ocular, pharyngeal or cough reflex present.

The spinal stretch reflexes were absent in only 8 cases of this group (TABLE 3). In 55 cases, one or more reflexes were present. Persistence of reflexes was clearly not simply a function of the initial examination since the incidence persisted or even increased throughout the 24-hour period. In individual cases, it was found that reflexes could be present early and disappear late or be absent early with late reappearance. In many cases, only one or two reflexes were present on either one or both sides of the body. They were, however, multiple in a significant number of cases, and even by 24 hours 19 cases showed three to five reflexes present. Biceps and triceps jerks were found more often than any other reflexes.

The spinal reflexes were then subjected to an even more rigorous test of relationship to brain death. Cases were selected with coma, apnea and ECS for 24 hours, no cephalic reflexes during this period, and a pathologic diagnosis of respirator brain, either complete or incomplete. There were 18 such cases (TABLE 4). In no case were the spinal reflexes completely absent throughout the 24-hour period. Again, the persistence of reflexes was not a phenomenon of early examination, but, in fact, showed a slight tendency to increase with time. In some cases, only one or two reflexes were present, but at the 24-hour period eight patients had three to five reflexes.

Spontaneous movements, induced movements and muscle tone were observed in the 63 patients having coma, apnea and ECS for 24 hours or more. While usually absent, it was remarkable that spontaneous movements were present in 14 cases and with a distribution throughout the time period. Induced movements were found even more frequently, in 36 cases. Muscle tone was reported present in 25 cases with an even distribution throughout the time period. Again, these criteria were examined in relationship to the most rigorous specification

TABLE 2

CEPHALIC REFLEXES IN NONSURVIVORS HAVING COMA, APNEA AND ECS
FOR 24 HOURS OR MORE *

Relation to Total 24-hour Period					
Total number of cases			63		
All cephalic reflexes absent from 0 hour			56		
One or more cephalic reflexes present			7		

	Hour				
Relation to Time	0	6	12	24	Total
Number of cases with one or more reflexes present	3	2	5	1	
Number of reflexes present, each reflex					
Pupillary	0	0	0	0	0
Corneal	1	0	0	1	2
Oculocephalic	0	0	0	0	0
Vestibular	0	0	0	1	1
Audio-ocular	0	0	0	0	0
Snout	2	1	3	0	6
Pharyngeal	0	0	0	0	0
Swallow	1	0	0	1	2
Cough	0	0	0	0	0
Jaw	1	1	2	1	5

* Timed from onset of three criteria.

TABLE 3

SPINAL REFLEXES IN NONSURVIVORS HAVING COMA, APNEA AND ECS
FOR 24 HOURS OR MORE *

Relation to Total 24-Hour Period				
Total number of cases			63	
All spinal reflexes absent from 0 hour			8	
One or more spinal reflexes present			55	

	Hour			
Relation to Time	0	6	12	24
Number of cases with one or more tendon reflexes present, either unilateral or bilateral	30	37	32	37
Number of tendon reflexes present				
1	9	10	8	10
2	12	13	7	7
3	3	5	7	8
4	3	5	4	3
5	3	4	6	8
Number of times present, each reflex				
Biceps	18	26	20	24
Triceps	21	27	22	27
Radial	13	15	17	19
Knee	8	8	13	13
Ankle	9	15	17	17

* Time from onset of three criteria.

of brain death in the 18 patients also having loss of cephalic reflexes and pathologic diagnosis of respirator brain (TABLE 5). Spontaneous movements were usually absent, but were present in 2 out of 18 cases, consisting of isolated jerks of one or both upper limbs. Induced movements were more often present than not. They consisted of flexor spasms of legs and, in two cases, of partial decerebrate spasms. Muscle tone was present in five cases.

The question of falling blood pressure was examined in the 63 presumptive cerebral death cases with coma, apnea and ECS for 24 hours. Recordings of systolic pressure below 80 mm Hg were made in only 25 instances in each of the time periods. There was no tendency for progressive hypotension.

Temporal Course of Clinical Signs in Presumptive Brain Death, Drug-Intoxicated Survivors, and Non-Drug-Intoxicated Survivors

In the expectation that major differences in patterns might be found, time courses of clinical signs were plotted for presumptive brain death cases and survivors at periods from 0 to 72 hours after entry into study. All of the 44 surviving patients from the major collaborative study were divided into those having drug-related and those having non-drug-related causes. On the first examination, there were 25 drug-intoxicated survivors, and as some of these gradually recovered, they left the examination sequence until by 48 hours

12 remained. Of the non-drug-related survivors, there were 19 at entry and 6 at 48 hours. A minor artifact in the plotting of survivor scores was caused by the examination protocol. Cases showing a return of respiration or consciousness were switched to a 24-hour examination schedule; hence, cases improving at 12 hours would next be reported at 36 hours rather than at 24. Consequently, 24-hour cases are weighted toward greater severity of disorder (less positive responses), and the 36-hour cases toward lesser severity (more positive responses).

Temporal patterns of the drug-intoxicated survivors are plotted in FIGURES 1–5. Electrocerebral silence was uncommonly present (one case at 0 hours and two at 6 hours) and was not present beyond 24 hours. The incidence of spontaneous respirations rose quite sharply until it was present in 67 percent of the cases by 12 hours and 93 percent by 48 hours (FIGURE 1). The percentage with cerebral responsivity rose steadily but less rapidly.

In plotting pupil size (FIGURE 2) it was considered that 2.5 to 5.5 mm constituted the normal range within the usual illumination of a hospital environment.[18] It was expected that intoxication including certain drugs such as atropine or glutethimide would be associated with large pupils, while opiates would be associated with small ones. Presumably reflecting the predominating intoxication with barbiturates [16] 61 percent of pupils examined were within the normal range at 0 hour and 55–81 percent later.

TABLE 4

SPINAL REFLEXES IN CASES HAVING:
(1) COMA, APNEA AND ECS FOR 24 HOURS OR MORE,
(2) NO CEPHALIC REFLEXES DURING THIS TIME, AND
(3) PATHOLOGIC DIAGNOSIS OF RESPIRATOR BRAIN (COMPLETE OR INCOMPLETE)

Relation to Total 24-Hour Period				
Total number of cases		18		
All spinal reflexes absent from 0 hour		0		
Spinal reflexes present one or more times		18		

	Hour			
Relation to Time	0	6	12	24
Number of cases with one or more reflexes present, either unilateral or bilateral	8	10	11	11
Number of tendon reflexes present				
1	2	4	2	2
2	3	2	2	1
3	1	1	2	4
4	1	2	2	1
5	1	1	3	3
Number of times present, each reflex				
Biceps	4	5	8	7
Triceps	6	6	8	8
Radial	5	5	7	8
Knee	3	4	5	5
Ankle	2	4	7	7

TABLE 5

MOVEMENTS AND MUSCLE TONE IN CASES HAVING:
COMA, APNEA AND ECS FOR 24 HOURS OR MORE
NO CEPHALIC REFLEXES DURING THIS TIME AND
PATHOLOGIC DIAGNOSIS OF RESPIRATOR BRAIN (COMPLETE OR INCOMPLETE)

Total number of cases			18	
Spontaneous movement				
Absent from 0 hour			16	
Present			2	
Time present (hr):	0	6	12	24
	1	0	0	1
Induced movement				
Absent from 0 hour			6	
Present			12	
Time present (hr):	0	6	12	24
	4	8	7	7
Muscle tone				
Absent from 0 hour			12	
Present			5	
Not examined			1	
Time present (hr):	0	6	12	24
	1	3	2	1

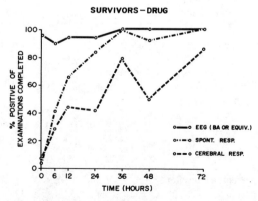

FIGURE 1. Graph of EEG, spontaneous respiration and cerebral responsiveness in relation to time after entry into study in drug-intoxicated survivors. The small percentage of patients with respiration and cerebral responsivity at 0 hour is accounted for by return of these functions before the first examination could be completed.

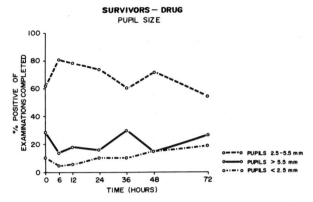

FIGURE 2. Graph of the pupil size in drug survivors showing high percentage of pupils in normal range.

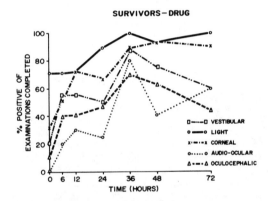

FIGURE 3. Percentage of positive responses for vestibular, pupillary, corneal and ocular reflexes over a 72-hour period after entry into study in drug-intoxicated survivors.

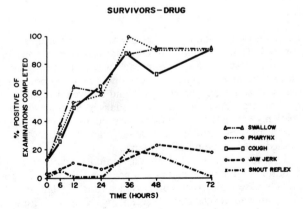

FIGURE 4. Percentage of positive responses for bulbar, jaw and snout reflexes over a 72-hour period after entry into study in drug-intoxicated survivors.

79

Pupillary light reflexes were present at high incidence on entry (71 percent) and increased further with time (FIGURE 3). Corneal reflexes were present in only 32 percent on entry but rose rapidly to 93 percent by 48 hours. The group of pharyngeal, swallow and cough responses were remarkable in that all were present at about 15 percent initially but returned at rapid rates to about 90 percent by 72 hours (FIGURE 4). The jaw jerk and snout reflexes departed from the course of other responses, remaining at quite low incidence throughout the 72-hour period. Tendon reflexes, muscle tone and induced and spontaneous movements followed a rather similar pattern with slow rates of return (FIGURE 5).

The non-drug-related survivors were characterized in general by much greater variability of temporal patterns and by generally delayed return of responses in comparison with drug intoxication. The incidence of spontaneous respirations did rise sharply to 54 percent by 6 hours but then showed little

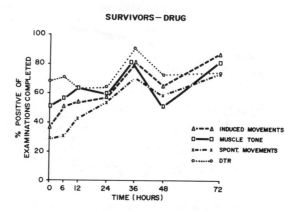

FIGURE 5. Percentage of positive responses for induced movements, muscle tone, spontaneous movements and deep tendon reflexes over a 72-hour period after entry into study in drug-intoxicated survivors.

change over the ensuing 42 hours. Pupil size was quite variable with 32 percent enlarged on initial examination and about equal percentages for equal and small pupils. With time there was a slow approach to the normal range. Among the cephalic reflexes, the light, corneal, oculocephalic and vestibular responses were present initially at about 50 percent level and showed irregular return to 100 percent by 72 hours. Audio-ocular and pharyngeal reflexes were absent in almost all patients on entry but returned gradually over 72 hours. Induced movements were present initially at a rather high incidence (62 percent) and steadily increased after six hours (FIGURE 6).

Striking differences were noted in the temporal pattern of patients with presumptive brain death defined as coma, apnea and ECS for 24 hours or more. Among these 63 cases, electrocerebral silence was present in 74 percent on initial examination and reached 100 percent by 72 hours (FIGURE 7). Spontaneous respirations and cerebral responsiveness were rarely present and remained at 0 incidence from 47 hours on. With regard to pupil size, it was

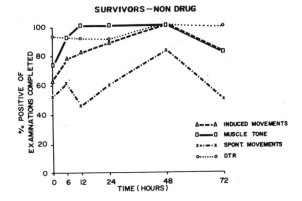

FIGURE 6. Relationship of positive responses for induced movements, spontaneous movements, muscle tone and deep-tendon reflexes to time in non-drug-intoxicated survivors.

observed in the total population of the collaborative study that no survivor had pupils in the extreme range of dilatation, greater than 8 mm. On the other hand, it is evident that not all cases of presumptive brain death have pupils dilated beyond 5.5 mm (FIGURE 8). Pupils within normal range varied between 25 and 40 percent and there was no major change with time. The pattern of cephalic reflexes differed markedly from that of the survivors (FIGURES 9 and 10). All were present in low incidence, well below 10 percent. None showed any definite recovery and most tended to approach 0 at some point between 24 and 72 hours. Some exceptions with late persistence at low incidence included corneal, swallow and jaw reflexes. Spinal reflexes were decidedly

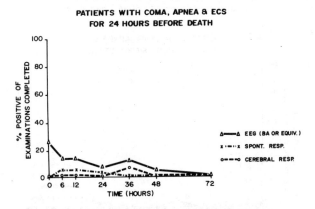

FIGURE 7. Positive responses for EEG (biological activity or equivocal), spontaneous respiration, and cerebral responsiveness after entry into study in patients with presumptive brain death (coma, apnea and ECS for a 24-hour period before cardiac death or cessation of resuscitation).

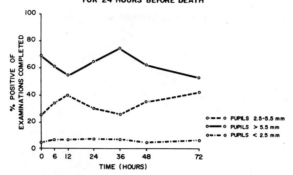

FIGURE 8. Relationship of pupil size to time in patients with presumptive brain death.

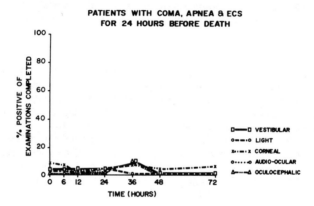

FIGURE 9. Relationship of positive responses for vestibular, pupillary, corneal and ocular reflexes to time in patients with presumptive brain death.

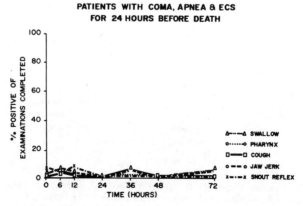

FIGURE 10. Relationship of positive responses for bulbar, jaw and snout reflexes to time in patients with presumptive brain death.

different (FIGURE 11). Stretch reflexes were present initially in about 50 percent of cases and did not fall off with time but, rather, tended to increase. A similar pattern was noted for induced movements. Spontaneous movements were present in low incidence and showed little tendency to change.

The marked differences in patterns between findings in presumptive brain death and the two groups of survivors are displayed in FIGURE 12. Spontaneous respirations, pupillary light reflex, pharyngeal reflex and corneal reflex have markedly different time courses in patients with cerebral death compared with survivors.

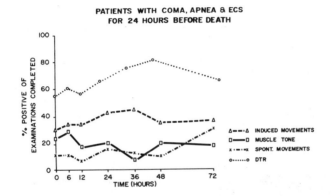

FIGURE 11. Relationship to positive responses for induced movements, spontaneous movements, muscle tone and deep-tendon reflexes to time in patients with presumptive brain death.

Discrimination Indices of Individual Clinical Tests in the Comparison of Presumptive Brain Death with Non-Brain Death Cases

In the clinical diagnosis of brain death, it is not only necessary to identify clinical responses which are absent in brain death cases, but also to determine whether these responses may be present in non-cerebral death cases and have significant discrimination value between the two outcomes. For evaluation of these discrimination powers, results of individual tests were correlated with case outcomes in which brain death was defined as coma, apnea and ECS for 24 hours or more and compared with cases having survival or cardiac death without ever developing ECS. Correlations were computed for the 0, 6 and 24 hour examinations (TABLE 6). It was found that pupil size showed a positive correlation with presumptive death but with low phi coefficients. Only at the 0 hour examination did the phi coefficient achieve a p value of $<.001$. Among other cephalic reflexes the following responses correlated well at 0-hour examination with presumptive brain death: light reflex at a coefficient of 0.502, oculocephalic at 0.556, and vestibular at 0.547. Other coefficients were positive but low. The audioocular and snout reflexes approached 0 correlation coefficient due to the fact that they tended to be absent not only in most cases of presumptive

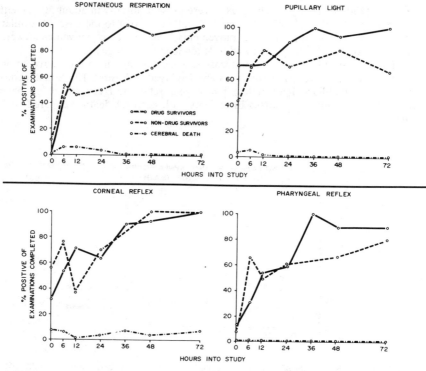

FIGURE 12. Comparison of the time courses of four selected clinical signs in drug-intoxicated survivors, non-drug-intoxicated survivors, and nonsurvivors with a presumptive diagnosis of brain death.

brain death but also in cases in coma without this outcome. At 6 hours, the best correlations were found for light reflex (0.626), corneal reflex (0.434), oculocephalic reflex (0.457), vestibular response (0.566), and swallowing reflex (0.481). At 24 hours the best reflexes were light (0.640), oculocephalic (0.423), and vestibular (0.540). Lowest coefficients were again found for audio-ocular and snout reflexes. Thus, the cephalic reflexes with consistently greatest correlation coefficients were light, oculocephalic and vestibular.

Among the spinal reflexes, the knee jerk showed fairly high correlations at 0, 6 and 24 hours with p values $<.01$. Phi coefficients of other spinal reflexes never exceeded 0.378 and tended to decrease at 24 hours. Abdominal and plantar reflexes were without value in discrimination between the two groups. The discrimination indices for spontaneous and induced movements and tone were somewhat inconsistent at the three examinations but were fairly high in the case of spontaneous movements and tone at 0 and 24 hours. Low blood pressure correlated positively with cerebral death but at quite low coefficients.

*Discrimination Indices for Selected Clinical Examinations
Singly and in Combination*

The following tests were selected for further statistical evaluations: pupillary light reflex, corneal reflex, oculocephalic response, vestibular response, knee jerk, spontaneous movements, induced movements and muscle tone. In these analyses, cases were limited to those in which complete data were available for all of the tests and time periods were extended to include 0, 6, 12 and 24 hours. In the first analysis, phi coefficients were computed for each examination period timed from the onset of entry into the study, i.e., initial examination after onset of coma and apnea. In combinations of tests, such results were classified as all responses negative versus the condition of one or more present. Highest discriminative values were still found most consistently for pupillary light and vestibular reflexes, either alone or in combination, followed by spontaneous movement, oculocephalic response and corneal reflex. The best com-

TABLE 6

PHI COEFFICIENTS FOR THE CORRELATIONS OF CLINICAL TEST RESULTS
WITH PATIENT OUTCOMES
(BRAIN DEATH VERSUS CARDIAC DEATH OR SURVIVAL)

Examination	Time after First Examination (hours)*		
	0	6	24
Pupil size	.376 †	.266	.396 ‡
Pupillary reflex	.502 †	.626 †	.640 †
Corneal	.293 ‡	.434 †	.333 ‡
Oculocephalic	.556 †	.457 †	.423 †
Vestibular	.547 †	.566 †	.540 †
Audio-ocular	—.061	—.057	.293
Snout	.023	.094	.332 ‡
Pharyngeal	.247	.304	.354
Swallow	.199	.481 †	.212
Cough	.262	.184	.290
Jaw	.209	.299 ‡	.293
Spinal			
Biceps	.285	.222	.209
Triceps	.139	.230	.161
Radial	.378	.246	.160
Knee	.314 ‡	.308 ‡	.384 ‡
Ankle	.285	.220	.030
Abdominal	—.029	—.177	—.169
Plantar	.061	.138	.123
Spontaneous	.395 †	.280	.464 †
Induced	.275	.375 †	.352 ‡
Tone	.387 †	.337 ‡	.544 †
Blood Pressure	.249	.275	.218

* Because of missing data, sample sizes range from 49 to 82.
† p <.001.
‡ p <.01.

binations of three tests were pupillary light, oculocephalic and vestibular reflexes and pupillary light, vestibular reflex and spontaneous movements.

Since the onset of ECS probably corresponds best with the time of onset of brain death, these cases were then compared in another way. Cases with presumptive death had initial examination time adjusted to begin at the onset of

TABLE 7

PHI COEFFICIENTS IN THE DISCRIMINATION OF BRAIN DEATH VERSUS
CARDIAC DEATH AND SURVIVAL, BRAIN DEATH CASES TIMED FROM
ONSET OF ECS AND NON-BRAIN DEATH CASES FROM
INITIAL EXAMINATION *

Examinations	Time (hours)			
	0	6	12	24
Individual:				
Pupillary	.6259	.7734	.7207	.6392
Corneal	.3966	.6187	.4949	.3372
Oculocephalic	.4601	.5611	.6691	.4449
Vestibular	.6259	.6728	.7207	.5536
Knee jerk	.3671	.3473 †	.3847	.4105
Spontaneous movement	.3936	.4404	.4771	.6140
Individual movement	.2949 †	.4078	.3506 †	.3878 †
Tone	.4474	.3840	.4744	.6746
Combination of two:				
Pupillary-vestibular	.7181	.8672	.8183	.7234
Pupillary-corneal	.6695	.8210	.7703	.6422
Pupillary-oculocephalic	.6217	.8210	.8183	.7205
Corneal-vestibular	.6217	.7734	.7207	.5536
Oculocephalic-vestibular	.5714	.6728	.7703	.5536
Vestibular-knee jerk	.5590	.5712	.6033	.5619
Vestibular-spontaneous movement	.6048	.7285	.7005	.7658
Combination of three:				
Pupillary-vestibular-spontaneous movement	.6980	.7786	.7521	.7658
Pupillary-corneal-vestibular	.6695	.8672	.8183	.7234
Pupillary-oculocephalic-vestibular	.6695	.8210	.8650	.7234
Corneal-vestibular-spontaneous movement	.6048	.7285	.7005	.6913
Oculocephalic-vestibular-spontaneous movement	.6048	.7285	.7005	.6913

* All values are significant at $p < .001$ except those with daggers (†) in which $p < .01$.

ECS, whereas those with other outcomes were timed from the onset of initial examination after entry into the study (TABLE 7). In this evaluation, pupillary light and vestibular reflexes still showed highest correlation coefficient followed by oculocephalic reflex, muscle tone, corneal reflex and spontaneous movements. The dual combination of pupillary light and vestibular reflexes showed highest values. The combination of three with highest values were pupillary light, corneal and vestibular reflexes; pupillary light, oculocephalic and vestibular reflexes; and pupillary light, vestibular reflex and spontaneous movements.

Frequency of Some Cephalic Reflexes in Normal Persons and Hospitalized Patients

To be valid indicators of brain death, cephalic reflexes should be present in all normal individuals. The experience of clinical examiners, however, has indicated that several of the reflexes are frequently absent but that the normal incidence is unknown.[19, 20] Consequently, a survey was made of 79 normal individuals between the ages of 3 and 63 years and 46 hospitalized patients. It was found that the audioocular reflexes could regularly be obtained in all but two of 79 normal subjects. No neurologic deficits could be identified in these two subjects. The snout reflex was frequently absent (65 absent out of 79) while the jaw jerk was occasionally absent (12 cases). In hospitalized patients, audio-ocular reflexes were present in all but a few instances, whereas the other two reflexes were often absent. No remarkable differences were noted among alert and drowsy patients. Consequently, both snout and jaw reflexes are frequently absent and audioocular responses are rarely absent in subjects without neurologic disease.

Predictive Value of Clinical Criteria in Relation to Pathologic Diagnosis

The predictive value of coma, apnea and ECS for 24 hours or more was evaluated in 27 cases in which autopsies were completed. In 22 instances, complete or incomplete respirator brain was diagnosed by the Center 6 neuro-pathologist (Leopold Liss, M.D.). In two cases, questionable or early respirator brain was recorded, one in a subject with intracerebral and intraventricular hemorrhages and secondary brain-stem hemorrhages, and the other in a case of severe edema and tonsillar herniation following surgical removal of a massive intracerebral hematoma. In three cases, respirator brain was not diagnosed but there were secondary brain-stem hemorrhages in each. Brain trauma was present in two cases and primary intracerebral hemorrhage in a third.

The relationship was then assessed for the following set of conditions present for any duration; coma, apnea, ECS and absence of all cephalic reflexes except the snout and jaw reflexes. There were 35 such cases in which autopsies were completed. In 27 cases, a positive diagnosis of respirator brain, either complete or incomplete, was made. Two questionable or early respirator brains were diagnosed. Respirator brain was considered not to be present in 6 cases. All of these had secondary brain-stem hemorrhages resulting from herniation syndromes with the following neuropathologic diagnoses: brain trauma (3), intracerebral and intraventricular hemorrhage (1), intracerebral hemorrhage (1), and meningitis with multiple cerebral abscesses (1). Thus, these criteria, present at any time in the sequence of observations, were associated either with pathologic diagnosis of respirator brain or a severe destructive process accompanied by brain-stem hemorrhages.

*Special Features in Patients with Cerebral Ischemia
Secondary to Cardiac Arrest*

Approximately 20 percent of the entire study group sustained an encephalopathy due to cardiac arrest without primary central nervous system disorder.
It seemed worthwhile to examine some details of the clinical findings and
courses of these cases since they might differ from the pattern of brain death
secondary to primary cerebral disorder. Inspection of results from the entire
study had not suggested any characteristic patterns for cerebral ischemia. Consequently, 15 cases with primary diagnosis of cerebral ischemia secondary to
cardiac arrest were analyzed from the Center 6 group. One of these cases
survived. Detailed data were also available on four other survivors of cardiac
arrest from the general study, making a total of 19 cases for analysis.

First, a group of 10 patients who developed ECS was selected for scrutiny.
It was remarkable that the pupils were dilated in most of these cases. None was
less than 2.5 mm at any examination. Pupil size greater than 5.5 mm was
noted in 80 percent at 0 hours, 90 percent at 6 hours and 100 percent at 12
hours. All of the cephalic reflexes were absent at 0, 6, 12, 24 and 48 hours,
except for the pupillary light reflex, which was present in a single case at 6
hours, and the snout and jaw jerks, which were present in 10 percent and 12.5
percent, respectively, at 0 hours with variable incidence thereafter. Tendon
reflexes were present at rates between 10 and 44 percent during the first 24
hours. Muscle tone was present in 10 percent and spontaneous movements in
20 percent at 0 hours. Consequently the pattern of findings differed from that
of all presumptive brain death cases only in respect to the uniform development
of dilated pupils.

Nine cases were then considered in which the patient either survived or
died of cardiac cause without ever developing ECS. The clinical pattern contrasted sharply with the above cases. Respirations returned by 6 hours in the
survivors but remained absent by 12 hours in the nonsurvivors. Cerebral responsivity returned in two out of five in six hours and in all survivors by 12 hours,
but remained absent in the nonsurvivors. Pupils did not tend to be dilated as
frequently as in cerebral death cases since at 0 hours 22 percent were greater
than 5.5 mm, 11 percent were in the normal range, and 66 percent were smaller
than 2.5 mm. By 24 hours, none was dilated. At 0 hours incidences of some
of the cephalic reflexes present were as follows: pupillary light 55 percent,
corneal 44 percent, oculocephalic 33 percent and vestibular 66 percent. The
audio-ocular was 0 as were pharyngeal and cough reflexes. The pupillary light
response returned to 100 percent incidence by 12 hours and the incidence of
pharyngeal, swallowing and cough reflexes also increased appreciably by this
time. Most of the other reflexes fluctuated irregularly in sequential examination,
with stretch reflexes present at 88 percent at 0 hour and between 66 and 75
percent thereafter.

In view of the possibility that the systemic blood pressures might differ in
cardiac arrest cases with ECS as opposed to cases of cardiac arrest without
presumptive brain death, the systolic and diastolic pressures of the Center 6
patients with cardiac arrest were examined. Ten cases of cardiac arrest with
ECS were compared with four having biological activity. The mean values for
systolic and diastolic pressures were consistently lower at each time interval
with cases of ECS as compared with those of biological activity. The numbers
analyzed were small and the standard deviations large, and significance was not

approached except for systolic pressures at 12-hour examination ($p < 0.05$) and at 6 hours ($p < 0.1$). Examined in another way, it was noted that none of the cases with biological activity had systolic pressures of 80 mm or less at 0 hours and 6 hours. At 12 hours and at 24 hours one of the four had a systolic pressure of 80. At 48 hours, all exceeded this level. Among those with ECS, values of systolic pressure of 80 or less were found in 6 out of 10 cases at 0 hours, 5 out of 9 at six hours, 5 out of 9 at 12 hours, 4 out of 7 at 24 hours, and 1 out of 4 at 48 hours.

Special Features in Primary Brain-Stem Lesions

In the Center 6 cases, three patients were observed having primary brain-stem hemorrhages in whom an autopsy was performed. Two were part of the major study, while one was a part of the modified study following the original series. All three were males of ages 54, 67 and 50 years.

In all three cases, there occurred the coexistence of coma, apnea and absence of cephalic reflexes on one or more examinations in which biological activity was present on the EEG. This was observed on two examinations in one case, two in another, and on one examination in a third. In the latter case, that of the modified study, only pupillary and corneal reflexes were tested in the cephalic group. In one case, respirations returned on the last two examinations. In another, biological activity on the original EEG changed to ECS on the last two recordings. Cardiac arrest developed in all cases.

On pathologic examination, the patient with persisting coma and absence of all cephalic reflexes for 36 hours, but with biological activity on EEG and return of respiration in the last 24 hours, showed only a primary brain-stem hemorrhage. In the patient with coma, apnea and absence of pupillary and corneal reflexes for 36 hours, with shift of initial biological activity to ECS for 24 hours, pathologic examination showed both the primary hemorrhage in the midbrain and pons and changes of respirator brain. In the patient with coma, apnea and absence of cephalic reflexes on the 24-hour examination, but with persisting biological activity, pathologic examination revealed a midbrain hemorrhage and incomplete respirator brain. Consequently, it would appear that the triad of coma, apnea and loss of cephalic reflexes may occur in some instances of primary brain-stem lesions without evidence of total brain death as indicated by EEG and pathologic examination.

DISCUSSION

In attempting to assess the validity of clinical signs in the diagnosis of brain death, the most difficult problem at present is the recognition of an alternate and incontrovertible end point against which all criteria may be compared. Standard neuropathologic examinations have not met this requirement. "Respirator brain," or the condition of necrosis and autolysis in the absence of inflammatory reaction, is still a relatively crude indicator. The passage of a period of hours after development of ECS and clinical signs of loss of brain function is necessary for the development of morphologic changes which can be detected at a gross or light microscopic level.[17] Thus, it is to be expected that some cases of brain death will escape detection by pathologic study. The outcome of eventual nonsurvival or somatic death from any cause is also a spurious end point. Patients, either with or without brain death, may reach somatic termination resulting from a number of immediate causes (toxemia, infection, vascular collapse) which may be fatal presently but are potentially controllable in the future.

Consequently, in the present study we have resorted to the use of multiple end points, all of which are related directly to the state of brain death. The definition of coma, apnea, loss of cephalic reflexes, and pathologic diagnosis of respirator brain (complete or incomplete) would exclude many cases of probable brain death but can scarcely be challenged for its validity or accuracy. This end point is quite useful in the negative approach of excluding clinical tests which fail to correlate with this definition. For other analyses, it is necessary to use a definition of broader range. The combination of coma, apnea, and ECS for 24 hours in absence of hypothermia or drug intoxication was considered suitable as a presumptive definition of brain death. It incorporates the elements considered essential in other definitions.[4, 14] The 24-hour requirement is a highly conservative stipulation. Moreover, the definition constitutes a reliable and objective set of observations which may readily be compared against any diagnostic procedure for brain death proposed in the future. With this definition, it is possible to examine suggested clinical signs for their concurrence rates. It is also feasible to follow the time course of clinical responses of cases having this end point as compared with the end point of survival. It is further possible to compute standard discrimination values for various tests in the comparison of presumptive brain death as opposed to a conservation definition of absence of brain death (patients surviving or dying of somatic mechanisms without developing ECS).

Using data from these approaches, we can first consider the vital signs of body temperature, heart rate, and blood pressure. Poikilothermia has been regularly observed in patients with brain death in whom resuscitative efforts have been maintained for several days.[11] During the early phases of observations, however, we have found body temperature to be of quite limited value in discrimination of brain death from any other groups studied. Heart rate also was of little value in reflecting outcome. No major trend for decline in blood pressure was detected in observations on the total group of 503 cases. Among 63 presumptive brain death cases, systolic pressures below 80 mm/Hg were recorded only 25 times among all of the time periods. Phi coefficients for estimation of discrimination value of blood pressure were quite low. Consequently, although blood pressure may well fall in patients with brain death after extended periods on the respirator,[1, 12] it appears that surviving spinal and peripheral mechanisms are adequate for maintenance of blood pressure in the supine position during the critical early period of observation.

The cephalic reflexes as a group showed clear correlations with the condition of presumptive brain death at any time period after development of ECS. In longitudinal analysis, cephalic reflexes were present at low incidences initially in presumptive cases of brain death and gradually approached 0 incidence with no trend toward recovery. In contrast, most of the reflexes returned within one to three days in the survivors. There were, however, important differences among the individual reflexes. The size of pupils was not a consistent or reliable indicator of brain death. In many cases of presumptive brain death, the patients had pupils in the normal or miotic range. There was no general trend toward increase in percentage of dilated pupils with time. Phi coefficients for pupil size were low. Only in the group of patients with cardiac arrest with ECS was dilatation regularly observed.

The pupillary light, vestibular, oculocephalic and corneal reflexes have been demonstrated to be of value by all methods of analysis. With only rare and transient exceptions, these reflexes are absent in cases of presumptive brain death. On the other hand, among drug-intoxicated survivors, the pupillary light reflex returns rapidly, followed by the corneal reflex. The highest phi coefficients were observed in these reflexes, either singly or in combination.

Some restrictions to general application were noted among all of the other cephalic reflexes. The audio-ocular reflex appeared to be excessively sensitive to abolition in any condition producing coma and apnea. It was, indeed, absent in cases of presumptive brain death but it was also absent in early phases of examination in individuals who survived. It may occasionally be found absent in normal subjects and in drowsy patients without neurologic disease. Its phi coefficients were extremely low. The jaw and snout reflexes were noted to be the two cephalic responses most likely to persist in cases of presumptive brain death. This occasional persistence might possibly be related to the survival of short latency monosynaptic components of these reflexes which could well occur if the lateral rim of the pons and midbrain were spared the process of necrosis. The technique of examination would not have distinguished between the monosynaptic component and the nociceptive bilateral polysynaptic component, which would require a wider distribution of neural connections in the brain stem and which would have been expected to have disappeared.[21, 22] Furthermore, it was noted that the jaw and snout reflexes tended to remain at low incidence even in drug survivors during recovery period. The snout reflex may be absent in normal persons and occasionally the jaw jerk is not present. All of these factors doubtless contributed to the low correlation coefficients of these two responses. The pharyngeal, swallowing and cough reflexes were of borderline value. The phi coefficients were variable but they did prove of value in the sequential examination of drug intoxication since they returned as a group usually within 36 hours.

With respect to the tendon reflexes, presence or absence of these responses bore little relationship to the identification of brain death. This was demonstrated conclusively by all methods of evaluation. In the cases of the major study group having ECS at any time period, tendon reflexes were retained in 41–51 percent at 0 and 12 hours. Among the presumptive cases of brain death with coma, apnea and ECS for 24 hours or more, one or more (usually multiple) tendon reflexes were present in all but 8 of 63 such cases. In the group characterized by the strict definition of coma, apnea and ECS for 24 hours, absence of cephalic reflexes and diagnosis of respirator brain at autopsy, tendon reflexes were present in all of these 18 cases. There was no tendency for loss of reflexes with the passage of time. On the contrary, the incidence of retained reflexes persisted or even increased with time. Phi coefficients were low for these reflexes at all time periods, with the possible exception of the knee jerk, and coefficients tended to decrease with late examinations. Consequently, it was concluded that the spinal-reflex arc may be preserved in brain death, probably as a reflection of the frequent independent survival of the spinal cord with its separate blood supply. This conclusion is consistent with the recent findings of Jørgensen.[11] The spinal-tendon reflexes should therefore not be used as clinical criteria for brain death.

Plantar responses also proved to be of no value in the recognition of brain death, confirming the original assertion of Mollaret and Goulon.[1] They were present in 66 instances on final examination among the 289 cases of the major study having ECS. Phi coefficients were low. There was a weak tendency for these reflexes to be extensor initially and flexor on final examination. The abdominal reflexes also proved to have no discrimination value.

In relation to movements, the category of spontaneous movements requires consideration. These movements were not identified as purposive or voluntary movements but rather were isolated muscle contractions, usually involving upper extremities and occurring without recorded stimulus. The absence of these movements did correlate with the outcome of brain death but with relatively weak phi coefficients. Furthermore, spontaneous movements were noted in 2 of 18 patients with our most rigorous definition of brain death. Based strictly on our data, the use of spontaneous movements in clinical criteria can only be considered as borderline in value. They may, however, be a source of

TABLE 8

CLINICAL CRITERIA IN THE IDENTIFICATION OF BRAIN DEATH

Criteria	Basis of Choice			
	Correlation Data	Rapid Return in Survivors	Lay Interpretation	High Completion Rate
Recommended				
Coma	(+)	+	+	+
Apnea	(+)	+	+	+
Light reflex	+	+		+
Vestibular reflex	+			
Oculocephalic reflex	+			+
Corneal reflex	+	+		+
Probable				
Spontaneous movements	+	+	+	+

considerable concern to lay observers, and this reason may justify their retention. Induced movements were generally fragments of complex spinal reflexes and were present more often than not in patients with the rigorous definition of brain death. They display generally low phi coefficients at the three examination intervals tested. Muscle tone proved to be somewhat better than induced movements, yet tone was still present in 5 of 18 patients with the rigorous definition of brain death. The phi coefficients tended to be variable although some were satisfactory. It was concluded, therefore, that induced movements and muscle tone need not be used in the diagnosis of brain death.

Clinical criteria that appear to be of greatest value are listed in TABLE 8. Coma and apnea were included by definition and could not be subjected to all of the analyses used for other responses. Yet it is clear that all cases of brain death by any definition were associated with coma and apnea and that no trend was noted for recovery of either function with time. Therefore these conditions are considered essential for the diagnosis. The four cephalic reflexes whose absence is of greatest value in identification of brain death are light, vestibular, oculocephalic and corneal reflexes. Absence of spontaneous movements is of intermediate value. The pupil size should not be considered a criterion, unless one is dealing with encephalopathy due to cardiac arrest. The pharyngeal, swallowing and cough reflexes should not be required to be absent; however, serial observations of these responses are of considerable value in the identification of potential survivors.

The question has been raised regarding the necessity of requiring electro-cerebral silence in addition to the clinical criteria.[6] We would contend that both are essential for the diagnosis of brain death. It is clear that the cephalic reflexes, consciousness and respirations may be lost in cases of severe brain-stem pathologic processes, while the cerebral hemispheres may remain intact. This was demonstrated in the present series in three cases of primary brain-stem hemorrhage. Brain-wave activity on EEG was demonstrated in these patients during periods in which the cephalic reflexes were lost. It is true that such patients are likely to die in the acute phase due to cardiac cause or may survive with overwhelming neurologic deficit, such as the pontine transection syndrome or the "locked-in" state. It is presently quite important that the definition of brain death be made with precision; therefore, it is important to avoid confusion of the brain-stem disorders with the condition of irreversible damage and necrosis in cerebral hemispheres as well as brain stem.

By means of the EEG as well as use of the selected clinical criteria, we have noted that the prediction can be made of massive central nervous system damage in all cases. In most instances, respirator brain can be recognized. In the remaining cases, there are extensive cerebral lesions with tentorial herniation and brain-stem hemorrhage. Further correlations cannot be made since current pathologic methods cannot confirm the existence of brain death in the latter cases. It is also probable that the clinical criteria have been analyzed as far as it is possible to do so. Further validation of these clinical criteria will very likely require additional instrumental approaches such as the demonstration of capillary flow failure [23] by practical isotopic techniques for recording of cerebral blood flow.[24]

Summary

Analyses have been performed upon data derived from 503 patients having coma and apnea in the Collaborative Study of Cerebral Survival and from subsets of 44 survivors and 102 cases in which details of temporal course and outcome were specified. Three methods of analysis were employed. The first consisted of correlation of proposed clinical signs with a series of presumptive definitions of brain death, the most rigorous of which included pathologic diagnosis. The second dealt with a conservative definition of brain death based upon the condition of electrocerebral silence with comparison of time course of clinical signs in patients having presumptive brain death versus that in patients who survived. Third, discrimination value of individual signs and combinations was evaluated by phi coefficients in relationship of presumptive brain death versus cases without evidence of brain death. These analyses lead to the exclusion of some of the proposed clinical signs. Body temperature and blood pressure showed no correlational trend and had no discriminative value. The spinal reflexes showed high persistence rates in cases of presumptive brain death and also had low phi coefficients. Some reflexes, the audio-ocular and abdominal, were excessively sensitive, being commonly absent both in brain death as well as in non-brain death cases and survivors. The snout and jaw reflexes were the two cephalic reflexes most likely to persist in presumptive brain death and to have low phi coefficients. The clinical signs recommended as diagnostic criteria include: coma, apnea, and the absence of the light, vestibular, oculocephalic and corneal reflexes. These criteria existed in the absence of severe hypothermia (below 90° F) or drug intoxication. The four cephalic reflexes were identified on the basis of prevailing absence in presumptive brain death, return in cases ultimately surviving, and high phi coefficients. Spontaneous movements are of borderline clinical value but may be retained in view of lay interpretations. Pupillary dilatation is not a criterion, except in the cases of brain death due to cardiac arrest. The pharyngeal, swallow and cough reflexes need not be criteria for brain death, but are of value in the sequential identification of drug-intoxicated survivors. EEG recording is necessary in addition to the clinical criteria in order to avoid incorrect identification of brain death in patients with primary brain-stem disorders and in potential survivors.

REFERENCES

1. MOLLARET, P. & M. GOULON. 1959. Le coma dépassé. Rev. Neurol. **101:** 3–15.
2. MOLLARET, P., I. BERTRAND & H. MOLLARET. 1959. Coma dépassé et necroses nerveuses centrales massives. Rev. Neurol. **101:** 116–139.
3. BEECHER, H. K. 1968. A definition of irreversible coma: Report of the Ad Hoc Committee of the Harvard Medical School to examine the definition of brain death. JAMA **205:** 337–340.
4. SILVERMAN, D., R. MASLAND, M. SAUNDERS & R. S. SCHWAB. 1970. Irreversible coma associated with electrocerebral silence. Neurology **20:** 525–533.
5. TASK FORCE ON DEATH AND DYING. 1972. Refinements in criteria for the determination of death: An appraisal. JAMA **221:** 48–53.
6. CONFERENCE OF ROYAL COLLEGES AND FACULTIES OF THE UNITED KINGDOM. 1976. Diagnosis of brain death. Lancet **2:** 1069–1070.
7. MOHANDAS, A. & S. N. CHOU. 1971. Brain death: A clinical and pathological study. J. Neurosurg. **35:** 211–218.
8. IVAN, L. P. 1973. Spinal reflexes in cerebral death. Neurology **23:** 650–652.
9. PLUM, F. & J. B. POSNER. 1972. Diagnosis of Stupor and Coma, 2nd ed. Contemporary Neurology Series. F. A. Davis Co. Philadelphia, Pa.
10. SIMS, J. K. 1971. Pupillary diameter in irreversible coma. New Engl. J. Med. **285:** 57.
11. JØRGENSEN, E. D. 1973. Spinal man after brain death. Acta. Neurochir. **28:** 258–273.
12. UEKI, K., K. TAKEUCHI & K. KATSURADA. 1973. Clinical study of brain death. Presentation No. 286, Fifth International Congress of Neurological Surgery, Tokyo, Japan.
13. WALKER, A. E. & G. F. MOLINARI. 1975. Criteria of cerebral death. Trans. Am. Neurol. Assoc. **100:** 29–35.
14. WALKER, A. E. 1977. An appraisal of the criteria of cerebral death. JAMA **237:** 982–986.
15. BENNETT, D. R., J. R. HUGHES, J. KOREIN, J. K. MERLIS & C. SUTER. 1976. Atlas of Electroencephalography in Coma and Cerebral Death. Raven Press. New York, N.Y.
16. WALKER, A. E. & G. F. MOLINARI. 1977. Sedative drug surveys in coma. Postgrad. Med. **61:** 105–109.

17. WALKER, A. E., E. L. DIAMOND & J. I. MOSELEY. 1975. The neuropathological findings in irreversible coma: A critique of the "respirator brain." J. Neuropath. Exp. Neurol. **34:** 295–323.
18. WALSH, F. D. & W. F. HOYT. 1969. Clinical Neuro-ophthalmology, 3rd ed. Vol. 1. Williams & Wilkins Co. Baltimore, Md.
19. WARTENBERG, R. 1945. The Examination of Reflexes. Yearbook Publishers, Inc. Chicago, Ill.
20. DEJONG, R. 1976. *In* Clinical Neurology. A. B. Baker & L. H. Baker, Eds. Vol. **1:** 1–83. Harper and Row. Hagerstown, Md.
21. KUGELBERG, E. 1952. Facial reflexes. Brain **75:** 385–396.
22. GANDIGLIO, G. & L. FRA. 1967. Further observations in facial reflexes. J. Neurol. Sci. **5:** 273–285.
23. MATAKAS, F., J. CERVOS-NAVARRO & H. SCHNEIDER. 1973. Experimental brain death. 1. Morphology and fine structure of the brain. J. Neurol. Neurosurg. Psych. **36:** 497–508.
24. BRAUNSTEIN, P., J. KOREIN, I. KRICHEFF, K. CAREY & N. CHASE. 1973. A simple bedside evaluation for cerebral blood flow in the study of cerebral death: A prospective study on 34 deeply comatose patients. Am. J. Roentgenol. Radium. Ther. Nucl. Med. **118:** 757–768.

DISCUSSION

J. CARONNA (*University of California, San Francisco, Calif.*): I'd like to ask for a clarification of the term cerebral death. The term cerebral death is frequently used interchangeably with brain death. Earlier Dr. Korein used the term cerebral death to mean something very different. As he defined it, all structures above the tentorium were necrotic. This entity has been called neocortical death by Brierley and associates; pathologically it's characterized by necrosis of the cortex but not of the brain stem. Clinically it's characterized by a flat EEG but with preservation of all brain-stem reflexes, and this condition looks more like a persistent vegetative state. Although I agree with you that their condition is hopeless and that this is an irreversible state, these patients fall under no existing set of criteria for brain death. So by equating them you are calling for a broadening of our understanding of what brain death is. Dr. Molinari and Dr. Allen both called for a very rigorous definition of brain death not as being a hopeless situation but rather as an affirmation that necrosis of both the cerebrum and the brain stem has occurred.

In addition, Dr. Allen, would you comment on the role of cortical evoked responses in determining cerebral nonviability?

KOREIN: The terms brain death and cerebral death have been used and are being used synonymously. However, I have attempted to differentiate these terms explicitly. It is hoped that this "purist" definition will be employed in the future. One should be cautious in using the pathologic term "necrotic," for reasons that will be discussed in this volume.

ALLEN: I am inclined to be a purist myself and urge that we seek to use the term brain death for the totality of necrosis of the cerebral hemispheres and brain stem. Unfortunately, in the evolution of our collaborative studies we used the term cerebral death. However, all of us who have previously used the terms brain death and cerebral death interchangeably would now rather use brain death in your context, Dr. Korein, and reserve the term cerebral death for the cases corresponding to those Dr. Caronna has described and which have been documented pathologically by such investigators as Brierley *et al.*, in which the brain stem indeed remains functional.

With respect to the question of evoked potentials, these studies were not carried out regularly in the study. Other researchers have done this in small groups of patients, and they do appear to be of validity in showing absence of cerebral function.

MOLINARI: In response to Dr. Caronna's comment, I must admit that I have been stung on the same abuse of the word. Having had a classical education, I balk at using a noun, brain, as an adjective, as in brain death. I have therefore fallen into the trap of using cerebral as the adjective derived from cerebrum. In this context we should be much more self-conscious about our use of words, and I propose a nomenclature that would include the pronunciation of death. There is only one death that is a legal event; and death may be pronounced by either neurologic or by cardiorespiratory criteria.

INGVAR: The semantic confusion under discussion exists in Scandinavia also, and we have tried to avoid it by emphasizing the pathoanatomic basis of such statements. Thus we call "conventional" brain death total brain infarction. What has been termed cerebral death in this discussion we call supratentorial infarction or an apallic state. I will discuss these problems in my paper.

GRENVIK (*Presbyterian University Hospital, Pittsburgh, Pa.*): I would like to ask Dr. Allen a question about the published criteria used in testing for apnea. If I understand it correctly, the criteria for apnea involved a 15-minute period of not overriding the respirator. There is a lot of confusion and disagreement on that point. I disagree wholeheartedly, unless I have misunderstood the publication, for I don't see how absence of overriding the respirator for 15 minutes would be a criterion of apnea.

ALLEN: I agree that this is an unsatisfactory test for apnea. This test was used initially in our collaborative study in order to avoid injury to possibly undamaged parts of the brain that might be caused by removing patients from the respirator.‡ Our methods for determination of apnea have evolved, and the one that has been proposed most recently has come out of studies in which oxygenation is used to prevent induced anoxia. Such techniques decrease the possibility of inducing further brain injury.

VAN TILL (*The Hague, The Netherlands*): I believe it is of the greatest importance that the terminology used be as precise as possible, and therefore agree to having separate definitions for brain death and cerebral death; cerebral death should only mean death of the cerebrum.

KOREIN: I agree to more precise nomenclature.

GLASS (*Downstate Medical Center, Brooklyn, New York*): Dr. Allen, will you describe the level of function in the group of patients that you describe as survivors, particularly the non-drug-intoxicated survivors?

ALLEN: They varied widely. A few were in an essentially persistent vegetative state. Some recovered to ambulation. However, there were a few with complete recovery without detectable neurologic deficits.

‡ Actually, the 15-minute test described was used as a criterion along with unresponsive coma to admit patients into the collaborative study. After they were admitted, most if not all patients in many centers did have an apnea test which required removal of the respirator. The problems with tests for apnea are discussed elsewhere in this volume.—*J. K.*

BRAIN ENERGETICS AND CEREBRAL DEATH *

Jack M. Fein

Department of Neurological Surgery
Albert Einstein College of Medicine—
Montefiore Hospital and Medical Center
Bronx, New York 10467

INTRODUCTION

Recent developments in the study of energy metabolism allow us to consider the process of brain death from a thermodynamic perspective. This provides an insight into two mechanisms of cerebral dysfunction which should be clearly differentiated if accurate prognosis of agonal states is to be made.

It is relatively simple to determine the presence of brain death using criteria such as those proposed in the NINCDS Collaborative Study.[1] However, there are various states of severe cerebral dysfunction in which prognosis is indeterminate. Finally, various conditions such as hypothermia or agents such as barbiturates may produce a selective suppression of electrophysiologic function and oxidative metabolism that mimics the agonal state.

Measurements of cerebral blood flow and metabolic rate as well as standardized EEG recordings are accurate parameters of the rates of nutrient supply and consumption in relation to the residual functional activity of the nervous system. A severe depression of cerebral blood flow may represent inadequate nutrient supply and contribute to the propagation of cerebral infarction. On the other hand it may simply reflect the decreased nutritional needs of tissue that is either transiently or permanently operating at a low functional level.

In purely thermodynamic terms the brain will tend toward a steady state appropriate to its functional level by keeping entropy production to a minimum. In the normal brain this requires a high rate of blood flow and oxidative metabolism to maintain the most efficient ratio of high-energy adenosine triphosphate (ATP) to the lower-energy adenosine diphosphate (ADP) and monophosphates (AMP). At the mitochondrial level the oxidation reduction potential changes at three points on the electron transport chain are large enough to provide the necessary energy for this ATP synthesis (FIGURE 1). The specific mechanism by which electron transport results in the production of ATP (oxidative phosphorylation) generates lively discussion, and it is still unsettled. The consensus now favors the thesis that mitochondria generate hydrogen gradients (chemiosmotic coupling hypothesis) due to substrate oxidation and that this gradient then serves as a driving force for the reversal of membrane-bound ATPase of the mitochondria. There is growing evidence to indicate that chemical and conformational mechanisms also contribute to the overall picture.

An immediate consequence of anoxia is that electrons cannot be transferred from cytochrome a-a_3, so that this system becomes more reduced. Because of the buffering effect of this carrier system the flavoprotein and NAD system will

* This work was supported by RCDA No. 5 KO4 NS00198–02 and Contract No. NO1 NS5–2305 from the National Institute of Health.

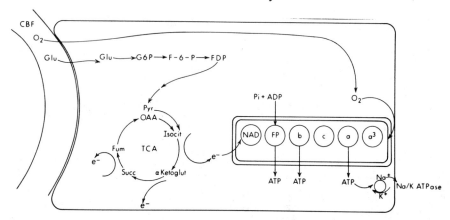

FIGURE 1. Major steps in glycolysis and generation of reducing equivalents. These enter the mitochondrial transport chain. The requisite energy for formation of high-energy phosphates is provided at three sites.

also tend to remain in the reduced redox couplet. Less ATP will be generated by the mitochondria and Pi and AMP will increase. The proportion of these phosphates that exist in a high-energy state may be expressed by the energy charge potential defined by Atkinson [2] as E.C.P.

$$= .5 \frac{(2\ ATP + ADP)}{(AMP + ADP + ATP)}$$

The E.C.P. is a convenient means of assessing the thermodynamic disequilbrium of the brain if we accept the premise that ATP is the main energy reserve of the system.

It was previously demonstrated [3] that cisternal subarachnoid hemorrhage may induce a primary suppression of cerebral oxidative metabolism and blood flow by two separate mechanisms. In the first instance the effect may be related to a suppression of cerebral functional activity, and in the second to ischemic injury. A biopsy technique to sample representative tissue was used to differentiate these.

This experimental design was utilized as a paradigm of the comatose state. It demonstrates the necessity for utilizing hemodynamic measurements in the context of brain energetics to differentiate nonfunctional from nonviable states.

METHODS

Sprague-Dawley rats weighing 200–300 grams were intubated, paralyzed with d-tubocurarine (.25 mg/kg), and maintained on a 65–75 percent nitrous oxide- 25–35 percent oxygen mixture. Arterial pH was maintained between 7.377 and 7.415, arterial pO_2 varied between 100 and 140 mm Hg, and arterial pCO_2 was maintained between 34 and 42 mm Hg. Aortic blood pressure was monitored by a PE 90 catheter passed transfemorally and connected to a P-23-Db Statham transducer. Cisternal pressure was monitored and controlled by a double-lumen scalp-vein needle, one arm of which was connected to a P23V Statham transducer (FIGURE 2). Plasma glucose levels were maintained between 115 and 140 mg percent by 5 percent dextrose and saline solution administered by intravenous infusion at a rate of 1 cc/kg/hr. Hydrogen gas was then administered by inhalation until saturation of the brain was achieved.[3] Its exponential washout was then detected polarographically by a single plati-nized-platinum electrode placed in the distal end of the sagittal sinus. Average total cerebral blood flow was obtained by resolving the biexponential decay into its initial weights and half-times.[2] Arteriovenous O_2 content and arteriovenous glucose as well as cerebrospinal fluid (CSF) glucose, pH, and lactate/pyruvate ratios were determined. Lactate concentration in CSF pyruvate was determined according to the method of Lowry *et al.* After control studies, the animals were divided into two groups: (1) Sixteen animals underwent unilateral trephination over the parietal cortex followed by isobaric injection (i.c.p. 5–10 mm Hg) of 0.2 cc of fresh isologous arterial blood into the cisterna magna (isobaric cisternal). (2) Seventeen animals underwent unilateral trephination over the parietal cortex followed by hyperbaric (i.c.p. 40–50 mm Hg) injection of 0.2 cc of isologous arterial blood into the cisterna magna (hyperbaric cisternal), and pressure was maintained by saline infusion.

Serial blood flow and metabolic consumption studies were then performed up to 12 hours after induced subarachnoid hemorrhage (SAH) in both groups. Approximately 6 hours after SAH a sample of the left parietal cortex was removed for regional analysis of energy metabolism. Substrate metabolism

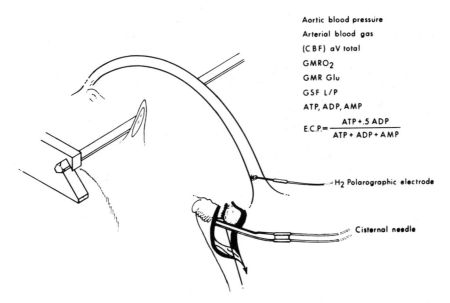

FIGURE 2. Schematic representation of experimental model used to simultaneously measure cerebral oxidative and energy metabolism. Parameters measured are indicated at right. Total cerebral blood flow was measured by a platinum polarographic electrode in the torcular Herophili. Cisternal needle allowed injection of arterial blood samples and simultaneous measurement of pressure.

was interrupted by excision of approximately 30 mg of tissue under the operating microscope into a cuvette containing liquid nitrogen. A freeze technique using a biopsy curette cooled with liquid nitrogen made it possible to do this bloodlessly. These chips were then weighed and extracted in 3M $HClO_4$ and neutralized with 2M $KHCO_3$. The supernatant was then assayed for levels of tissue glucose, lactate, pyruvate, phosphocreatine (PCr), adenosinetriphosphate (ATP), adenosinediphosphate (ADP), and adenosinemonophosphate (AMP), according to methods described by Lowry et al.[4] The energy charge potential was calculated. After microdissection of the parietal lobe specimen the average total cerebral blood flow and average total oxygen and glucose consumption rates were repeatedly measured to elicit evidence of recovery. EEG was measured using bipolar leads inserted over the right and left frontal regions using Brush couplers for each channel.

RESULTS

The control values for CBF, CMR, CMR glu, and $CMRO_2$ before SAH were not significantly different in the two experimental groups. Control cerebral blood flow (47.2 cc/100 g/min), cerebral metabolic consumption rates for oxygen (3.5 cc/100 g/min) and glucose (5.6 cc/100 g/min), and lactate/pyruvate ratios (13.6) were obtained by pooling the means of all three groups. The changes in these values in subsequent measurements are expressed as percentage change from control measurement.

I. In the isobaric cisternal group, the metabolic consumption rates of oxygen and glucose decreased during the first hour after hemorrhage. This was primarily related to a depression of the extraction rates of these substrates (FIGURE 3). A depression in cerebral blood flow seen in the first hour ($p < .01$) was most significant at the second hour after SAH, when the standard deviation of mean values was considered ($p < .001$). The CSF lactate/pyruvate ratios remained unchanged initially, although the concentration of both substrates promptly increased after SAH.

Six hours after SAH when CBF, $CMRO_2$ and CMR glu were, respectively, 28 percent, 34 percent and 41 percent of control, the energy charge potential in the parietal biopsy specimen was 80 ± 4 percent of control values. ATP concentration was 90 percent, ADP 92 percent and AMP 105 percent of control values. CBF and $CMRO_2$ and CMR glucose showed a variable pattern thereafter, with eleven of the sixteen animals showing recovery to near normal hemodynamic values.

II. In the hyperbaric cisternal group, the mean cerebral perfusion pressure was approximately 40 mm Hg lower than in the previous two groups. Loss of autoregulation was evident in the early decrease of CBF (FIGURE 4). The $CMRO_2$ decreased after SAH. By five hours after SAH, the $CMRO_2$ also fell to 32 percent of control values. Glucose extraction and CMR glucose initially increased, but by one and one-half hours after SAH had returned to normal and was consistently depressed thereafter. The inadequate perfusion and resulting ischemia were also evident in a rapid and sustained rise of CSF lactate/pyruvate ratio. ATP values had fallen to 30 ± 4 percent, ADP values decreased to 50 ± 7 percent, and AMP had risen to 14 percent of control values. The cerebral energy charge potential was $.365 \pm .189$. Serial CBF, $CMRO_2$, and CMR glu measurements made after biopsy showed progressive falls to a near no-flow state in all seventeen animals.

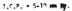

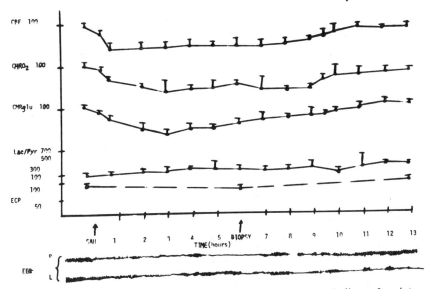

FIGURE 3. Measurements of serial oxidative and energy metabolism after intra-cisternal hemorrhage at normal pressure. An early suppression of oxidative metabolism is seen. The lower blood flow is appropriate to the metabolic state as indicated by the unchanged lactate/pyruvate ratio and the normal energy charge potential. Bipolar EEG leads show intermittent suppression of spontaneous organized discharges with eventual recovery.

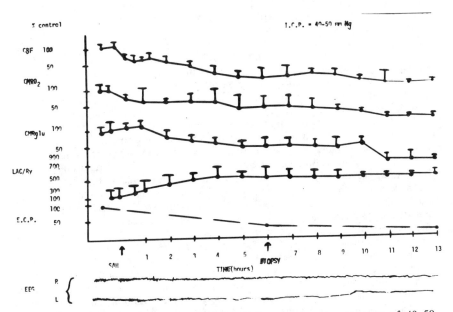

FIGURE 4. After intracisternal subarachnoid hemorrhage at a pressure of 40–50 mm Hg. A marked reduction in CBF occurs as well as a depression of $CMRO_2$, which is primarily related to a decrease of AVO_2, and a slight increase in anaerobic metabolism of glucose. A profound tissue lactoacidosis occurs associated with an increase in the lactate/pyruvate ratio. There is a secondary fall in ECP confirming the presence of a dysergic metabolic state.

Discussion

The experimental model utilized here provides the basic paradigm for understanding the difference between loss of function and loss of viability in the nervous system.

To study the primary effects of subarachnoid blood on brain metabolism it became necessary to assure a constant perfusion pressure, which, in the model used here, is mainly dependent on the control of intracranial hypertension. When that variable was adequately controlled, hemodynamic and metabolic effects of SAH appear to be related to some primary effect on brain-stem structures. Although there is no substantial evidence that a brain-stem center regulates oxidative metabolism of the cerebral convexities directly, a more indirect influence may be exerted by stimulation of cerebral functional activity.

Most of the previous literature in brain energetics has regarded the level of brain ATP as the essential fuel upon which all energy-requiring processes are dependent. However, determinations of the energy-rich phosphate compound ATP are usually performed as terminal analysis in the small-animal brain. It has therefore been difficult to correlate the energy level with recovery of function. The application of this limited biopsy technique to survival experiments is the first we know of in which such correlations have been attempted. Two immediate problems of utilizing the technique are (1) its accuracy and (2) the question of whether the biopsy is representative of brain energetics. The accuracy of the technique was tested by comparing the energy charge potential obtained from the biopsy through the trephine opening compared with that obtained by pouring liquid nitrogen over the exposed homotopic cortex in the opposite hemisphere. No significant difference ($N = 14$, $p > .2$) in energy charge potential was found with these alternate methods of sampling tissue.

In making a diagnosis of cerebral death we are presuming to indicate that the loss of function that we perceive on clinical examination is correlated to a very high degree with loss of viability. The experimental model utilized here provides the basic paradigm for understanding the difference between loss of function and loss of viability in the nervous system. The important point to be made here is that clinical methods of diagnosis are all based on parameters that assess function, not viability. It is only by collating measurements of loss of function with states incompatible with recovery that these parameters become clinically useful. This insight can be gained by assessing the hemodynamic and functional parameters of brain activity in association with the brain energy state. It has been estimated by Sundt and others[5] that a reduction of ATP levels to approximately 30 percent of normal is incompatible with tissue viability.

Severe and rapidly progressive cerebral infarction may be induced by injection under pressure and maintaining this pressure so that cerebral perfusion pressure is compromised. After hyperbaric cisternal subarachnoid hemorrhage, there was a 40 mm decrease in cerebral perfusion pressure which produced a dramatic decrease in blood flow because of the loss of autoregulation in the brain. Although both glucose and oxygen supply fall equally in ischemia, a relatively anaerobic metabolism was seen with a slight increase in glucose consumption and a decrease in oxygen consumption. The extreme ischemia induced a progressive fall in phosphate stores with an eventual fall to 20 percent of control values. This dramatic fall in energy state is the net result of consumption of available high-energy phosphates by the brain to maintain the essential functions of the cell membranes. As this is exhausted and cell membranes degenerate, cell death is predictable. There was no recovery in animals in whom flow was persistently low and in whom energy charge potential was less than 20 percent of control. The engine "has run out of fuel and then destroys itself." Thus these parameters may be a useful index of irreversibility and a diagnosis of brain death can be made. By contrast, when subarachnoid blood is injected under normal pressure, there is a primary suppression of brain metabolic rate. The mechanism for this is unknown. This also was seen and separately reported in cats.[3] This was not seen when blood was injected over the cat cerebral convexity. This suppression of both glucose and oxygen metabolism appeared to be a primary effect with secondary decreases in cerebral blood flow in response to the decreased metabolic need of the brain for nutrients. This is a situation that may be likened to an idling engine which is not consuming much fuel but is also not producing much work. The energy charge potential was maintained at about 75 percent of normal level in this situation and after a while there was recovery of the functional and hemodynamic parameters. This situation may also be likened to the clinical state in which brain metabolism is primarily suppressed by agents such as barbiturates and conditions such as hypothermia.

This then is the basic problem in making the diagnosis of brain death. If we are to use secondary elaborated functions of the brain in assessing viability or nonviability, we must utilize correlations that are either related to a function of the cell which is unquestionably essential or to retrospective correlation of outcome.

Earlier research by Woodhall et al.[6] sought to explain the early functional loss seen in ischemia in terms of loss of energy stores, specifically ATP concentration. Later workers,[7] however, have shown that alterations in functional activity occur at a threshold of perfusion pressure and oxygen partial pressure in brain which is above that inducing ATP decreases. The energy level of tissue may, however, be a sufficient determinant of the possibility of recovery from ischemia.

Obtaining representative tissue will continue to be the major obstacle to direct clinical measurement of brain energetics. It is hoped that the insights gained from such correlations in animals will make prognoses on the basis of agonal measurements of flow, metabolism, and EEG more accurate.

SUMMARY

The energy-charge potential of the brain, defined as the ratio of high- and low-energy phosphate levels, may be correlated with brain viability after injury. Two different states of dysergic brain metabolism may be induced by subarachnoid hemorrhage, depending on the intracranial pressure. Simultaneous measurements of oxidative metabolism and ATP, ADP, and AMP levels were made in rats after cisternal injection of fresh arterial blood under high (>50 mm Hg) and normal (5–10 mm Hg) intracranial pressure. The hyperbaric injections were uniformly associated with progressive and severe cerebral infarctions. These were correlated with low flow and depressed energy charge potential. A low rate of blood flow and metabolism persisted and the animals showed no signs of recovery postoperatively. Injections under normal pressure were associated with an equally severe suppression of brain blood flow and metabolic rates, but energy charge potential was preserved and clinical function, flow and metabolism were eventually recovered. Despite the cerebral dysfunction, which may appear similar in both cases, the prognosis for viability in the two instances is quite different. These paradigms are useful in formulating concepts of the energy state necessary for functional brain survival.

REFERENCES

1. WALKER, A. E. ET AL. 1977. An appraisal of the criteria of cerebral death. A summary statement. A collaborative study. JAMA 237: 892–896.
2. ATKINSON, D. E. 1968. The energy charge of the adenylate pool as a regulatory parameter: Interaction with feedback monitors. Biochemistry 7: 4030–4034.
3. FEIN, J. M. 1975. Cerebral energy metabolism after subarachnoid hemorrhage. Stroke 6: 1–8.
4. LOWRY, O. H., J. V. PASSONNEAU, F. X. HASSELBERG & D. N. SCHULTZ. 1964. Effect of ischemia on known substrates and cofactors of the glucolytic pathway in brain. J. Biol. Chem. 239: 18–30.
5. SUNDT, T. ET AL. 1972. Focal transient cerebral ischemia in the squirrel monkey. Circ. Res. 30: 703–712.
6. WOODHALL, B. ET AL. 1971. Brain energetics and neurosurgery. J. Neurosurg. 34: 3–14.
7. SHUTZ, H. ET AL. 1973. Brain mitochondrial function after ischemia and hypoxia. II. Normotensive systemic hypoxemia. Arch. Neurol. 29: 417.

BILATERAL RETICULAR FORMATION LESIONS CAUSING COMA: THEIR EFFECTS ON REGIONAL CEREBRAL BLOOD FLOW, GLUCOSE UTILIZATION AND OXIDATIVE METABOLISM *

W. K. Hass and R. A. Hawkins

Departments of Neurology and Neurosurgery
New York University Medical Center
New York, New York 10016

Much of the discussion at this Conference will concern the reliability of clinical electrophysiologic and limited cerebral blood flow (CBF) observations which may assist the clinician in the prediction and diagnosis of that irreversible state known as "brain death." Dr. Allen has pointed out that bilateral absence of the pupillary light reflex as well as the absence of vestibulo-ocular, oculo-cephalic, and corneal reflexes correlate highly with brain death and persistent vegetative state.

The paradigm for brain death leading to systemic death has been the description of a chain of neurologic events which follow acute reduction or cessation of CBF, leading to diffuse hypoxia and ischemia. This acute reduction to less than 20 percent of normal blood flow is classically related to failure of cardiac output or to peripheral vasomotor collapse.

We shall, in contrast, address those events following traumatic head injury that in association with primary or secondary brain-stem damage may lead to the persistent vegetative state or brain death. Attempts to predict these tragic outcomes shortly after head injury according to carefully designed protocols are not yet entirely satisfactory.[1] Accuracy of prediction improves *pari passu* with the number of hours after the moment of injury. More complex quantitative estimates of CBF prove reliable in the prediction of brain death only if no flow at all can be recorded.[2]

Ten years ago, therefore, we turned to the use of the clinical mass spectrometer to estimate CBF and, in particular, cerebral oxidative metabolism ($CMRO_2$).[3, 4] At an average study period of seven days after head injury we noted that death subsequently occurred without recovery of consciousness in all patients whose $CMRO_2$ was less than one-third of normal. If the $CMRO_2$ was between one-third and two-thirds of normal, 75 percent of all patients died without recovery of consciousness. Almost all patients with a $CMRO_2$ that was greater than two-thirds of normal recovered consciousness and survived the cerebral aspect of their injury.[5]

The lowest mean values for $CMRO_2$ noted in those patients who demonstrated prominent impairment of brain-stem function were akin to those described by Dr. Allen. There was a significant difference in mean $CMRO_2$ values between the alert or "alert-with-deficit" patients and those with moderate to severe brain-stem dysfunction. On the other hand in the entire group of 45 patients there were no significant differences in mean CBF, arterial pH, arterial

* This work was supported by Grant No. NS 07366 from the National Institute of Neurological Disease and Stroke.

0077–8923/78/0315–0105 $01.75/0 © 1978, NYAS

pCO_2 and arterial pO_2. Attempts in those patients to increase $CMRO_2$ by increasing arterial pO_2, mean arterial pressure, or arterial pCO_2 were unsuccessful. The rate of $CMRO_2$ appeared fixed. This suggested that brain-stem injury per se profoundly reduced $CMRO_2$ by at least 40 percent.

This observation was reinforced by the observations of Ingvar and associates of a single patient with isolated upper midbrain infarction. Their patient presented in coma and has remained so for three years.[6] He exhibited a reduction of both $CMRO_2$ and CBF to one-fourth of the normal levels. In addition, Heiss and Jellinger have found that it is the amount of *brain-stem injury* and *not* of telencephalic injury that correlates with the level of CBF in patients with established persistent coma at a time (> 23 days) after the cerebral insult when one may assume that the metabolism-flow couple has been restored.[7] It appears therefore that the reduction in CBF presumably coupled to a reduction in $CMRO_2$ is not merely the algebraic sum of areas of ischemia throughout the brain and brain stem, but, more likely, in large part a reflection of the impairment of a metabolic regulatory mechanism within the brain stem itself.

The work of Lindsley *et al.* on the midbrain reticular formation lesions suggested to us that symmetrical, bilateral 7-mm³ mesencephalic radiofrequency lesions placed in the rostral reticular formation of the rat between the superior portion of the inferior colliculus and the inferior portion of the medial geniculate body would produce an animal model similar to that previously described in the cat.[8] Indeed, rats with these lesions lie immobile in one position and respond, at most, to painful stimuli with feeble nonpurposeful limb movements lasting 1–2 seconds. The pupils are meiotic and the rats neither eat nor drink; their electroencephalograms show marked slowing of activity with fast desyncronized activity occurring only for periods of 1–2 seconds after painful stimuli.

Using ^{14}C antipyrine to study changes in the regional blood flow in the brains of "lesioned" rats in contrast to their "sham-lesioned" controls we found no consistant reduction of regional CBF after one hour. After six hours, however, there was a 35–66 percent reduction in mean regional CBF in all grey-matter regions and 26–47 percent reduction in all white-matter regions. After 24 hours CBF was reduced 41–55 percent in all grey- and 30–41 percent in all white-matter regions. These results were significant to $p < 0.01$–0.001, depending on the region studied. In separate studies of the difference in oxygen content between arterial blood and cavernous sinus blood we found a mean reduction of $CMRO_2$ in lesioned rats of 40 percent or more at 6 and 24 hours.[9]

Use of a regional glucose metabolism technique employing (^{2-14}C) glucose, developed by Dr. Hawkins, as early as one hour after lesion placement produced a consistent significant reduction of regional brain glucose metabolism (rCMR-glu) of 40–55 percent in all grey-matter areas and of 31–46 percent in all white-matter regions.[9, 10] At 6 and 24 hours a marked and significant reduction in *both* rCMRglu and regional CBF was present and persistent in the lesioned animals. These changes do not occur when lesions are placed elsewhere, for example, in the occipital cortex or in the superior colliculus; nor in the case of the extrareticular lesions is the experimental animal reduced to the nonadaptive state I have described after the simultaneous bilateral reticular formation lesions.

In contrast to the bilateral simultaneous lesions described, *unilateral* reticular formation lesions result only in a failure of the animal to eat or drink during the first 24 hours. During this time the rat appears alert and will often exhibit circling behavior, a mild contralateral hemiparesis, and a 10–30 percent reduction in regional CBF. Subsequently animals with unilateral reticular formation lesions begin to eat, drink, and thrive. They are indistinguishable in terms of function and CBF from normal animals after one month.

Serial *sequential* lesions, placed 1–7 days after an initial unilateral reticular formation lesion has been created on the contralateral side, will produce with less predictability the nonadaptive state described after simultaneous bilateral reticular formation lesions for up to only three days after the placement of the first unilateral reticular formation lesion. If the between-lesion interval is greater than three days, the rats remain alert. These observations parallel those of Adametz in cats.[11] They suggest that it is not the volume of tissue destroyed in the brain stem per se, but the volume of tissue destroyed at a given moment in time that determines the development of the nonadaptive state and the accompanying reduction in regional CBF, rCMRglu, and $CMRO_2$.

More importantly the sequential lesion experiments strongly suggest that there is a capacity for functional and anatomic plasticity in the nervous system. This is presumably a rostral reorganization at the level of the thalamus, perhaps in or near the parafascicular nucleus, which points to what may be a potential "road back" from the effects of major brain-stem lesions.

Conventional knowledge today dictates that the capacity for regeneration in the central nervous system is highly limited. On the other hand, the difference between the effects of simultaneous bilateral reticular formation lesions and bilateral sequential lesions placed more than three days apart suggests that as we begin to know more about this problem, we may learn how to modify the effects of severe brain-stem trauma by enhancing or encouraging the natural tendency toward rostral reorganization illustrated by the sequential lesion studies. It is our hope that such an effort will lead to a conference in the future on brain recovery after head injury rather than this all to sad consideration of "brain death."

REFERENCES

1. JENNETT, B. & M. BOND. 1975. Assessment of outcome after severe brain damage. Lancet **1**: 480–484.
2. KOREIN, J., P. BRAUNSTEIN, I. KRICHEFF, A. LIEBERMAN & N. CHASE. 1975. Radioisotopic bolus technique as a test to detect circulatory deficit associated with cerebral death. Circulation **51**: 924–939.
3. WALD, A., W. K. HASS & J. RANSOHOFF. 1971. Experience with a mass spectrometer system for blood gas analysis in humans. J. Assoc. Adv. Med. Instrum. **5**: 325–342.
4. HASS, W. K., A. WALD, J. RANSOHOFF & P. DOROGI. 1972. Argon and nitrous oxide cerebral blood flows simultaneously monitored by mass spectrometry in patients with head injury. Eur. Neurol. **8**: 164–168.
5. HASS, W. K. 1976. Prognostic value of cerebral oxidative metabolism in head trauma. *In* Head Injuries. R. L. McLaurin, Ed. Grune & Stratton Inc. New York, N.Y.
6. INGVAR, D. H. & P. SORANDER. 1970. Destruction of the reticular core of the brain stem; a pathoanatomical follow up of a case of coma of three years duration. Arch. Neurol. **23**: 1–8.
7. HEISS, W. D. & K. JELLINGER. 1972. Cerebral blood flow and brain stem lesion. Z. Neurol. **203**: 197–209.
8. LINDSLEY, D. B., L. H. SCHREINER, W. B. KNOWLES & H. W. MAGOUN. 1950. Behavioral and EEG changes following chronic brain stem lesions in the cat. Electroencephalogr. Clin. Neurophysiol. **2**: 483–498.

9. HASS, W. K., R. A. HAWKINS & J. RANSOHOFF. 1977. Cerebral blood flow, glucose utilization, and oxidative metabolism after bilateral reticular formation lesions. Acta Neurol. Scand. 56(Suppl. 64): 240–241.

10. HAWKINS, R., W. K. HASS & J. RANSOHOFF. 1977. Advantages of 2-14C glucose for regional cerebral glucose utilization. Acta Neurol. Scand. 56(Suppl. 65): 436–437.

11. ADAMETZ, J. H. 1959. Rate of recovery of functioning in cats with rostral reticular lesions. J. Neurosurg. 16: 85–98.

DISCUSSION

R. SATRAN (*University of Rochester Medical School, Rochester, N.Y.*): Dr. Hass, do you know what is happening between hour 1 and hour 6? It is not unusual in these days of rapid transportation to encounter people who have brain-stem strokes within a few hours. Perhaps some of the results you have derived may be used therapeutically. Do you have any ideas or data about this?

HASS: By the first hour glucose metabolism is down and after 6 hours glucose metabolism is decreased in tandem with blood flow. During that time there is brain-stem swelling about the necrotic centers of the radiofrequency lesion, no doubt due to traumatic ischemia. The acute treatment problem, therefore, is one of treatment of regional traumatic ischemia and associated edema of the brain stem. This treatment problem seems now to be on the verge of a partial solution. Recent work with ethycrinic acid by the Albany neurosurgical group reveals that injuries caused by a combination of hypoxia and head vibration are limited by the use of this diuretic and similar drugs which inhibit potassium-mediated chloride transport. Preliminary studies in brain-injured humans with ethycrinic acid are similarly promising.

Thus, the real clinical problem in the crucial hours you refer to is treatment to limit the extent of the local tissue injury. In addition we are also going to have to learn how to speed up rostral reorganization by other means, which we are working on now.

INGVAR: I have a question for Dr. Fein about the limitation of the brain biopsy which is unique in these cases. Is it not possible that the brain biopsy specimen you get may be from a region that has a reduced energy charge potential and that there still may be other regions where this has not been the case? Secondly, could a decrease of the energy charge be reversible if the case becomes chronic?

FEIN: The brain certainly is nonhomogeneous, but all I can say is that cortical tissue appears to have the lowest energy-charge potential consistently, with intracisternal hemorrhage under pressure.

PEARSON: Dr. Korein has suggested that we are working towards a definition of death that may be based on the lack of an organism or its individual cells to maintain an internal energy level above that of their environment.†

---

† I believe that Dr. Pearson is referring to the energy requirements of the organism in relation to maintaining its maximal organizational structure or negentropy at the expense of the environment.—*J. K.*

We have now been told that we can have an irreversible state if the internal energy falls below a level of about 20 percent. Apparently then the cell can no longer maintain the membrane it requires to keep itself separate from its environment, across which it must transport essential metabolic substrates in order to survive. What is the minimal time it takes to reach that state after the circulation ceases? In a subsequent paper we will present data that show that if cerebral circulation is absent for approximately 25–60 minutes, no recovery will occur. It seems that we must know how long after the circulation ceases it takes for this metabolically irreversible state to occur. Does anybody know how long that is?

HASS: At the recent meeting in Copenhagen there developed what I'd like to call the 20–20 rule. It is likely that there will be irreversible injury locally, and presumably globally, when (a) under conditions of normal or inhomogeneous blood flow pO_2 is 20 Torr (20 mm Hg or less) or (b) pO_2 is normal and cerebral blood flow is reduced to the region of 20 percent of normal or below. The duration of time that one or both of these circumstances must be present in order to result in irreversibility remains a problem. Very often when we get down to one or the other of these thresholds of ischemia, both factors are operating.

INGVAR: These figures that we just heard quoted are of limited value. They only pertain to the acute state. In a subsequent paper in this volume I will describe patients in whom the supratentorial cerebral metabolic rate is 10 percent of normal. These patients have survived for many years and some have supratentorial CBF of 7, 8, or 9 ml/gm, which is significantly below the figures mentioned. Indeed, I agree that if you drop below certain thresholds in the acute state, the deleterious effects to cerebral tissue would be enormous. But there are chronic states with gliotic scars supratentorially where the metabolic demands become very low indeed. We shall come back to this.‡

HASS: What's operating there is precisely what I was talking about— that we turn down the thermostats with brain-stem injuries and therefore reduce the threshold of ischemia. It's like an anesthetic effect or perhaps like the effect seen in part with barbiturate treatment, and that is, I think, the fundamental question.

‡ This interesting problem, which may involve the metabolic activity of non-neural tissue in Dr. Ingvar's cases, is discussed elsewhere in this volume. Some of Dr. Ingvar's own work suggests that the minimal metabolic rate that a neuron requires just to maintain its own integrity is about 20 percent of normal.—*J. K.*

THE EEG IN DETERMINATION OF BRAIN DEATH

Donald R. Bennett

Departments of Neurology
University of Nebraska College of Medicine and
Creighton University School of Medicine
Omaha, Nebraska 68105

Brain death is a state in which cortical, subcortical, and brain-stem functions are permanently lost. It is equated with destruction of neurons within these structures, i.e., "total brain infarction."[1] Brain death is one form of irreversible coma. All patients in irreversible coma are not brain-dead. The generation of spontaneous as well as evoked potentials is a basic biological property of neurons. Brain waves recorded from the scalp (EEG) reflect activity in postsynaptic dendritic and somatic membranes of neurons in the cerebral cortex. Although these intrinsic spontaneous oscillations are modified by impulses originating in deeper structures, the absence of brain waves for a significant period of time indicates the loss of this particular cortical neuronal function. In deeply comatose patients, the presence or absence of cerebral cortical function cannot be adequately evaluated by the conventional neurologic examination. In this situation, the electroencephalogram (EEG) can be a definite aid. Other neurophysiologic techniques such as steady (DC) recordings and evoked potentials will be discussed elsewhere in this volume.

In 1959, Mollaret and Goulon described the clinical and electroencephalographic findings in twenty-three cases of brain death which they called "coma dépassé" (a state beyond coma).[2] In this condition the patient is deeply comatose, apneic, and with absent brain-stem reflexes. They also included loss of deep-tendon reflexes and vegetative functions, criteria that have not been considered by several groups as a necessary prerequisite for the determination of brain death.[3] Mollaret and Goulon described the EEG in this state as devoid of brain waves.[2] Since these investigators, as well as Fishgold and Mathis,[4] called attention to the value of electroencephalography in the determination of brain death, its exact role has been somewhat controversial. There are those who feel that it is not necessary and that the determination of brain death can be made on the basis of clinical assessment alone, groups who recommend it as an aid or confirmatory test, and, finally, others who consider it a definite requirement.[3] The reasons for this controversy can be divided into the following categories: definition and technical reasons, interpretative reasons, and electroclinical correlations. The data to be presented are derived in part from the National Institutes of Health (NIH)-sponsored study on Cerebral Survival (CS)[5] as well as from my work in this field.[6]

DEFINITION AND TECHNICAL REASONS

EEGs that show an absence of brain waves have been called flat, isoelectric, null, equipotential, or as showing electrocerebral silence (ECS). Although

0077-8923/78/0315-0110 $01.75/0 © 1978, NYAS

semantic debate exists, all investigators agree that the definition must be an operational one, i.e., specifying the techniques as well as the duration of recording. In the Cerebral Survival Study the term "electrocerebral silence" was used and considered present when the record showed an absence of cerebral potentials over 2 μV during a period of at least 30 minutes from symmetrically placed electrode pairs ≥ 10 cm apart and with interelectrode resistances between 100 and 10,000 ohms. In exceptional cases a satisfactory EEG may be obtained with a resistance below 25,000 ohms, but the resistance should be noted. An example of an ECS record is shown in FIGURE 1. For further detail regarding recording techniques the reader is referred to the American EEG Society Guidelines.[7]

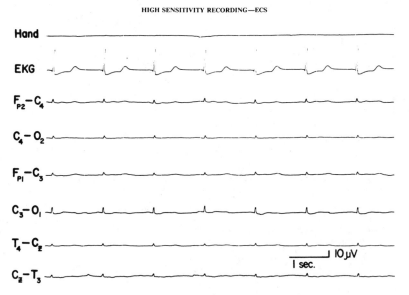

FIGURE 1. An example of an ECS tracing recorded at the required high sensitivity. (From Bennett, D. R. et al.[6] Reprinted by permission.)

The absence of potentials over 2 μV was selected because at the required high gains (sensitivity at least 2.5–3.5 μV/mm) the tracing may be contaminated by the intrinsic noise level of the recording machine. This, together with the thickness of the pen line, makes it extremely difficult to state with any certainty that brain waves under 2 μV are present. In addition to equipment limitations, there are other technical problems, particularly artifacts which can be very troublesome when recording in intensive care units or at the bedside. In the Cerebral Survival Study, approximately 6 percent of 2,256 EEGs were classified as unsatisfactory because of technical difficulties.[5] In some of these tracings a diagnosis of the presence of brain waves could be made despite recording problems, while in others an interpretation could not be given.

The opponents of the EEG as a required test in the determination of brain death rightfully stress these technical problems. In 1969 the Ad Hoc Committee of the American Electroencephalographic Society on EEG Criteria for Determination of Cerebral Death reported their findings on a questionnaire survey sent to their members.[8] Of the 176 who answered, 43 percent had no experience with this type of problem. It was noted that many electroencephalographers were using little more than average recording sensitivity (median 5.0 μV/mm) in determining electrocerebral silence, and there were great variations in technique and duration of recording. Because of a vigorous educational program sponsored by this Society over the last nine years, it is assumed that many of these problems have been corrected. However, a follow-up survey has not been made.

In the United States telephone transmission of the EEG has become popular. Because of unpredictable telephone-line noise and other artefacts, the American EEG Society does not recommend at this time telephone transmission of EEGs for the determination of ECS in suspected brain death cases.[7] The technical limitations will be addressed in somewhat greater detail by Dr. Hughes in this volume.

Also of importance, because the scalp recorded voltage is less than that recorded from the underlying cerebral cortex, are studies comparing scalp ECS with electrocorticography. These have shown that this is not a limitation, i.e., ECS exists in both,[9-12] although in one patient low-amplitude potentials were noted from the cortex.[11] In several cases of deep coma of diverse etiologies, depth recordings have shown absent diencephalic activity.[9-12] In one case potentials were noted in the posterior thalamus.[10]

TABLE 1

CEREBRAL SURVIVAL STUDY (CSS): EEG READER CONCURRENCE

Number of EEGs Reviewed *	Center Interpretation	Panel Interpretation			Percentage of Concurrence
		ECS	Equivocal	B.A.	
133	ECS	115	9	9	86%
27	Equivocal	1	18	8	67%
143	Brain activity	11	1	131	82%
Total 303					

* Total number of ECGs was 2,256.

INTERPRETATIVE REASONS

Because of technical problems as well as the experience of the electroencephalographer, it is natural that there will be some differences in interpretation. Although reader concurrence was not critically evaluated in the Cerebral Survival Study, a panel of expert electroencephalographers reviewed 303 of 2,256 records (13 percent). These tracings were selected by the Project Coordinator because he disagreed with the original reading or found them interesting. Random records were also reviewed. In TABLE 1 the results of the panel survey are tabulated. There was a difference of opinion on 39 records. The most important disagreement was between the nine records called ECS by the project electroencephalographer but noted as showing definite brain waves (brain activity; BA) by the panel. On the other hand the difference of interpretation between the 12 tracings diagnosed by the center electroencephalographer as having brain waves and either ECS[11] or equivocal (one) by the panel has less serious clinical implications. Although the percentage of concurrence in all categories by the panel is not as high as one would expect, the project coordinator who reviewed all the records (2,256) agreed on the diagnosis in 1,953 tracings. If all the EEGs were reviewed by the panel, it is probable that concurrence would have been approximately 2 percent. In the present state of electroencephalography, this is about the best one can expect.*

TERMINOLOGY

The following terms used in the Cerebral Survival Study are defined as follows:

1. *Cerebral Unresponsivity.* The patient has no apparent awareness of externally applied stimuli, obeys no commands, and does not phonate, either spontaneously or secondary to a painful stimulus.

2. *Apnea.* This is the absence in a cerebrally unresponsive patient on controlled ventilation of any attempt to override the respirator. It should be emphasized that this definition does not in any way imply absent respiratory center function. Because of the critical condition of the patients it was decided that a period of observation with the patient off the respirator might be harmful although such tests were used on the basis of the physician's clinical judgment.

3. *Cephalic Reflexes.* These include the following brain-stem reflexes: pupillary, corneal, oculocephalic, vestibular, audio-ocular, snout, cough, pharyngeal, swallowing and jaw jerk.

ELECTROCLINICAL CORRELATIONS

(1.) *Primary diagnoses.* In TABLE 2 the primary diagnoses correlated with the initial EEG interpretations in 500 cases from the CS Study are listed.[5] Fifty-six percent of the records showed brain waves and 37 percent ECS; and approximately 7 percent were equivocal, i.e., because of technical problems, particularly artefacts, a definite interpretation on the presence or absence of brain waves could not be made. ECS was most frequent in the initial EEGs from patients with cerebral trauma or CNS infections, approximately equal with records showing definite brain waves in intracranial hemorrhage and comprised 23 percent of the tracings from patients with primary cardiac disease. Patients under one year of age were excluded from the study. The criteria for brain death in infants and young children have not been established. Further study of this group is presented in this volume by Pampiglione *et al.*

(2.) *Vital signs (blood pressure, pulse and temperature).* The data from the CS Study suggest that these vegetative functions have little predictive value as to ultimate outcome. However, a comparison of these vital sign values

---

* If the EEGs are read conservatively and *any* doubt exists, it may be repeated; furthermore, we are not considering the EEG to be *the* criterion of brain death by any means, but *one* of the criteria tempered by the clinical judgment of the physician.— *J. K.*

between patients with brain waves and ECS has not been made. It is emphasized that in a hypothermic or hypotensive patient with an ECS record, therapeutic measures to correct these deficiencies are required before an interpretation can be made.[5]

(3.) *Cerebral unresponsivity and apnea.* One-hundred eighty-seven patients with ECS were in this state at the time of the initial examination. It should be mentioned that on rare occasions in patients with ECS spontaneous respirations may be present; however, these are insufficient to maintain adequate oxygenation (Ref. 13 and personal observations). Recovery of spontaneous respiration in patients with ECS has been reported, mainly in those in whom the cerebral insult produced primarily cortical and subcortical damage with relative preservation of brain-stem function (apallic syndrome [14, 15] or neocortical death [16]). Some of these patients may recover from coma and appear to be "awake," although they are not aware of their surroundings nor do they behave

TABLE 2

CSS: CORRELATION OF PRIMARY DIAGNOSES WITH INITIAL EEG FINDINGS

Primary Diagnosis	Total	Brain Activity	ECS	Equivocal
Cardiac disease	103	74	24	5
Cerebral trauma	94	31	55	8
Cerebral vascular disease				
Thrombosis or embolism	33	22	10	1
Subarachnoid hemorrhage	34	13	18	3
Intracerebral hemorrhage	74	35	33	6
Other	9	7	1	1
CNS infection	17	6	11	0
Exogenous intoxications	36	33	3	0
Metabolic disorders	36	25	9	2
CNS neoplasms	12	4	8	0
Other	52	33	15	4
Total	500	283	187	30

in a purposeful manner. In this state the EEG may continue to show ECS.[14–16]

(4.) *Cephalic reflexes.* One-hundred forty-four of the 187 patients in the CS Study with *initial* ECS showed absence of all cephalic reflexes. Pupillary reflexes were present in three, corneal in one, oculocephalic in one and vestibular in one. In the remainder all of the reflexes were not tested. Allen *et al.* in a study of 63 cases with cerebral unresponsivity, apnea and ECS of diverse etiologies found all ten cephalic reflexes absent for 24 hours in 56 cases on serial examinations six hours apart.[17] The rare detection of brain-stem reflexes in this group is in marked contrast to the study by Jørgensen.[18] Testing the pupillary, vestibular, oculocephalic, swallowing and cough reflexes, he found some of these to be present in 29 of 77 patients with ECS secondary to primary intracranial lesions. Twenty-two of 38 patients whose ECS was secondary to extracranial disorders retained their cranial-nerve reflexes until a few hours before death. Of the 13 patients with drug-induced ECS one-half retained or regained their cranial-nerve reflexes. The reason for this discrepancy is difficult to evaluate. In this study the EEGs were performed soon after resuscitation, which may be a factor. However, in my experience, only one patient of 20 with an ECS or equivocal EEG record obtained within four hours of qualification (cerebral unresponsitivity and apnea) demonstrated a cephalic reflex (corneal). In the series by Allen et al. the majority of cases were examined within five hours of qualification.[17]

(5.) *Movements and spinal reflexes.* Occasionally spontaneous and evoked "movements" may be seen. In the study by Allen et al. the former were noted in 14 cases and the latter in 36 patients.[17] A description of the type of movement was not given. Spinal reflexes were present in 71 of the 187 cases in the CS Study with cerebral unresponsitivity, apnea, and ECS. Ivan,[19] in a study of 52 patients considered cerebrally † dead, noted the preservation of muscle stretch reflexes in 35 percent. He also noted tonic neck reflexes (neck-arm flexion and neck-hip flexion) in 25 and 45 percent, respectively. Perhaps some of the induced movements reported by Allen were of this type.

(6.) *Recovery of EEG activity and survival.* Recovery from coma associated with ECS secondary to hypnotic or sedative drugs is now well known.[20] ECS can last as long as 28 hours with complete recovery.[21] Drugs that may produce reversible coma and ECS are barbiturates, methaqualone, diazepam, mecloqualone, meprobamate, and trichloroethylene.[20] Other potential reversible conditions are hypothermia and endogenous intoxication; however, the former appears to be based more on experimental evidence than actual clinical cases. In the latter, it is most likely that hypoxia caused by an associated cardiac and/or respiratory arrest accounts for the ECS rather than the electrolyte abnormality. In the last 20 years a number of authors have reported the return of brain waves in non-drug-induced comas. These are summarized by Prior in her book *The EEG in Acute Cerebral Anoxia.*[22] As she noted, inadequate techniques gave the record the appearance of being flat. Even when proper procedures are used the author's interpretation of ECS may not be shared by other electroencephalographers. In the CS Study there were seven cases reported by the center electroencephalographers to have ECS in one record with subsequent return of brain waves.[5] Three of these were secondary to drug intoxication, and *two of these patients survived.* In two patients, one with Reye's syndrome and the other with hydrocephalus, the review panel disagreed with the project electroencephalographer and stated that brain waves were present. However, in another patient with hepatic encephalopathy the panel diagnosed a return of activity while the center electroencephalographer did not. The EEGs from the last case, a patient with subarachnoid hemorrhage, were not reviewed by the panel. With the exception of two drug-intoxicated cases the others died. Silverman et al. in 1970 reported their review of 23 patients who were said to have survived following ECS.[23] In five cases there was an error about recovery. Of the remaining 18 patients, the etiology of the coma was as follows: CNS depressants, eleven; cardiac arrest or vascular collapse, four; insulin coma, one; hyponatremia, one; and measles encephalitis, one. Of the nine records available for review, these authors agreed on the interpretation of ECS in only three, all from patients with drug-induced coma. However, despite these technical and interpretative

---

† These patients may have had brain-stem function, that is, they were not necessarily brain-dead.—*J. K.*

problems, it is possible that in non-drug-intoxicated cases, brain waves may return after an initial period of ECS.[18, 24] This may occur when the recording is performed soon after the catastrophe, such as a cardiac and/or respiratory arrest. What this means in terms of ultimate prognosis remains to be determined.

VALUE OF ELECTROENCEPHALOGRAPHY IN SUSPECTED BRAIN DEATH

In the preceding sections the limitations of electroencephalography have perhaps been somewhat overemphasized; however, before one can appreciate the value of the procedure these have to be known. ECS has a high degree of correlation with the other tests used to evaluate brain death, i.e., clinical examination and isotope and angiographic studies. ECS has a high degree of correlation with mortality. Of the 187 patients whose initial EEG showed ECS, only two survived and both cases were those of drug intoxication (TABLE 3). Seventy-five patients were declared brain-dead and resuscitation was discontinued. Seventy-nine percent of the remaining patients suffered cardiac death within 24 hours of the first ECS record. One patient survived 144 hours before cardiac death. In contrast, 48 of the 241 patients whose initial record showed definite brain waves recovered sufficiently to be discharged from the study. The remaining patients died, although the duration of life was more prolonged, in some cases to more than four weeks.

Of equal and perhaps greater importance is a statement by the electroencephalographer that the brain is generating electrical activity and thus alerting the physician to the possibility that a remedial lesion may be present in patients who satisfy the clinical criteria of brain death, i.e., cerebral unresponsivity, apnea, and absent brain-stem reflexes. There are several causes of deep coma that can mimic the state of brain death. Drug intoxication with or without ECS has been previously mentioned. Walker and Molinari have documented the problems of sedative drug blood determinations in coma.[26] Bolton et al. reported a patient in deep coma with apnea and absent cephalic reflexes secondary to hypoxia from cardiac arrest who survived without neurologic deficits.[25] Brain-stem injury from trauma, infarction, or hemorrhage can also simulate brain death. Although the patients reported by Allen et al.[17] and the

TABLE 3

CSS: CEREBRAL UNRESPONSIVITY, APNEA AND ABSENT CEPHALIC REFLEXES ON INITIAL EXAMINATION

EEG Classification	Number of Cases	Number in Whom All 10 Cephalic Reflexes Were Tested and Absent	Number of Survivors *
ECS	187	144	2
Brain activity or equivocal findings	313	137	48
Total	500	281	50

* Discharged from study.

TABLE 4

CSS: Initial Examination—Cephalic Reflexes Not Examined in 503 Patients

Reflex	Number of Cases
Pupillary	2
Corneal	2
Oculocephalic	8
Vestibular	44
Audioocular	12
Snout	15
Pharyngeal	79
Swallowing	85
Cough	72
Jaw jerk	24
Total	343

one by Deliyannakis and coauthors[27] did not survive, in these conditions simulation of brain death remains a possibility. A patient with tetanus treated with curare clinically satisfied the criteria for brain death.[28]

Another point in favor of including the EEG as a definite test before brain death can be declared is the reliability of the tests used to examine the brain-stem reflexes. The techniques for examining these reflexes are certainly qualitative and not as well standardized as the EEG. Although peer review of EEGs and pathologic specimens was done in the CS study, interexaminer reliability of the neurologic examination was not assessed. Other considerations are iatrogenically induced areflexias, for example by the use of mydriatic agents. Some brain-stem reflexes may not be accessible for examination because of traumatic injuries about the head and face or for other legitimate reasons. Noteworthy are the number of cephalic reflexes not examined in the CS study (TABLE 4). Three-hundred forty-three (7 percent) of 5,030 reflexes (503 patients × ten reflexes) were not tested. Either the pupillary, corneal, oculocephalic, vestibular or pharyngeal reflexes, which physicians might routinely test, were not examined in 56 cases. Allen has concluded that tests of the first four reflexes have the greatest diagnostic value.[17] The EEG thus provides an additional safeguard.

Since the outcome of patients with coma, apnea and absent cephalic reflexes with definite brain waves on serial examinations was not specifically analyzed in the CS Study, the cases from Center 8 (University of Utah) were reviewed. Ninety-four patients qualified (67 included in the 503 cases of the CS Study), but five were excluded because either they were not apneic at the time of the initial examination, the EEG was technically unsatisfactory, or the neurologic examination was not performed within two hours of the EEG. In TABLE 5, the primary diagnosis is correlated with the EEG interpretation at the first and second examinations. Sixty-four of the initial evaluations were performed within four hours of qualification (cerebral unresponsivity and apnea), 16 within eight hours, five before 12 hours, and four after this time. Forty-one patients died or regained spontaneous respiration before the second evaluation. Of the remaining patients 90 percent of the tests were accomplished within six to eight hours of the initial examination. The presence or absence of the following reflexes was noted: pupillary, corneal, oculocephalic, oculovestibular, and pharyngeal. Of the 56 patients whose initial EEGs showed brain waves, 16 had absence of four or five of the cephalic reflexes tested. Four of these patients survived (one with cardiac arrest and three with drug intoxication). In contrast,

TABLE 5

CORRELATION OF INITIAL AND SECOND-EXAMINATION EEGs IN 89 PATIENTS
WITH CEREBRAL UNRESPONSITIVITY AND APNEA

Primary Diagnosis	EEG	First Examination *	Second Examination †
Cardiac and/or respiratory arrest	Brain activity	24	11
	ECS	5	2
	Equivocal	1	1
Total		30	14
Cerebral vascular disease			
Intracranial hemorrhage	Brain activity	5	2
	ECS	6	7
	Equivocal	6	4
Total		17	13
Thrombosis or embolism	Brain activity	4	1
	ECS	0	0
	Equivocal	0	0
Total		4	1
Drug intoxication	Brain activity	17	8
	ECS	0	0
	Equivocal	0	0
Total		17	8
Cerebral trauma	Brain activity	5	2
	ECS	10	0
	Equivocal	1	6
Total		16	8
Brain tumors	Brain activity	1	1
	ECS	4	3
	Equivocal	0	0
Total		5	4

* First examination—89 patients.
† Second examination—48 patients.

there was a group of eight patients with brain waves who had absence of all but one cephalic reflex at the initial examination (five pupillary, two vestibular, and one pharyngeal). If these tests had been omitted, the patients would have satisfied the *clinical* criteria for brain death on the basis of a single examination. Five of these eight patients survived (one with cardiac arrest and four with drug intoxication).

The cases presented, although certainly not large in number, indicate that reliance only on the clinical criteria for brain death may result in missing occasional cases who might recover. Of the nine survivors in the two groups, coma was secondary to drug overdose in seven. Two patients recovered completely following a cardiac arrest.

Guidelines for determination of brain death are implicit in emphasizing that there be adequate knowledge of the nature and extent of the intracranial pathology in order to rule out remediable lesions, and that the patient be observed over a sufficient period of time to assure a complete evaluation and appropriate treatment. This time interval has ranged from six to 24 hours. If one accepts the definition of brain death as discussed in the beginning of this paper, then other studies in addition to the neurologic examination are required. The EEG can provide critical information if one recognizes the limitations, as previously discussed. If brain waves are present in a patient with cerebral unresponsivity, apnea and absent cephalic reflexes, a remediable cause may be present. Other ancillary tests and their specificity in brain death will be discussed elsewhere in this volume.

SUMMARY

The values and limitations of electroencephalography in the determination of brain death have been reviewed. Electrocerebral silence per se does not necessarily mean total or irreversible brain dysfunction. *In the state of brain death the EEG is always silent; however, ECS does not always mean brain death.* Electroencephalography, when properly used, can be a most helpful aid to the physician. Clinical criteria alone for the establishment of brain death may lack specificity, and occasional cases with potentially remediable lesions may be overlooked. The diagnosis of brain death cannot be made by only one test. The physician has to make his decision based on the entire clinical picture and results of the studies that are available to him.

REFERENCES

1. INGVAR, D. H. 1971. Total brain infarction. Acta Anaesthesiol. Scand. (Suppl.) **45:** 129–140.
2. MOLLARET, P. & M. GOULON. 1959. Le coma dépassé. Rev. Neurol. (Paris) **101:** 3–15.
3. WALKER, A. E. 1975. Cerebral death. *In* The Nervous System. The Clinical Neurosciences. D. B. Tower, Ed. Vol. **2:** 75–87. Raven Press. New York, N.Y.
4. FISHGOLD, H. & P. MATHIS. 1959. Obnubilations, comas et stupeurs: Études electroencephalographique. Electroencephalogr. Clin. Neurophysiol. Suppl. **11:** 1–124.
5. An appraisal of the criteria of cerebral death—a summary statement. (Final report: Collaborative Study of Cerebral Survival. HEW, NIH, NINDS, Contract 1–NS–1–2316. Bethesda, Md., April 1974.) JAMA **237:** 982–986, 1977.
6. BENNETT, D. R., J. R. HUGHES, J. KOREIN, J. K. MERLIS & C. SUTER. 1976. Atlas of Electroencephalography in Coma and Cerebral Death. Raven Press. New York, N.Y.
7. AMERICAN ELECTROENCEPHALOGRAPHIC SOCIETY. 1976. Minimum Technical Standards for EEG Recording in Suspected Cerebral Death. Willoughby, Ohio.

8. SILVERMAN, D., M. G. SAUNDERS, R. S. SCHWAB & R. L. MASLAND. 1969. Cerebral death and the electroencephalogram. Report of ad hoc committee of the American Electroencephalographic Society on EEG criteria for determination of cerebral death. JAMA **209:** 1505–1510.
9. JOUVET, M. 1959. Diagnostic électro-sous-cortico-graphique de la mort du système nerveux central au cours de certains coma. Electroencephalogr. Clin. Neurophysiol **11:** 805–808.
10. CARBONELL, J., R. CARRASCOAA, G. DIERSSEN, S. OBRADUR, J. C. OLIVEROS & M. SEVILLANO. 1963. Some electrophysiological observations in a case of deep coma secondary to cardiac arrest. Electroencephalogr. Clin. Neurophysiol. **15:** 520–524.
11. FINDJI, J., J. GACHES, J. P. HOUTTEVILLE, P. CREISSARD & A. CALISKAN. 1970. Cortical, transcortical, and subcortical electroencephalographic recordings in ten cases of profound irreversible coma. Neurochirurgia **13:** 211–219.
12. VELASCO, M., M. LOPEZ-PORTILLO, J. E. OLVERA-RABIELA & F. VELASCO. 1971. EEG and deep recoring in cases of irreversible coma. Arch. Invest. Med. (Mexico). **2:** 1–14.
13. PRIOR, P. 1973. The EEG in Acute Cerebral Anoxia. : 101. Elsevier. New York, N.Y.
14. INGVAR, D. M. & A. BRUN. 1972. Das komplette appallische syndrom. Arch. Psychiat. Nerven Kr. **215:** 219–239.
15. BENNETT, D. R., N. M. NORD, T. S. ROBERTS & H. MAVOR. 1971. Prolonged survival with flat electroencephalogram following cardiac arrest. Electroencephalogr. Clin. Neurophysiol. **30:** 94.
16. BRIERLEY, J. B., D. I. GRAHAM, J. H. ADAMS & J. A. SIMPSON. 1971. Neocortical death after cardiac arrest. A clinical neurophysiological and neuropathological report of two cases. Lancet **ii:** 560–565.
17. ALLEN, N., J. D. BURKHOLDER & G. F. MOLINARI. 1975. Clinical criteria of cerebral death. *In* Final Report, Collaborative Study of Cerebral Survival. National Institute of Neurological Diseases and Stroke.
18. JØRGENSEN, E. O. 1974. EEG without detectable cortical activity and cranial nerve areflexia as parameters of brain death. Electroencephalogr. Clin. Neurophysiol. **36:** 70–75.
19. IVAN, L. P. 1973. Spinal reflexes in cerebral death. Neurology. **23:** 650–652.
20. POWNER, D. J. 1976. Drug associated isoelectric EEG's. JAMA **236:** 1123.
21. HAIDER, I., H. MATTHEW & I. OSWALD. 1971. Electroencephalographic changes in acute drug poisoning. Electroencephalogr. Clin. Neurophysiol. **30:** 23–31.
22. PRIOR, P.[13] : 128–131, 134.
23. SILVERMAN, D., .R. L. MASLAND, M. G. SAUNDERS & R. S. SCHWAB. 1970. Irreversible coma associated with electrocerebral silence. Neurology **20:** 525–533.
24. BENNETT, D. R. *et al.*[6] : 151–154.
25. BOLTON, C. F., J. D. BROWN, E. CHOLOD & K. WARREN. 1976. EEG and "brain life." Lancet **i:** 535.
26. WALKER, A. E. & G. F. MOLINARI. 1977. Sedative drug surveys in coma. Postgraduate Medicine. **61:** 105–109.
27. DELIYANNAKIS, E., F. IOANNOV & A. DAVAROVKAS. 1975. Brain stem death with persistence of bioelectric activity of the cerebral hemispheres. Clinical Electroencephalogr. **6:** 75–79.
28. BENNETT, D. R. *et al.*[6] : 183.

LIMITATIONS OF THE EEG IN COMA AND BRAIN DEATH

John R. Hughes

Department of Neurology
University of Illinois Medical Center
Chicago, Illinois 60612

INTRODUCTION

The Committee on Cessation of Cerebral Function of the International Federation of Societies for Electroencephalography and Clinical Neurophysiology has provided a definition of brain death. As chairman of that committee, Ingvar [1] has stated that "brain death is . . . an irreversible cessation of function of all cerebral structures, including the cerebellum and brain stem down to the spinal segment C-1." If brain death is defined in this particular manner and refers to the cessation of function throughout the *entire* brain down to the spinal cord, the electroencephalogram (EEG) obviously has various limitations. These limitations of the EEG can be conveniently divided into (1) technical (and avoidable) difficulties and (2) poor prediction of eventual life or death from misleading data.

TECHNICAL DIFFICULTIES

The technical difficulties include relatively high amounts of noise from either an electrode or amplifier, so that low-level brain activity may not be delineated from the noise if the latter is more than 2 μV in amplitude. Examples of this are well illustrated in the *Atlas of Electroencephalography* by Bennett and his colleagues. [2] One other technical difficulty arises from high, but especially *unequal* resistances between electrodes, producing artefacts, especially of the 60-Hz variety. Widely spaced electrodes are recommended in the case of questionable brain death by most experts in the field of electroencephalography in order to increase the probabilities of recording low-amplitude activity, but Jung [3] has reported that the area explored by one scalp electrode may have a radius of approximately 4 cm. In this case electrodes placed more than 8 cm from each other could fail to pick up focal activity of low amplitude; Jørgensen [4] has concluded that cortical activity could be present in a single region only and that such focal activity would then be missed if the recording electrodes were sufficiently far from each other, say 10 cm, as recommended by the American EEG Society. [5] This latter technical difficulty seems theoretically possible, but convincing examples are not found in the literature. One other technical difficulty is that a brief EEG may fail to record activity appearing only sporadically. Jørgensen and Bitsch [6] continuously recorded at high gain for up to 8 hours in one patient and found intermixed cortical activity with amplitudes down to 2 μV appearing at intervals up to 20 minutes. Therefore, their recommendation was that a 30-minute recording was required in order to determine that electrocerebral silence (ECS) is valid. In his summary of the experiences and recommendations from the Collaborative Study on Coma

121

0077-8923/78/0315-0121 $01.75/0 © 1978, NYAS

and Cerebral Death, supported by the National Institutes of Health, Walker [7] states that a 30-minute recording is required. However, the Committee on the Cessation of Cerebral Function of the International Federation has recommended that the tracing continue for as long as 60 minutes,[1] but the standard length of time in the United States would seem to be 30 minutes. One obvious technical difficulty occurs from the use of low gains in tracings with only minimal activity that cannot be detected without the use of the highest possible amplification of the machine. Excellent examples of this "pseudo-electrocerebral silence" are found in the *Atlas* by Bennett and his colleagues.[2] Finally, one other technical difficulty arises from the preservation of function of extracranial organs and therefore, the electro-oculogram (EOG), electroretinogram (ERG), electromyogram (EMG) and electrocardiogram (EKG) must be properly identified by the electroencephalographer. In the case of the EMG, Pavulon® or Anectine® usually resolves the problem of the records uninterpretable from muscle artefact, since these drugs can usually be safely given to patients already on respirators, permitting electroencephalographers to view the EEG without overwhelming artefacts. In the great majority of instances, experienced technicians can overcome the difficulties mentioned in this section.

MISLEADING DATA

ECS and Drug Intoxication

The EEG may be misleading in a number of ways and possibly the most important and significant example is the record showing electrocerebral silence in a patient who later shows a recovery with clear biological activity. Although certain studies, like those of Prior [8] and Kimura et al.,[9] have indicated that all patients showing ECS eventually died within a relatively short period of time, there are some well-known examples of patients with ECS who recovered. The best known examples are those involving drug intoxication.[10-12] In his report of the American EEG Society's Ad Hoc Committee on EEG Criteria for the determination of cerebral death, Silverman and his colleagues [13] reported that 1,665 records had been reviewed and that only three represented genuine electrocerebral silence (ECS) with later recovery of some cerebral function. Two of these instances were in patients with barbiturate intoxication and one was in a patient with meprobamate intoxication who then died from other causes. One comment in the paper was that recovery of EEG activity in one patient occurred at 72 hours, but one cannot be certain of the number of electroencephalographic records taken within that three-day period, so that it seems uncertain whether or not ECS was repeatedly observed throughout and actually did *continue* for the 72-hour period. During the next year (1970) Silverman and his colleagues [14] reported on 2,650 patients who provided 279 EEGs with presumed ECS for as long as a 24-hour duration, and only three (likely the same three as reported in the previous year) recovered cerebral function. One emphasis in this article was that there were many "pseudo-isoelectric recordings," referring to those that looked flat, but recorded at low-gain settings rather than at the highest possible gain of the EEG machine.

In the collaborative study on coma supported by the NIH [7] 61 patients with drug intoxication were entered into the study; survival was 44 percent with two complete recoveries in patients who had had electrocerebral silence for

12 and 21 hours, respectively. Jørgensen [15] has reported ECS for a 14-hour period, but with eventual recovery, and has suggested that 24 hours be the limit for ECS and possible recovery. Haider et al. [16] have reported on 15 patients with drug intoxication who had ECS lasting 3–28 hours and recorded with gain settings of 2 μV/mm. These investigators reported that 11 of the patients made a full recovery, but the report does not indicate whether or not the one with 28 hours of ECS actually did recover. Kirshbaum and Carollo [17] studied a patient in barbiturate coma with ECS (no gains indicated) whose second record three days later showed delta waves and whose third record six days later was normal. Mantz and his colleagues [18] reported on a 47-year-old female who had been in coma for 110 hours and for 24 hours showed ECS and later fully recovered. The one example of ECS shown was at a gain setting of approximately 2 μV/mm. During the next day and also one hour before ECS the EEG showed the suppression burst pattern. Bird and Plum [19] reported on a patient with barbiturate intoxication whose EEG showed ECS for at least 23 hours, but normal gains using 50-μV calibration signals apparently were used. This latter patient did recover clinically. Thus, the literature shows some instances of apparent ECS which are actually "pseudo-isoelectric" recordings without the use of the highest gain settings, but some recordings can be found in patients with drug intoxication with actual ECS and later full clinical recovery. The limit for recovery would seem to be approximately 24 hours of ECS.*

ECS and Hypothermia

Hypothermia is one other condition that is well known to have some effect on electrical activity of the central nervous system. In one case presented by Tentler and his colleagues [20] a "flat" record was noted for 19½ minutes in a patient under hypothermia who also had chlorpromazine and anesthesia for a surgical operation. Since there was such an extended period of time during which the EEG was "flat," the clinical expectation was that some form of cerebral damage would be evident, but no impairment was noted upon awakening of this patient. Later, a normal EEG was reported one week after the surgery. The authors reported that both hypothermia and the chlorpromazine likely protected both the vital centers of the brain and also the cerebral cortex, explaining the recovery of this patient. It seems possible that hypothermia may have contributed toward the loss of amplitude in the record, but the statement in the report is "The complete absence of cortical rhythms was shown as a *practically* flat line." Therefore, the authors did not seem certain that complete ECS had actually occurred and no calibration signals are shown in the examples provided in the article to determine the sensitivity setting. Therefore, this example may be more illustrative of diminished EEG activity from hypothermia and *also* cerebral ischemia related to blood loss occurring during the operation when a hemorrhage occurred, but this case is not a good example of definite ECS.

Williams and Spencer [21] reported on four patients who had suffered a cardiac arrest and had signs of severe neurologic injury; they were treated with hypothermia of 30–34° C for 72 hours. Since three of these patients had shown

---

* This limit is based on the current literature, but longer duration of drug-induced ECS should be considered as a possibility if full life support is maintained.—*J. K.*

full recovery, the authors concluded that the hypothermia likely reduced cerebral swelling, permitting such recovery, but no EEGs were actually recorded in this study. Nevertheless, the hypothermia was considered to have an effect on the central nervous system. Prior[8] has reported that temperatures must be below 30° C to be significant for an EEG change and that ECS will likely not occur until the temperature is at least below 20° C. Some of the data from the latter conclusions may have come from the work of Pearcy and Virtue.[22] These investigators studied 108 human subjects with hypothermia; in one-half a tendency toward slowing of frequencies was noted, but it was not usually greater than a 25 percent change. In only five patients were the temperatures below 29° C, and in four of those there was a decrease in frequency and in one an increase in frequency of the EEG. A careful inspection of the data from this report reveals that all the frequencies seen in those five patients were in the theta or alpha range, and there was a voltage *increase* in two of those patients in whom a decrease in frequency had been found, and *no change* in voltage in the others. Studies in dogs were also included and 12 animals were "cooled" below 28° C. The beginning of significant loss of EEG in the dog was at approximately 24° C, and one example showed a "flat" record at 17° C; however, standard calibrations of 50 μV were used in this latter example so that actual ECS cannot be verified. Nevertheless, these studies do show that in man temperatures under 29° C would seem to be required before a significant effect is seen on the EEG, and in dogs temperatures possibly under 20° C are required before very significant loss of amplitude approaching ECS can be found. Since both drug intoxication and hypothermia may play a role in the amplitudes recorded on the EEG, Prior[8] has suggested that one cannot predict the outcome in patients whose EEG record shows ECS if there is a history of drug overdose or hypothermia. The former condition represents an important practical consideration, but the latter is mainly theoretical.

ECS without Drug Intoxication and Hypothermia

The literature contains a number of examples of ECS (or presumed ECS) without involving drug intoxication or hypothermia in which later there was recovery of activity. In some instances the ECS must be considered questionable. In Prior's series[8] all patients with ECS died within a short period of time, although one of these patients with ECS during the first hour or two showed a transient lightening of coma and return of EEG activity. However, close inspection of the example shows that short interelectrode distances were used and standard gains from only four channels were also utilized. This example seems to show some questionable activity in three of the channels and muscle activity is predominant in the other. Levin and Kinnell[23] reported a case of ventricular fibrillation with general anesthesia in which the patient survived despite a "prolonged flat EEG." The cardiac resuscitation took 45 minutes and the EEG was considered to be flat in the recovery room, although it was not clear whether or not the EEG was really flat for the full 45 minutes. The examples shown include only one channel of EEG without any calibrations to indicate the gain used and the only example on the thirteenth day with calibrations was one in which a 100-μV calibration signal was used. The patient described by Houtteville et al.[24] had encephalitis and recovered, but the authors reported that one could not see definite rhythms in this EEG. However, the gains were so low that a standard calibration signal of 50 μV was used and also questionable rhythms seemed to appear in the example shown. In the report by Cloche et al.[25] there were five cases of anoxia after cardiac arrest, and electrical reactivity was reported to appear after a silence of several hours. Jørgensen[4] reported that without drug involvement ECS can exist for eight hours with recovery of consciousness nevertheless, but the examples shown are not totally convincing as to the presence or absence of cerebral activity. Riehl and McIntyre[26] claimed in two cases that there was a near complete recovery of EEG activity following an ECS record. One patient was reported to have ECS for seven hours, but inspection of the protocol shows that the first EEG was done at 1:30 P.M. and the second one at 3:00 P.M., the latter being recorded for 30 minutes and considered flat. The patient was in the hospital at 8:20 A.M., but no EEG was reported as having been done then, so the actual duration of ECS seems questionable. The other case was one in which the EEG was considered flat for two hours, but the example shown uses a standard 50-μV calibration signal. The authors do conclude that brain death must rest on a combination of a flat EEG and also specific clinical deficits, all of which must persist for at least 24 hours.

In other instances ECS did exist, but other variables raised questions regarding the ECS. One case presented by Hughes and his colleagues[27] showed in the first recording only muscle artefact which was eliminated by 60 mg of succinylcholine (Anectine), then revealing only ECS at the highest possible gain settings of 2 μV/mm. However, clear activity appeared 22 hours later and again four days after the first record, although within a few days cardiac death occurred. Nevertheless, this example is one in which clear ECS occurred followed later by definite EEG activity. However, a few questions do remain in this case: (1) only 17 minutes of record showing ECS could be run (rather than the usual 30 minutes) because of the medical emergencies that were occurring with the patient at that time of recording; and (2) the succinylcholine that was given, although usually considered to have an effect on the periphery, could possibly have an effect on some remaining low-amplitude EEG activity, since one report[28] exists suggesting an additional central effect from this drug.† Green and Lauber[29] reported on a five-year-old child with ECS (with maximal gains) whose record 24 hours later showed fast activity, but was described as only 2–4 μV in amplitude. The patient then died 7 hours later. A second patient, six weeks old, had ECS and in 24 hours showed 12–18/sec-rhythms, slow waves and sharp waves with clear rhythms also seen at 72 and 96 hours after ECS. This second patient, regaining spontaneous respiration and eye movement also, but dying in 3 weeks, is a clearer example of genuine EEG recovery after ECS.

In other cases ECS without significant complications seemed to have occurred. Leenstra-Borsje et al.[30] reported on two patients with ECS in whom follow-up studies showed some cerebral activity after seven hours in one and after two days in the other, but these patients did die within a short period of time. Their conclusion was that ECS alone was not absolute proof of cerebral death. Jonkman[31] used the gain setting of 2–3 μV/mm and reported on two cases with ECS that did not represent complete cerebral death. In one patient with ECS there was an external hydrocephalus, but EEG activity returned after

---

† Clinical studies by Suter and others indicate that this muscle paralysant never causes ECS in dosages used.—J. K.

removal of the extracerebral fluid. Mental impairment was only mild in this child. The second case was in a two-year-old child with acute encephalitis, leading to massive cerebral edema and decortication, but swallowing and other subcortical functions did remain. Jonkman reported that the EEG showed only an ECS for five months, but depth electrode studies did reveal the presence of subcortical activity. One of the most interesting cases of this type was presented by Bricolo *et al.*[32] who reported on a 14-year-old who had a severe head injury producing a subdural hematoma, then decerebrate rigidity for 3 months, and who was considered alive with an "apallic syndrome." A complete disappearance of all EEG activity was reported for the first 120 days, but in the next months very slow activity appeared first on the right and then on the left side and after 16 months organized 8–9/-sec rhythms were seen, persisting until the reporting of this case. These authors also concluded that ECS *alone* does not, therefore, determine cerebral death.

In the hundreds of EEGs surveyed by Silverman and his group,[14] all in patients with presumed ECS and also recovery, there were only three in which the patient truly did recover cerebral function and that were actually representative of electrocerebral silence. These investigators concluded that ECS, when properly recorded, together with a neurologic picture of total unresponsiveness and coma with absent reflexes and absent spontaneous respiration, represents strong presumptive evidence of total brain death, except after administration of central nervous system depressant drugs and the theoretical example of hibernation. However, some of the examples mentioned in this section do suggest the possibility of ECS without drug intoxication and hypothermia, but with definite recovery of activity and in some instances recovery of clinical function. Clearly, these examples are very rare and the reviewer could find no illustrated reports in which EEGs had been done frequently enough to determine the exact number of hours (2–8?) of clear ECS with later recovery of activity.

Subcortical Activity and ECS in EEG

One of the major limitations of the EEG in the determination of brain death is the inability of the scalp electrodes to record all subcortical activity. Various investigators have attempted to attack this problem directly by implantation of electrodes into subcortical structures. Silverman[33] has reminded us that there may be an 80 percent attenuation of activity by the dura, skull and scalp, and if ECS is defined by the presence of no more than 2 μV of activity, this possibility would suggest that 10 μV could be seen on the surface of the cerebral cortex. The logical extension of this argument would be that even greater amplitude might be found in the depths. Jouvet[34] reported a flat EEG in one patient, but also failed to detect any activity from the median thalamus of that same patient. However, in another case Carbanell and his colleagues[35] reported a flat tracing from the scalp (without designating gain settings) and also directly from the parietal and temporal cortex, amygdala, putamen and globus pallidus, but activity *was* recorded in the median dorsal nucleus and ventral lateral nucleus of the thalamus. One tracing fails to show any activity in the cortex, but in the thalamus, subthalamus and pons 40–60 μV of activity is noted. Also, stimulating the pons produced an evoked response in the inferior caudal thalamus, but not when the stimulation and recording points were reversed. Vissor[36] reported a 27-year-old female who had been in coma for 47 days, in whom ECS was recorded from the twelfth to the forty-seventh day. Depth electrode studies on the thirty-seventh day, however, showed theta and delta rhythms in the thalamic region. The conclusion of this investigator was that a silent scalp EEG did not mean that subcortical regions were also silent. The author also concluded that it is better to speak of statistics on the chance of fatal prognosis rather than on brain death per se. Finally, Findji and his colleagues [37] reported on 10 patients with subcortical implanted electrodes in addition to EEG recordings. Three patients showed "flat" EEGs with two reported to show no activity, but one showing only slight cortical activity; however, the examples included either 50- or 100-μV calibration signals, likely representing low gain settings. In the other seven patients, scalp EEGs were said to show "barely perceptible" activity, but in all of these ten patients the authors reported that there were signs of activity within the thalamic structures. Thus, these cases point to the possibility of subcortical activity with ECS recorded from scalp electrodes, but good examples with proper gain settings are difficult to find in the literature.

Evoked Potentials and ECS

In the search for examples of subcortical activity remaining in patients who show ECS in their scalp EEGs, a number of investigators have reported on evoked responses as one means of assessing subcortical function. For example, Arfel [38] reported that patients with ECS may show some type of visual responses (VER), but only from the anterior frontal regions. Upon more careful investigation these responses were considered by that author to be only retinal in origin, persisting for many hours after the extinction of spontaneous cerebral rhythms. Also, Poole [39] reported that the VER was not usually seen in cases of ECS, but did mention the exceptions of patients with clinical survival without a VER and those with clinical deficits with a preserved evoked cerebral response. A more complete study was done by Trojaberg and Jørgensen,[40] who reported on 50 patients with ECS who also were tested for evoked responses. In 19 of these patients cranial nerve reflexes did persist and then both the visual and the somatosensory evoked responses (SER) were found, but with long latency and without late components. Angiograms were taken on six of these patients and intracranial circulation was found to exist in all six. Three of these patients did recover consciousness and one actually was sent home. In the other 31 patients no cranial nerve reflexes were found at the time of ECS and there were no VERs or SERs, except for one patient who showed a visual evoked response. Angiograms in 20 of these patients showed only one with some type of circulation, and that was in the carotid branches of the patient who had the VER. The general conclusion of these authors was that since there were 19 patients with ECS, but also with evoked responses, although simple in form and late in latency, these data did suggest some type of life within the cerebrum. The authors also reported on eight patients with stagnant anoxia and one with hepatic cirrhosis who regained cortical activity 4–24 hours after ECS. Three of these patients did recover consciousness and one was actually out of the hospital at the time of writing of that report.

In a more recent study, Starr [41] followed the demise of comatose patients to the state of cerebral death with brain-stem auditory evoked responses. When cerebral death occurred the characteristic seven wavelets were missing, except that wavelet #I (from the auditory nerve) was at times seen with a long latency. In 11 of 27 patients with ECS who met all other criteria for brain death, wavelet I could be found at a latency of 1.8–2.1 msec, compared to the normal of 1.4 msec.

Mehta and Seshia [42] investigated the orbicularis oculi reflex in three children with brain death by stimulating the supraorbital nerve and recording from the orbicularis oculi. By this means of evaluating brain-stem function, both early and late components of this reflex were absent, but the response to the peripheral facial nerve was present.

Clinical Signs and ECS

Other examples of an ECS recording representing a misleading sign of cerebral death are instances in which ECS is found with *clinical* signs of brain-stem life. Arfel [43] claims that all EMG activity (or eye-blinks) recorded by scalp electrodes is evidence of residual brain-stem function. Jørgensen [4] alludes to this same type of problem in claiming that the brain is dead only when ECS is recorded in the absence of all cranial nerve reflexes, spontaneous respiration, and spontaneous blood pressure. In a case reported by Vissor [36] in which ECS was recorded for seven days, respiration did remain and the conclusion of the author was that the scalp-recorded ECS did not represent silent subcortical functioning. Similarly, in the case reported by Jonkman [31] also involving ECS for a long period of time, the patient did continue to show swallowing and other subcortical functions at the time a depth electrode recorded subcortical activity. One interesting case was reported by Bennett *et al.*[44] in which cardio-pulmonary arrest resulted in coma with EEG recordings during the first three days showing primarily muscle artefact, but an ECS was reported on the fourth day. Four weeks later the patient was said to show akinetic mutism, continuing to show the same clinical picture two years later. However, annual EEGs were said to show only ECS. Epidural and also cortical bipolar recordings from the right parietal cortex in this patient failed to show any spontaneous activity.

Other interesting cases of ECS and residual clinical functions were reported by Brierley *et al.*[45] These authors reported on two patients with ECS, said to be "strictly defined," with at least a five-month survival. The authors reported that neurologic and neurophysiologic studies led to the conclusion that the neocortex was in fact dead while the lower visual, auditory, and spinal reflex path were intact. Neuropathologic examination later confirmed the *in vivo* prediction of the extent of cerebral damage. In case 1 there was eye-opening, yawning, spontaneous respiration and reflexes of brain-stem function such as reactive pupils, and in case 2 there was spontaneous respiration with other brain-stem reflexes remaining. In case 1 ECS was recorded on days 3, 6, 7, 12, 13, 20, 21, 34 and 85; in case 2 ECS was found on days 2, 6, 7, 10, 13, 14, 21, 35, 61 and 87. The later neuropathologic studies showed that up to four of the outer layers of the neocortex could be identified in the frontal lobes, but these latter areas were likely isolated from white matter by a band of necrosis and therefore were devoid of subcortical connections. The authors discussed the problem that a patient in whom spontaneous respiration is resumed after cardiac arrest, yet ECS is seen in the EEG, is usually regarded as "alive," while another surviving the same accident who also has an ECS recording, but whose respiratory function depends on mechanical ventilation, would likely be regarded

as "dead." The authors pointed out that clearly this distinction between alive
and dead attaches cardinal importance to the function of respiration and not
to those higher functions of the nervous system that demarcate man from lower
primates and all other verebrates. However, other than the interesting philosophical point, these studies do emphasize that ECS from scalp recordings may
be clearly limited in failing to show subcortical functioning which can be determined by clinical findings. The studies also emphasize the lengthy period
of time (e.g., 87 days) during which ECS can be recorded with continuation
of brain-stem functions. Bental and Leibowicz [46] reported on a so-called flat
record for 28 days, but actually referred to the recordings as *almost* flat and
also *almost completely* flat; inspection of the report shows that 50-μV calibration
signals were actually used. Also, Lundervold [47] reported on a flat tracing for
14 days after an arrest in one patient. However, the calibration signal in the
example shows a sensitivity setting of 14 μV/mm, and therefore ECS would
not have been proven in this patient.

Brain-Stem Death and Cortical Life

The condition of brain-stem death and cortical life also may lead to poor
prediction on the basis of the EEG. Korein and Maccario [48] reported on two
patients who did have ECS, but on neuropathologic investigation showed only
minimal neuronal changes within the cerebral cortex and had large intraventricular hemorrhages and bilateral destruction of the thalamus and central
diencephalic structures down to the lower brain-stem levels. Although ECS
was recorded in these patients, they demonstrate that the cortex may be mini-
mally involved in instances of nearly total brain-stem destruction. Jørgensen
and his colleagues [49] allude to the possibility of EEG activity with brain-stem
death by reporting on two patients who did show EEG rhythms for four and
eight hours, respectively, after all cranial nerve reflexes had disappeared. Bolton
et al.[50] discussed a patient with clinical signs of brain death, including the
absence of brain-stem reflexes, but a suppression burst pattern was recorded in
the EEG. In 24 hours the patient improved clinically and electrographically,
and in 72 hours the EEG was nearly normal. Deliyannakis *et al.*[51] reported on
a patient whose bioelectric activity was said to exist 48 hours prior to death,
but who had dilated, fixed pupils and other signs of brain-stem death. Neuropathologic investigation revealed that only some pieces from the peduncle, pons
and medulla remained, but that the gray and white matter of the hemispheres
were distinguishable in most places. These latter instances are not clear examples
of remaining cortical function in the face of brain-stem death, but they theoretically point to this possibility and suggest that the EEG activity that might
remain could be misleading in predicting an overly optimistic outcome of
patients with this condition.

Blood-Flow Studies versus EEG

Since EEG has some limitations in the determination of cerebral death, as
discussed in the previous sections, many investigators have addressed themselves
to the question of the usefulness of blood-flow studies (compared to the EEG)
in order to determine precisely the death of the entire brain. In the report by

Ingvar[1] from the Committee on Cessation of Cerebral Function of the International Federation brain death was considered to require the absence of blood flow to the central nervous system structures down to spinal segment C-1. A general review of the angiographic technique used in cerebral blood-flow studies was presented by Smith and Walker,[52] and later Korein et al.[53] described a specific radioisotopic bolus technique. Ketz[54] claimed that cessation of blood flow determined by angiographic studies was clearly the most reliable sign of cerebral death, and Jørgensen et al.[49] have added that the absence of brain circulation demonstrated at intervals of 20 minutes by the angiographic technique documents brain death. Miyazaki et al.[55] maintained that cerebral death should mean irreversible loss of function of the entire brain, including the brain stem, so that nonfilling of cerebral arteries in bilateral carotid and vertebral angiograms is an absolute criterion for the determination of cerebral death, and ECS is only an incidental criterion. Pendl et al.[56] reported on one patient with ECS, in whom circulation was angiographically demonstrated. In addition, in one patient described by Hughes and his colleagues[27] ECS was shown on the first record, but electrical activity was seen later on the next day; at the time ECS was recorded a positive cerebroradioangiogram showed circulation within the brain. On the other hand, Ouaknine et al.[57] reported that more sophisticated tests, such as cerebral-blood flow studies, are not more exact than bedside tests such as the EEG.

The studies of Okada[58] are perhaps of some theoretical interest with regard to blood flow and cerebral activity. This investigator used guinea-pig olfactory cortex, made completely ischemic for 45 minutes, after which the neurons within this tissue were physiologically and biochemically investigated. The results showed considerable resistance to ischemia in that the neurons still had the ability to recover even after 45 minutes without blood flow. After the slices were incubated for 20 minutes in an oxygenated medium with glucose, electrical activity was actually observed and high-energy compounds like ATP were also found. Okada concluded that these studies call attention to the problem of brain death, as indicated by loss of electrical activity or flat EEGs, but possibly also to a question of the significance of positive and negative angiographic findings. Nevertheless, there is no case known to me of absence of blood flow within the cerebrum for a significant period of time and recovery of either electrical activity or clinical signs.

Other Misleading Signs in the EEG

The EEG in comatose patients can be misleading in other ways. For example, Lundervold[59] points out that herniation usually produces bilaterally slow activity and therefore may obscure an original focus, and that the slow waves are, at times, higher in voltage on the unaffected side. Therefore, since the slowing of lower amplitude is found on the affected side, the EEG may be misleading in these patients. Lundervold also mentioned the well-known fact that parietal lesions are often seen best in the EEG as slow waves maximal on the temporal areas, leading to a slight inaccuracy of localization of the lesion. The limited value of EEG in lesions of the posterior fossa is also well known in that determination of lateralization from the EEG is most difficult in these patients. Furthermore, focal changes are not uncommon in patients with hypoglycemia.[60] Serafetinides et al.[61] have reported that intracarotid sodium amytal may produce loss of consciousness from interference of function within a *given* hemisphere, usually the dominant one. Thus, coma may be associated with sudden ipsilateral EEG changes, implying a disconnection of the dominant hemisphere from its subcortical base. These studies emphasize that it is possible to see only unilateral slow waves in patients who are in coma, a finding that is unexpected and therefore potentially misleading. Triphasic waves are occasionally noted in comatose patients, and Simsarian and Harner[62] reported that these triphasic waves were seen in 20 percent of patients with hepatic disease, but in 22 percent with renal disease. These data emphasize that triphasic waves are not specifically associated with hepatic disease. Silverman[63] has stressed that *triphasic-like* patterns are occasionally seen in comatose patients without metabolic disorders, but these same patterns are usually found in deeper stages than the more classical triphasic waves associated with hepatic or renal coma, which usually appear in a light stage. Therefore, one may easily predict a light comatose stage on the basis of this triphasic-like pattern, but a much deeper state may exist. Other examples of the EEG possibly misleading the electroencephalographer's prediction of clinical outcome come from some patients with carbon monoxide poisoning who had normal EEGs, but who did not recover, and some with abnormal EEGs, who had complete clinical recovery.[64] Other examples of "normal-appearing" records are the well-known EEGs of alpha coma, in which alternating "sleeping" and "waking" patterns may be seen according to the time of day or night.[65, 66] Finally, Westmoreland and her colleagues[67] have pointed out that alpha coma may be associated not only with pontine lesions, but also with diffuse cerebral pathology. These latter examples represent other ways in which the EEG does have limitations in patients in coma and may lead to incorrect predictions.

EEG as a Predictor of Life or Death

The EEG may be a poor predictor of life or death under certain circumstances. It seems at least possible that the crucial areas subserving consciousness may be so far from the scalp electrodes that lesions involving those same areas leading to coma may have little or no electrographic expression. Therefore, the EEG will record either a normal-looking tracing if only the latter area and no other brain areas are involved or a very great range of abnormalities depending on what *other* areas are also involved. Thus, nearly every conceivable EEG pattern has been reported in coma and the type of reactivity of these patterns varies considerably.[61, 63, 65, 68-70] Notwithstanding, on the basis of the EEG, Prior[8] attempted to predict life or death or a large number of comatose patients who had suffered cardiac or respiratory arrest. She graded the EEG from #1–#5 and the rating #3 represented continuous delta (or) continuous spike activity (or) records with episodic reduction in voltage (or) complete isoelectric records of less than 1 second's duration. In all of the other grades of the EEG, the electrographic recording did well in predicting the outcome of the patient, but in the instance of grade #3, 13 patients recovered and 30 suffered either significant brain damage or death. On the basis of the first tracing alone, 11 patients recovered and 12 suffered brain damage or death, so that serial tracings were required in order that a reasonable prediction could be made. Prior also mentioned the progression towards a normal EEG in patients with anoxic coma, whose sudden demise may therefore be surprising.

In these cases the diseased organ, namely the heart, was the actual limiting factor so that the improvement of the EEG may be misleading in offering too optimistic an outcome.

POSITIVE CORRELATIONS

Despite the clear limitations of the EEG in dealing with comatose patients, in general, and in brain death, in particular, the scalp recordings have rendered a number of clear positive correlations. In one study [27] an EEG index was calculated based on the incidence and amplitude of all the different rhythms noted, and a neurologic index was calculated also, based on all reflex changes. The EEG index was significantly related to the neurologic index in all patients except those in alpha coma ($p < 0.0001$). Also, Meyers and Stockard [71] found good correlations between the frequency and reactivity of the EEG and the level of brain-stem function based on an index evaluating 10 different reflexes. The statistics presented by Prior [8] are also optimistic. All patients with ECS did die, although the previous sections of this review reveal that this outcome does not necessarily occur. However, on the basis of the *first* EEG of the comatose patients that Prior studied, there was an 85.3 percent concordance between the EEG prediction and the clinical outcome of the patient, and in addition there was an 83.3 percent concordance for *all* reports. Only 13 percent of the records showed an intermediate grade #3 type of abnormality, which required serial recordings to provide a judgment on prognosis. Prior used a linear discriminant functional analysis, which resulted in a set of weights with which to multiply each variable, and the results were then summed to produce a discriminant score. The 93 EEGs were then classified with discriminant scores with the values predicting either recovery or death. Only one EEG was misclassified as suggesting death, but the patient did recover. These patients had a history of cardiac arrest and no other kind of associated disorder with histologic studies of those who died. In 42 other EEGs from 19 patients who had no other complications than the cardiac arrest, but in whom there was no histologic confirmation, 10 of the 42 EEGs were misclassified. Finally, in another group in which other complications did occur other than cardiac and respiratory arrest, the EEG predicted death in two survivors and survival in two that died, with uncertain prediction in four others. However, in 54 other cases a correct prediction was made. These studies of Prior do, however, tend to leave a positive note of optimism on the usefulness of the EEG in predicting the outcome in comatose patients. Nevertheless, this review has addressed itself primarily to the limitations of the scalp-recorded EEG in the determination of brain death.‡

REFERENCES

1. INGVAR, D. H. 1974. Report of the Committee on Cessation of Cerebral Function. Electroenceph. Clin. Neurophysiol. 37: 530–531.

‡ It should be kept in mind that these statistics are based on using the EEG as the *only* criterion to predict death or brain death. Multiple criteria, including the clinical criteria and the physician's medical judgment, must also be used. Then the significance of ECS in the EEG is far more meaningful than the statistics would suggest. —*J. K.*

2. BENNETT, D. R., J. R. HUGHES, J. KOREIN, J. K. MERLIS & C. SUTER. 1976. Atlas of Electroencephalography in Coma and Cerebral Death. Raven Press. New York, N.Y.

3. JUNG, R. 1953. Handbuch Inn Med. bd. V/I. Springer. Berlin.

4. JØRGENSEN, E. O. 1974. EEG without detectable cortical activity and cranial nerve areflexia as parameters of brain death. Electroenceph. Clin. Neurophysiol. 36: 70–75.

5. AMERICAN EEG SOCIETY. 1976. Guidelines in EEG, minimum technical standards for EEG recording in suspected cerebral death.

6. JØRGENSEN, E. O. & V. BITSCH. 1973. Acute glutethimide poisoning. Ageskr. Laeg. 135: 802–809.

7. WALKER, A. E. 1975. Cerebral death. In The Nervous System, The Clinical Neurosciences. T. N. Chase, Ed., Vol. 2: 75–87. Raven Press. New York, N.Y.

8. PRIOR, P. 1973. The EEG in Acute Cerebral Anoxia. Excerpta Medica. Amsterdam.

9. KIMURA, J., H. W. GERBER & W. F. McCORMICK. 1968. The isoelectric electroencephalogram. Significance in establishing death in patients maintained on mechanical ventilation. Arch. Intern. Med. 121: 511.

10. BILIKIEWICZ, A. & S. SMOCZYNSKI. 1970. Electroencephalographic changes during atropine-induced coma. Pol. Med. J. 9: 926–931.

11. MELLARIO, F., M. GAULTIER, E. FOURNIER, P. GERVAIS & J-P. FREJAVILLE. 1973. Contributions of electroencephalography to resuscitation in toxicology. Clin. Toxic 6(2): 271–285.

12. POWNER, D. J. 1976. Drug-associated isoelectric EEGs. JAMA 236(10): 1123.

13. SILVERMAN, D., M. SAUNDERS, R. SCHWAB & R. MASLAND. 1969. Cerebral death and the electroencephalogram. Report of the Ad Hoc Committee of the American Electroencephalographic Society on EEG criteria for determination of cerebral death. JAMA 209: 1505–1510.

14. SILVERMAN, D., R. L. MASLAND, M. G. SAUNDERS & R. S. SCHWAB. 1970. Irreversible coma associated with electrocerebral silence. Neurology 20: 525–533.

15. JØRGENSEN, E. O. 1974. Requirements for recording the EEG at high sensitivity in suspected brain death. Electroenceph. Clin. Neurophysiol. 36: 65–69.

16. HAIDER, J., H. MATTHEW & I. OSWALD. 1971. Electroencephalographic changes in acute drug poisoning. Electroenceph. Clin. Neurophysiol. 30: 23–31.

17. KIRSHBAUM, R. J. & V. J. CAROLLO. 1970. Reversible iso-electric EEG in barbiturate coma. JAMA 212: 1215.

18. MANTZ, J. M., J. D. TEMPE, D. KURTZE, A. LOBSTEIN & G. MACK. 1971. Twenty-four hour cerebral electrical silence during a massive poisoning with 10 grams of pentobarbital. Hemodialysis cure. Presse Med. 79: 1243–1246.

19. BIRD, T. D. & F. PLUM. 1968. Recovery from barbiturate overdose coma with a prolonged isoelectric electroencephalogram. Neurology 18: 456–468.

20. TENTLER, R. L., M. SADOVE, D. R. BECKA & R. C. TAYLOR. 1957. Electroencephalographic evidence of cortical "death" followed by full recovery: Protective action of hypothermia. JAMA 164: 1667–1670.

21. WILLIAMS, G. R., JR. & F. C. SPENCER. 1958. The clinical use of hypothermia following cardiac arrest. Ann. Surg. 148: 462–468.

22. PEARCY, W. C. & R. W. VIRTUE. 1959. The electroencephalogram in hypothermia with circulatory arrest. Anesthesiology 20: 341–347.

23. LEVIN, P. & J. KINNELL. 1966. Successful cardiac resuscitation despite prolonged silence of EEG. Arch. Intern. Med. 117: 557–560.

24. HOUTTEVILLE, J. P., J. GACHES, J. GARREAU & G. TEMEN. 1970. Severe meningoencephalitis with total EEG silence during infectious mononucleosis: Recovery. Ann. Med. Intern. 121: 347–353.

25. CLOCHE, R., J. M. DESMONTS, G. HENNETIER & F. ROBERT. 1968. Morphology and evolution of the EEG in acute cerebral anoxia (42 cases). Electroenceph. Clin. Neurophysiol. 25: 89.

26. RIEHL, J. L. & H. B. McINTYRE. 1968. Reliability of the EEG in the determina-

tion of cerebral death: Report of a case with recovery of an isoelectric tracing. Bull. Los Angeles Neurol. Soc. **33:** 86–89.
27. HUGHES, J. R., B. BOSHES & J. LEESTMA. 1976. Electro-clinical and pathologic correlations in comatose patients. Clin. EEG **7:** 13–30.
28. ELLIS, C. H., S. NORTON & W. V. MORGAN. 1952. Central depression by drugs which block neuromuscular transmission. Fed. Proc. **11:** 42–43.
29. GREEN, J. B. & A. LAUBER. 1972. Return of EEG activity after electrocerebral silence: Two case reports. J. Neur. Neurosurg. Psychiat. **35:** 103–107.
30. LEENSTRA-BORSJE, H., S. BOONSTRA, E. J. BLOKZUL & S. L. H. NOTERMANS. 1969. A retrospective investigation of the clinical symptoms and course of patients with a complete or incomplete isoelectric EEG. Electroenceph. Clin. Neurophysiol. **27:** 215.
31. JONKMAN, E. J. 1969. Cerebral death and the isoelectric EEG (Review of literature). Electroenceph. Clin. Neurophysiol. **27:** 215.
32. BRICOLO, A., A. BENATI, C. MAZZA & A. P. BRICOLO. 1971. Prolonged isoelectric EEG in a case of post-traumatic coma. Electroenceph. Clin. Neurophysiol. **31:** 174.
33. SILVERMAN, D. 1975. Electrographic recording techniques for suspected cerebral death. *In* Handbook of Electroencephalography and Clinical Neurophysiology. R. Harner & R. Naquet, Eds., Vol. **12:** 122–129. Elsevier. Amsterdam.
34. JOUVET, M. 1959. Diagnostic electro-sous-corticographique de la mort du systeme nerveux central au cours de certains coma. Electroenceph. Clin. Neurophysiol. **11:** 805–808.
35. CARBONELL, J., R. CARRASCOSA, G. DIERSSEN, S. OBRADOR, J. C. OLIVEROS & M. SEVILLANO. 1963. Some electrophysiological observations in a case of deep coma secondary to cardiac arrest. Electroenceph. Clin. Neurophysiol. **15:** 520–525.
36. VISSOR, S. L. 1969. Two cases of isoelectric EEGs (apparent exceptions proving the rule). Electroenceph. Clin. Neurophysiol. **27:** 215.
37. FINDJI, F., J. GACHES, J. P. HOUTTEVILLE, P. CREISSARD & A. CALISKAN. 1970. Cortical, transcortical, and subcortical electroencephalographic recordings in ten cases of profound irreversible coma. Neurochirurgia **13:** 211–219.
38. ARFEL, G. 1967. Stimulations visuelles et silence cerebral. Electroenceph. Clin. Neurophysiol. **23:** 172–175.
39. POOLE, E. W., J. CHARTRES & E. K. WITTRICK. 1970. Evoked cerebral sensory responses in the assessment of surviving function in cerebral disaster. Electroenceph. Clin. Neurophysiol. **29:** 705.
40. TROJABERG, W. & E. O. JØRGENSEN. 1973. Evoked cortical potentials in patients with "isoelectric" EEGs. Electroenceph. Clin. Neurophysiol. **35:** 301–309.
41. STARR, A. 1976. Auditory brain stem responses in brain death. Brain **99:** 543–554.
42. MEHTA, A. J. & S. S. SESHIA. 1976. Orbicularis oculi reflex in brain death. J. Neur. Neurosurg. Psychiat. **39:** 784–787.
43. ARFEL, G. 1975. Brain death evidence contributed by laboratory studies other than surface EEGs. *In* Handbook of Electroencephalography and Clinical Neurophysiology. R. Harner & R. Naquet, Eds. Vol. **12:** 116–121. Elsevier. Amsterdam.
44. BENNETT, D. R., N. M. NORD, J. S. ROBERTS & H. MAVOR. 1971. Prolonged survival with flat electroencephalogram following cardiac arrest. Electroenceph. Clin. Neurophysiol. **30:** 94.
45. BRIERLEY, V. B., D. I. GRAHAM, J. H. ADAMS & J. A. SIMPSON. 1971. Neocortical death after cardiac arrest. A clinical neurophysiological report of two cases. Lancet **ii:** 560–565.
46. BENTAL, E. & U. LEIBOWITZ. 1961. Flat electroencephalograms during 28 days in a case of "encephalitis." Electroenceph. Clin. Neurophysiol. **13:** 457–460.
47. LUNDERVOLD, A. 1954. Electroencephalographic changes in a case of acute

cerebral anoxia unconscious for about three years. Electroenceph. Clin. Neurophysiol. **6:** 311–315.

48. KOREIN, J. & M. MACCARIO. 1971. On the diagnosis of cerebral death: A prospective study of 55 patients to define irreversible coma. Clin. EEG **2:** 178–199.

49. JØRGENSEN, P. B., E. O. JØRGENSEN & A. ROSENKLINT. 1973. Brain death pathogenesis and diagnosis. Acta Neurol. Scandinav. **49:** 355–367.

50. BOLTON, C. F., J. D. BROWN, E. CHOLOD & K. WARREN. 1976. EEG and "brain death." Lancet **i**(7958)**:** 535.

51. DELIYANNAKIS, E., F. JOANNOU & A. DAVAROUKAS. 1975. Brain stem death with persistence of bioelectric activity of the cerebral hemispheres. Clin. EEG **6:** 75–79.

52. SMTIH, A. J. K. & A. E. WALKER. 1973. Cerebral blood flow and brain metabolism as indicators of cerebral death. A review. Johns Hopkins Med. J. **133:** 107–119.

53. KOREIN, J., P. BRAUNSTEIN, I. KRICHEFF, A. LIEBERMAN & N. CHASE. 1975. Radioisotopic bolus technique as a test to detect circulatory deficit associated with cerebral death. 142 studies on 80 patients of an innocuous IV procedure as an adjunct in the diagnosis of cerebral death. Circulation **57:** 924–939.

54. KETZ, E. 1974. Beitrag zum Problem de Hirntodes. Schweiz. Arch. Neur. Neurochir. Psych. **110:** 205–221.

55. MIYAZAKI, Y., H. TAKAMATSU, Y. TANAKA, N. MIKAMI, S. AKAGAWA & T. SOHMA. 1972. Criteria of cerebral death. Acta Radiol. **13:** 318–328.

56. PENDL, G., J. A. GANGLBERGER, K. STEINBEREITHNER & C. TSCHAKALOFF. 1972. Cerebraler Zirkulationsstillstand in Korrelation mit EEG—und pO₂—AVD Untersuchungen. Acta Radiol. **13:** 329–333.

57. OUAKNINE, G., I. Z. KOSARY, J. BRAHAM, P. CZERNIAK & N. HILLEL. 1973. Laboratory criteria of brain death. J. Neurosurg. **39:** 429–433.

58. OKADA, Y. 1974. Recovery of neuronal activity and high-energy compound level after complete and prolonged brain ischemia. Brain Res. **72:** 346–349.

59. LUNDERVOLD, A. 1975. EEG in patients with coma due to localized brain lesions. *In* Handbook of Electroencephalography and Clinical Neurophysiology. R. Harner & R. Naquet, Eds. Vol. **12:** 37–46. Elsevier. Amsterdam.

60. HARNER, R. N. & R. I. KATZ. 1975. Electroencephalography in metabolic coma. *In* Handbook of Electroencephalography and Clinical Neurophysiology. R. Harner & R. Naquet, Eds. Vol. **12:** 47–62. Elsevier. Amsterdam.

61. SERAFETINIDES, E. A., M. V. DRIVER & R. D. HOARE. 1965. EEG patterns induced by intracarotid injection of sodium amytal. Electroenceph. Clin. Neurophysiol. **18:** 170–175.

62. SIMSARIAN, J. P. & R. N. HARNER. 1972. Diagnosis of metabolic encephalopathy: Significance of triphasic waves in the electroencephalogram. Neurology. **22:** 456.

63. SILVERMAN, D. 1975. The electroencephalogram in anoxic coma. *In* Handbook of Electroencephalography and Clinical Neurophysiology. R. Harner & R. Naquet, Eds. Vol. **12:** 81–94. Elsevier. Amsterdam.

64. BOKONJIC, N. 1963. Stagnant anoxia and carbon monoxide poisoning: A clinical and electroencephalographic study on humans. Electroenceph. Clin. Neurophysiol. Suppl. **21**.

65. CHATRIAN, G. E. 1975. Electroencephalographic and behavioral signs of sleep in comatose states. *In* Handbook of Electroencephalography and Clinical Neurophysiology. R. Harner & R. Naquet, Eds. Vol. **12:** 63–77. Elsevier. Amsterdam.

66. HUGHES, J. R., J. CAYAFFA, J. LEESTMA & Y. MIZUNO. 1972. Alternating "waking" and "sleep" patterns in a deeply comatose patient. Clin. EEG **3:** 86–93.

67. WESTMORELAND, B., D. W. KLASS, F. W. SHARBROUGH & T. J. REGAN. 1974. "Alpha coma" : EEG, clinical, pathological and etiologic correlations. Electroenceph. Clin. Neurophysiol. **37:** 202.

68. MATHIS, P., H. TORRUBIA & H. FISCHGOLD. 1957. Réactivité périodicité et corré-lation cortico-cardio-respiratoire dans le coma. Electroenceph. Clin. Neuro-physiol. Suppl. **6:** 453–462.
69. ARFEL, G. 1975. Introduction to clinical and EEG studies in coma. *In* Hand-book of Electroencephalography and Clinical Neurophysiology. R. Harner & R. Naquet, Eds. Vol. **12:** 5–23. Elsevier. Amsterdam.
70. LOEB, C. 1975. Correlative EEG and clinicopathological studies of patients in coma. *In* Handbook of Electroencephalography and Clinical Neurophysiology. R. Harner & R. Naquet, Eds. Vol. **12:** 24–36. Elsevier. Amsterdam.
71. MYERS, R. R. & J. J. STOCKARD. 1975. Neurologic and electroencephalographic correlates in glutethimide intoxication. Clin. Pharm. Ther. **17:** 212–220.

THE RELATIONSHIP OF THE EEG TO THE CLINICAL EXAMINATION IN DETERMINING BRAIN DEATH

Eli S. Goldensohn

Department of Neurology
College of Physicians & Surgeons
Columbia University
New York, New York 10032

Both of the preceding papers on the use and limitations of the electro-encephalogram (EEG) in the diagnosis of brain death correctly emphasize that the EEG examination cannot stand alone as decisive in the diagnosis of brain death and that EEG information must be evaluated in conjunction with the history and neurologic examination. This approach to the use of the EEG is in accord with the Interagency Brain Death Committee, whose recommendations were approved by the American Neurological Association membership in June of 1976.[1] The earlier report of the Ad Hoc Committee of the Harvard Medical School[2] also stresses the important confirmatory value of the electroencephalo-gram in cerebral death, but both state that the EEG examination is not essential in establishing brain death. The recent Conference of the Royal Colleges and Faculties of the United Kingdom[3] stresses the clinical examination and mini-mizes the value of the EEG. Similarly the Ad Hoc Committee on Death of the Minnesota State Medical Association[4] mentions the EEG as a confirmatory test and recommends that the decision of whether or not to use the EEG should be made by the attending physician. Although often described as not an essential criterion, in actual practice, however, it appears that the use of the EEG to confirm cerebral death is practically universal.

There is a strong and justified bias on the part of practicing physicians not to de-emphasize the clinical examination in favor of laboratory data in reaching decisions. They correctly emphasize that the final decision rests upon clinical judgment. In seems to me, however, that in the case of cerebral survival the reliability of information from the clinical examination performed with the aid of instruments (pin, tuning fork, syringe with cold water, percussion hammer, flashlight, otoscope, and ophthalmoscope) is no greater than that obtained from more complicated and sensitive instruments such as the electroencephalograph. Experience in the Collaborative Study, supported by the National Institute of Neurologic Diseases and Stroke,[5] has shown that there is little justification for suspecting laboratory error when the minimal technical standards of EEG recording, which have been widely circulated since 1971 by the American Electroencephalographic Society,[6] are applied and when interpretation is made by a qualified electroencephalographer. The Conference of the Royal Colleges and Faculties of the United Kingdom,[3] which downplays the value of the EEG, recommends as an essential diagnostic test the routine application of 20 ml of ice water to each tympanum through external auditory meati after establishing that there is clear access to the tympanic membranes by the use of an otoscope. The chances of error in this technique are self-evident. The Royal Colleges Conference's major point against requiring the use of the EEG is that it may not be available where needed. Usually, however, the early diagnosis of brain

137

0077-8923/78/0315-0137 $01.75/0 © 1978, NYAS

death is undertaken in hospitals with complex technical facilities for maintaining life and where EEGs are available.

In order to view the role of the EEG in proper prospective and to clearly define its limitations, it is necessary to compare its relative accuracy with other criteria used to establish cerebral death. In the Collaborative Study [5] purposeful movements were confused with movements of spinal-reflex origin in 9 percent of the 503 patients suspected of being brain-dead. Apnea, which usually continued after temporarily disconnecting the patient from the respirator, was sometimes followed by transient respiratory efforts. In 1 percent of the EEG examinations the original reader diagnosed electrocerebral silence but the review panel considered that cerebral activity was present. A total of 3 percent disagreement between a review panel and the original reader of the electro-encephalogram was reported in this series of 503 cases. If all drug-induced comas were eliminated, none of the patients who had a 30-minute long isoelectric record recovered. This confirmed the findings of the American Electroencephalographic Society Committee on Cerebral Death,[6] who found that only three patients, all with drug intoxication, recovered in a series of 1,665 patients with a flat record. Prior's study came to a similar conclusion.[7] It should also be recalled that cases have been reported of recovery after a single isoelectric EEG recording.[8-10] Thus, neither coma with absent cephalic reflexes and apnea nor the EEG can be considered adequate single criteria to establish brain death. A combination of the three criteria, namely, cerebral unresponsivity, apnea, and electrocerebral silence combined were 99 percent correct. It is of interest that in the collaborative study the absence of cephalic reflexes did not improve the accuracy of the diagnosis of brain death. On the basis of the findings of the Collaborative Study of the National Institutes of Neurological Diseases and Stroke,[5] it has been suggested that the criteria for brain death may include coma with cerebral unresponsivity, apnea, dilated fixed pupils, absent cephalic reflexes, and electrocerebral silence for 30 minutes recorded at least six hours after the onset of coma and apnea.

In spite of an apparent majority who feel that the EEG need not be included in the essential criteria, but be used optionally for confirmation, there are good reasons to use the EEG in all cases of suspected brain death. The concept should be applied that a laboratory test is just as essential as clinical criteria when the probability of its result substantially adds to obtaining the correct diagnosis. Perhaps the failure to include the EEG as part of the required information in determining brain death is related to the physician's desire to be free to use his own judgment in evaluating all the information. This can be accomplished by having no absolute criteria, but only guidelines. This allows the EEG examination, which is a highly reliable, noninvasive benign technique, to remain one of the foremost considerations in establishing cerebral death. Its use should not be as an isolated piece of information to make the diagnosis, but rather to demonstrate inactivity and to rule out the possibility that cerebral cortical activity exists. Bolton et al.,[8] among others,[9, 10] describe patients who showed clinical signs suggesting brain death at 12 hours after acute cerebral anoxia, but the EEG at that time showed cerebral electrical activity and the patient recovered. Whenever the EEG shows that cerebral cortical activity is present, all the other criteria for brain death must be re-evaluated and be considered inconclusive!

On the basis of these considerations on applicability of EEG information we offer guidelines to assist staff physicians at our hospital in determining cerebral death. The guidelines that follow are not presented as a rigid set of rules, for no set of criteria can replace the physician's evaluation of the total circumstances surrounding a given case, and the final decision regarding death must continue to depend on the physician's judgment. The patient will be shown to have experienced brain death when: (1) there is cerebral unresponsivity; (2) there is no spontaneous respiration; (3) the brain-stem reflexes are absent and (4) the EEG run according to the special protocol of the department, which follows the recommendations of the guidelines of the American Electroencephalographic Society, shows no cerebral activity; (5) the patient has been observed for a period of time sufficient to ensure knowledge of the pertinent circumstances of the case and to permit appropriate effort to correct deviations of respiration, circulation, and body temperature; (6) the possibility that the condition is due to intoxication from exogenous and endogenous toxins has been excluded; and (7) there is adequate knowledge of the nature and extent of any intracranial pathology

Thus, we consider the EEG as a highly valuable piece of information on a par with the various clinical criteria in importance in establishing brain death. If the patient is either cerebrally responsive or cerebral activity is seen on the EEG, he cannot be considered brain-dead. The accuracy of the EEG examination depends on proper performance and proper interpretation. Perhaps the EEG should be used only in those cases in which the electroencephalographer is Board-qualified and therefore known to be able to interpret the recording. There is general agreement that when the EEG is flat, according to proper standards of recording, the brain may or may not be dead, but that if the EEG shows electrocortical activity, the brain cannot be said to be dead. The law of Britain, as it stands, says that a person is dead when a doctor states that he is dead; it gives no indication of how a doctor should reach that conclusion. The laws in the United States will undoubtedly not be unduly specific about the decision that brain death has occurred. Nevertheless, in making a decision of such magnitude, we should lean heavily on a properly run and interpreted EEG, which has a probability of correctness that matches the expert clinical neurologic examination.

REFERENCES

1. INTERAGENCY COMMITTEE ON BRAIN DEATH. 1976. Report to American Neurological Association, Box 520875, Biscayne Annex, Miami, Florida 33152.
2. AD HOC COMMITTEE OF THE HARVARD MEDICAL SCHOOL. 1968. A definition of irreversible coma. Report of the Ad Hoc Committee of the Harvard Medical School to Examine the Definition of Brain Death. JAMA 205: 337–340.
3. CONFERENCE OF ROYAL COLLEGES AND FACULTIES OF THE UNITED KINGDOM. 1976. Diagnosis of brain death. Lancet, November 13 : 1069–1070.
4. AD HOC COMMITTEE ON DEATH. 1976. Criteria for the Determination of Brain Death, Recommendation of the Ad Hoc Committee on Death. Minnesota State Medical Association, 101 East 5th Street, Suite 900, St. Paul, Minnesota 55102.
5. A Collaborative Study. 1977. An appraisal of the criteria of cerebral death. JAMA 237(10): 982–986.
6. AD HOC COMMITTEE OF THE AMERICAN ELECTROENCEPHALOGRAPHIC SOCIETY. 1969. Cerebral death and the electroencephalogram. Report of the Ad Hoc Committee on EEG Criteria for Determination of Cerebral Death. JAMA 209: 1505–1510.

7. Prior, P. F. 1973. The EEG in acute cerebral anoxia. Assessment of cerebral function and prognosis in patients resuscitated after cardiorespiratory arrest. Excerpta Med. **811:** 314.
8. Bolton, D. F., J. D. Brown, E. Cholod & K. Warren. 1976. EEG and "brain life." Lancet, March 6 : 535.
9. Bricolo, A., A. Benati, C. Mazza, et al. 1971. Prolonged isoelectric EEG in a case of post-traumatic coma. Electroencephalogr. Clin. Neurophysiol. **31:** 174.
10. Tentler, R. L., M. Sadove, R. Becka, et al. 1957. Electroencephalographic evidence of cortical death followed by full recovery: Protective action of hypothermia. JAMA **164:** 1667–1670.

Discussion

L. P. Hinterbuchner: Perhaps the best way of presenting this question is to describe an actual incident. I received a call from my hospital, where a physician requested an immediate EEG to determine brain death on a patient wno had undergone surgery several days ago, had an episode of respiratory arrest, was resuscitated, and remained in coma. No neurologic consultation was called. We have one technician and electroencephalographer in the hospital. I placed a call to the technician and she was fully booked with outpatients. This is a practical problem; what do we do under these circumstances? I wish it had been possible to disrupt the schedule and perform an EEG on this comatose patient. If I understand correctly, even if ECS is present, the patient is not necessarily brain-dead. My feeling is that many physicians have a great desire to pass the buck to the neurologist in determining brain death, and leave all further responsibility to him. This question is directed to Dr. Goldensohn in terms of "practical aspects." Do we ask for an x-ray or EEG, do we drop everything else and disrupt all the schedules in the hospital, neglecting ill patients who can benefit from these services? What should we do?

Goldensohn: You are asking multiple questions. The real problem may be that there is a tendency to avoid responsibility. Many times when we have to make a diagnosis pertaining to brain death, the decision is required in a short time. This is especially so if the patient is a potential donor for organ transplantation. In such circumstances, the extra equipment and personnel are usually available. I don't know what size hospital you are referring to.

Most often the EEG is not an emergency procedure requiring cessation of all other activity. Therefore, practically speaking, time is usually available. However, if the situation is such that the patient's family is suffering because of a lingering situation, then a portable instrument and technician may be brought in from another facility or the patient should be moved to another facility. There may even be those situations in which routine examinations on other patients should be delayed. This is a matter of clinical judgment and the neurologist should see the patient first.

Hughes: Perhaps I could add a comment, and attempt to answer part of the question. Even though my topic was the limitations of EEG in cases of brain death and coma, I hope nobody leaves the room with the attitude that EEG really plays no role at all. I think Dr. Bennett and I accentuated the problem of rare exceptions when we were discussing patients whose EEG activity returned after it was once flat. We most often refer to the exceptions of drug intoxication. I wouldn't like the questioner to think that the point of the previous papers has been that the EEG is of no value because ECS is not meaningful. The presence of ECS is extremely significant, and as Dr. Goldensohn has indicated and all of you are aware, one combines the result of the EEG with the clinical picture. Despite the fact that there are exceptions in the significance of ECS pertaining to brain death as noted by Dr. Bennett and myself, the value of the EEG as one of the criteria for diagnosing brain death cannot be minimized. One must not conclude on the basis of these papers that ECS on an EEG is not a highly meaningful criterion in the diagnosis of brain death.

The second point I'd like to make regarding the practical issue is what I tell my own technicians, which is, "the most important EEGs run are these records. You just must, in my view, do everything possible in order to get them done right."

GRENVIK: I have a practical question in regard to the use of drugs in these patients and I'd like to take the example of barbiturates. We commonly use barbiturates in the treatment of seizure disorders. There are many other conditions for which barbiturates are used. In addition, we have patients with an overdose of barbiturates. We have patients in whom we use a relatively small dose repeatedly for control of intracranial pressure. There are other therapeutic situations in which barbiturates are also used. So, if we now have one of these patients developing signs of brain death, he or she may or may not have measurable concentrations of barbiturates in the serum. Do you see any problem with brain death certification in such a case? As far as I know there should be no higher concentration of barbiturates in brain cells than in the serum.

GOLDENSOHN: There is no study that I am aware of in this regard. We find that most patients have received some medication, as you indicated. Many patients already have drugs in their serum and tissues. Drugs are not metabolized very rapidly in patients in this state. We have the clinical impression that if the drugs are below therapeutic levels this is not important in electrocerebral silence. We have had to deal with the problem in this manner because traces of barbiturates or diazapam are often found in such patients.

BENNETT: The reverse of this situation would be in a patient who is on therapeutic drugs and meets the clinical criteria for brain death, that is, cerebral unresponsivity, apnea, and absent cephalic reflexes. If blood levels of the drugs are not available and you perform an EEG and find brain activity, the problem of turning off the respirator does not arise.

PAMPIGLIONE: I would like to clarify one relatively minor point. The report quoted by Dr. Goldensohn is an important one and was published in the *Lancet*. However, on the panel there was no member of the EEG Society and no member of the British Clinical Neurophysiology Association. I believe that the individuals who made that particular statement were not accustomed to any clinical neurophysiology service that is worth calling such.

GOLDENSOHN: I accept that completely. I am sure that you are correct.

GOLDMAN (*Naval Medical Research Institute, Bethesda, Md.*): I'd like to ask the discussants a relatively practical question. Concerning organ transplantation we often encounter the anencephalic donor, i.e., the newborn baby who is anencephalic. How do you approach the problem of determining death in these donors?

BENNETT: Studies on anencephalic and on hydroanencephalic patients with

EEGs are not that prevalent. Even in those cases reported, where there is no evidence of scalp-recorded EEG activity, respirations and brain-stem reflexes are present. They may have what is considered an ECS scalp recording, but with preservation of brain-stem functions.

GOLDMAN: Where do we go from there in determining whether they are organ donors?

BENNETT: The answer to that is based on one's criteria for brain death. If your criteria include destruction of cortical, subcortical, and brain-stem structures, these malformed infants would not satisfy these criteria. They do have brain-stem reflexes. However, if you consider them to be cerebrally dead, that is, the cortex and subcortical structures are not present in these cases, but the brain stem is, you could use that definition.*

SUTER: I just wanted to make a comment on Dr. Hughes' reference to succinylcholine because this has come up repeatedly. There is no evidence available that succinylcholine alters brain waves in normal individuals. This drug has been used innumerable times as a routine procedure. I have evaluated patients with brain damage and very little EEG activity, and have administered succinylcholine in these patients for 30 to 60 minutes. I have never been able to demonstrate any diminution of EEG activity nor have I produced ECS.

KOREIN: One must not gain the impression on the basis of this discussion and the preceding papers that the EEG is *not* of enormous value in the diagnosis of brain death. All the patients that were described with ECS that were not brain-dead fall into three categories. The first had brain-stem function reflected by cephalic reflexes; even Brierley's two patients who survived more than 80 days consistently had pupillary responses. The second group with reversible ECS was comprised mainly of patients with exogenous intoxication and included a relatively small number of individuals with other disorders such as endogenous intoxication and encephalitis. Finally, the third group of patients with reversible ECS consisted of those in whom the EEG was taken early, usually within six hours, after the intracranial insult. Therefore the clinical evaluation of the patient, including the determination of unresponsive coma, apnea and absent cephalic reflexes in combination with unequivocal ECS in the EEG, as stated in current criteria, allows the physician to arrive at a diagnosis of brain death in most situations. There are infrequent circumstances in which the physician's clinical judgment, based on all the findings, dictates that examinations or tests should be repeated or additional tests be performed to eliminate any uncertainty. For example, repeating the neurologic examination and the EEG after six hours, or performance of a confirmatory test to determine the absence of CBF, may be indicated. Although a variety of ancillary procedures have been recommended and are being explored, as will be discussed elsewhere in this volume, especially to identify patients with reversible drug intoxication, most patients can be diagnosed as being brain-dead on the basis of criteria thus far presented.

---

* This represents an illustration of the critical controversy that clearly separates brain from cerebral death. The topic will be discussed in a limited manner in this volume, but should be extensively explored. The problem is compounded by the observation of anencephalic monsters surviving beyond the age of 17 years (personal communication, Dr. C. Suter; see also Lemire, R., J. Beckwith & J. Warkany. 1978. Anencephaly. Raven Press. New York, N.Y.)—*J. K.*

EVALUATION OF THE CRITICAL DEFICIT OF CEREBRAL CIRCULATION USING RADIOACTIVE TRACERS (BOLUS TECHNIQUE)*

Philip Braunstein,† Julius Korein,‡ Irvin I. Kricheff,†
and Abraham Lieberman ‡

*Departments of † Radiology and ‡ Neurology
New York University Medical Center
New York, New York 10016*

Technological and medical advances now often make it possible to sustain life in deeply comatose patients who would previously have died. These same advances at times also make possible prolongation of life in a body when the brain of that individual has died. In as far as the brain is the essence and substance of individual human existence, the undue prolongation of life in a body with a dead brain is futile. Such efforts prolong the anguish of relatives and drain resources which could be used for individuals still able to benefit from them. The advent of transplant surgery has created a need for viable organs; these tend to deteriorate after cessation of the heartbeat. Therefore, individuals with brain death are a source of such organs if they can be removed before the heart stops.

The above factors may result in a situation that requires a relatively rapid decision regarding the question of brain death. It should be clearly borne in mind that under certain circumstances, comatose states, including those that are reversible, may temporarily mimic brain death in all clinical and electro-encephalographic studies.[1-6] Situations that may transiently simulate brain death may occur in patients with drug intoxication, but have also been reported in other conditions, such as induced hypothermia, encephalitis, and metabolic disorders.

The Harvard criteria [7] require 24 hours of observation plus the absence of drugs and hypothermia in order to make a judgment of brain death. The problem of drug intoxication is often a difficult one to deal with since there may be no detailed history available in such patients. Moreover, the laboratory search for drugs is not rapid, especially when the nature of the drug is not known.[8] It is particularly noteworthy that a collaborative study on cerebral survival (CSCS),[9, 10] based on the study of 503 comatose and apneic patients, found a significant proportion of these patients had drug levels in the blood compatible with coma, even when other more obvious causes of coma were known.[8, 11]

A significant additional parameter, stressed primarily by European investigators [12] and that can greatly increase the reliability and decrease the time required to diagnose brain death, is the demonstration of the virtual absence of cerebral circulation. It has been shown angiographically that individuals

* This work was supported in part by NINCDS Contracts No. 71–2319 and No. 1–NS–2307 from The National Institutes of Health and by Neurology Research Fund No. 8–0168–708 from New York University Medical Center.

with "cerebral death" § have effectively lost cerebral circulation.[13, 14] This loss has been demonstrated by four-vessel angiography. Cerebral circulatory deficit has also been verified by the intracarotid injection of a radionuclide.[1, 12, 15]

Other procedures using arteriovenous differences in blood gases, e.g., argon or nitrous oxide employing the Fick principle,[16, 17] have also been used to measure such abnormal reduction in blood flow. This deficit in cerebral circulation is probably associated with severe degrees of cerebral edema [12, 13, 18, 19] followed by degeneration or necrosis of neurons of the cerebral hemispheres, brain stem, and cerebellum. Other mechanisms and patterns of cerebral destruction are possible as well.

The demonstration of such cerebral circulatory deficit has hitherto required transportation of these desperately ill patients, who may or may not be in irreversible coma, to fixed central facilities where radionuclides or angiographic procedures may be performed. There is justifiable reluctance to submit patients to such procedures, with their associated risks, when these procedures are not primarily intended for their personal benefit but, rather, to determine if they have brain death. Certain European investigators consider demonstration of absent intracranial circulation alone as the sine qua non of brain death.

The clinical criteria and procedures detailed in other parts of this volume most certainly always remain the fundamental guidelines in the consideration of brain death. Only if and when these criteria are met, considering their limitations at times, such as the occasional difficulty in obtaining an unequivocally isoelectric EEG, is it appropriate to even consider confirmatory tests.

The need for such confirmatory tests is pointed out in the summary statement of the CSCS.[20] This need arises basically because the clinical and EEG findings may not be clear-cut sometimes. In any event, if the discontinuance of life support in a relatively short time is being considered, it becomes imperative that confirmatory tests be available. As pointed out elsewhere, certain types of coma, including reversible coma, may not be distinguishable from brain death by conventional means for a prolonged period. It is, of course, unthinkable to cease life support in a patient who may possibly be in a reversible coma.

Since the brain cannot long survive a critical deficit in cerebral circulation, no matter what the cause, a test that proves such a deficit would be most useful. The summary statement of the CSCS states that the confirmatory test should be one that tests for the absence of cerebral blood flow (CBF).[20]

It is desirable that such a confirmatory test be available at the bedside and be innocuous so that the fragile life of a comatose patient who is not brain-dead is not further imperiled. The test should be readily repeatable after a suitable interval for confirmation of the findings. It is important that such a confirmatory test never indicates brain death mistakenly; however, an occasional mistaken diagnosis of life in a dead brain is acceptable. We believe the confirmatory bedside radioisotopic "bolus study" to be described meets all these requirements. Evidence for this will be presented in this report.

TECHNIQUE [8, 9, 21, 22]

The principle of the bolus technique is the detection of the passage of a rapidly injected intravenous bolus of radioactive material by one or two probes

§ The term here is used as a synonym for brain death.—*J. K.*

placed so as to detect radioactivity in the head and to display this as a time/activity curve. The appearance of such curves in the presence of cerebral circulation has been well documented.[23-27]

In practice the material used was either ^{99m}technetium pertechnetate (^{99m}TcO$_4$) or ^{99m}technetium sulfur colloid (^{99m}Tc SC). ^{99m}TcO$_4$ is used routinely for brain scanning, and ^{99m}Tc SC is used routinely for liver imaging. The required dose for each study, 2 mCi, is well within the limits for ordinary diagnostic use; and the resultant radiation doses are low. No side effects have been reported from either agent in their present forms. The advantage of ^{99m}Tc SC is that it is cleared rapidly from the blood by the reticuloendothelial system; therefore, if the test needs to be repeated again very soon, the background activity is minimal.

The agent is most efficiently injected through an intravenous line, which these patients invariably have in place for other reasons. The material is diluted with saline to 2 cc in order to obviate the dead space of this line, which may be up to 0.5 cc.

During the pilot phase of the early studies, it was found that a control probe to monitor the adequacy of the radioactive bolus injection was essential. This extra probe is placed directly over a palpated major artery, a femoral artery if at all possible. As will become obvious later, if the time/activity curve from this control probe does not document an adequate bolus response, no reliance can be placed on its absence from the head tracing.

Two types of instruments were used. One instrument was a twin-probe, modified renogram apparatus with the probes balanced; and each probe was set at a sensitivity of 100,000 counts/minute at full deflection of the chart recorder pen. The tracing was a record of the linear response.[8, 9] This two-probe apparatus was used, as illustrated in FIGURES 1A, B, and C,[28] with one probe placed in contact with the midline of the forehead and positioned so as to detect radioisotopic activity from vessels within the supratentorial part of the intracranial cavity. Meanwhile, the other probe was placed directly over the femoral artery as a control.

The second instrument—a three-probe machine (developed by the Phillips Instrument Corporation)—was also used for linear readout.[21] With the three-probe instrument, two probes were placed on either side of the head; and the third probe was used for femoral-artery control (FIGURES 2A, B, and C).[20] The sensitivity of the settings was adjusted so that the single probe over the femoral artery was 100,000 counts/minute at full deflection. The output from the two head probes was summated, and the tracing was recorded at a sensitivity of 300,000 counts/minute at full pen deflection. This amplification was used because the volume from which the isotopic activity was detected by the two head probes resulted in an approximately three-fold increase of pen deflection. The collimators of both instruments were designed in a manner so as to limit the field of view of the adult head.

Both types of instruments were placed adjacent to the head in a manner that excluded the posterior fossa from the field of detection. If the posterior fossa was included in the field of detection, significant activity from extracranial vessels in the neck would invariably occur with resultant artifact. Restrictions in design and characteristics of these radioisotope detectors limited their use to the adult head size.

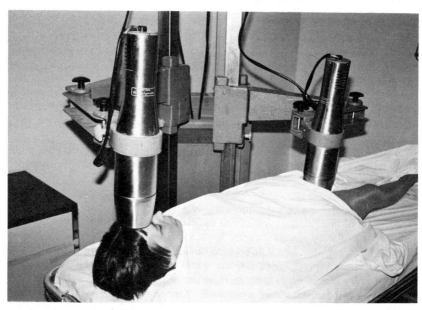

FIGURE 1A. Illustration of two-probe (single-head probe) apparatus in use. Control probe is directly over palpated femoral artery.

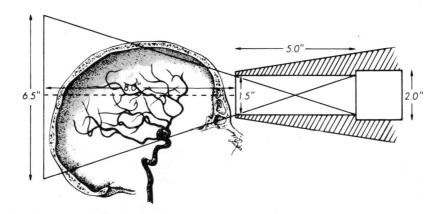

FIGURE 1B. Lateral view of the field of detection of the single-head probe. Note that the field excludes most of the posterior fossa but incorporates most of the major components of the cerebral circulation.

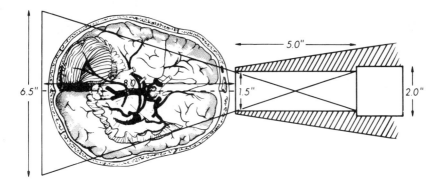

FIGURE 1C. Top view of the field of detection of the single-head probe. Note that the major cerebral vessels are within the field of detection. The anterolateral portion of the skull is excluded bilaterally, including components of the middle meningeal and superficial temporal arteries.

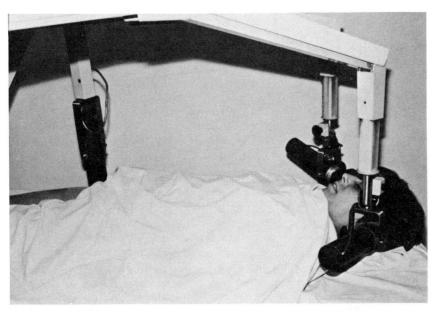

FIGURE 2A. Illustration of three-probe machine (dual-head probe) in use. Control probe is also directly over femoral artery.

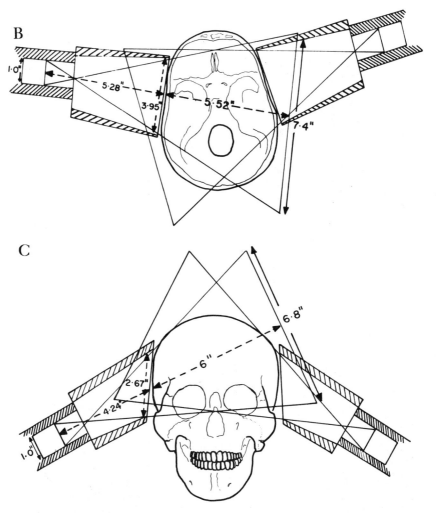

FIGURE 2B and C. Top (B) and frontal (C) views of placement of the twin-head probes and their fields of detection. Although the posterior fossa is excluded, virtually the entire contents of the cranial cavity, skull, and scalp are incorporated.

METHOD

During the period of this study, all patients above the age of 18 admitted to the Bellevue Hospital Center, who were for whatever reason, or who subsequently became, comatose and apneic, were evaluated. All patients received a complete physical and neurologic examination and a diagnostic workup, which included toxicologic examinations of the blood and urine. Appropriate treatment was instituted in all patients, as indicated. If the patient's level of coma persisted or increased despite treatment to the point where he remained cerebrally unresponsive to all stimuli with no purposeful movements, and if he remained on a respirator which he was not triggering for at least 15 minutes, he was considered to fulfill the criteria for admission to the study.

At this juncture the patient received a complete neurologic re-evaluation, with special emphasis being placed on pupillary size, reactivity, oculocephalic reflexes, ice-water calorics, and respirator dependence. If at this time the patient was still in unresponsive coma, was apneic, had no cephalic reflexes with fixed dilated pupils, and met the criteria of respirator dependency, he was entered into the next phase of the study.

Respirator dependency was diagnosed by the absence of spontaneous respiration with the respirator shut off while 100 percent oxygen was delivered passively through the endotrachial tube at the rate of 6 liters per minute for up to 6 minutes. The specifics of this latter criterion may vary depending on the decision of the clinician; [29] it should be noted that this only tests reaction to an increase of arterial pCO_2. At this time, an electroencephalogram (EEG) was performed according to previously described criteria.[30-33] An intravenous radioisotope bolus study was then performed using 2 mCi of $^{99m}TcO_4$ or ^{99m}Tc SC, utilizing modifications of the techniques previously described.[8, 9, 22] The bolus study was always interpreted without knowledge of the EEG findings.

In most cases where the initial radioisotopic study did not show a clear head bolus, the EEG was repeated. A second bolus study was then performed after one hour in all patients who did not have prior cardiac arrest. The primary diagnosis of the 100 patients in this study is shown in TABLE 1.

In the first 80 patients studied in this manner, the results of the bolus examination were assessed by correlation with all the clinical and laboratory findings, including EEG, after the patients were followed until cessation of the heartbeat or it was clear that they were not brain-dead. Some patients, of course, who on initial studies did have a head bolus and EEG activity, remained in a coma requiring subsequent reassessment. In the results, only their final studies are evaluated.

After studying 80 deeply comatose, apneic patients in this way,[9] a prospective study was undertaken to validate, by means of four-vessel angiography, the significance of a bolus study showing absence of a clear head bolus. Details of the angiographic methods, criteria, and findings are given elsewhere in these proceedings.[34]

TABLE 1

PRIMARY DIAGNOSIS OF THE 100 PATIENTS IN THIS STUDY

Diagnosis	Number of Patients
Intracranial hemorrhage	30
Cranial cerebral trauma	20
Primary cardiac arrest	13
Drug intoxication	13
Respiratory arrest *	24

* These include patients with metabolic disorders, CNS infarction, CNS infection, shock, neoplasm, and other disorders with anoxia, and often with secondary cardiac arrest.

Since cerebral angiography can only be justified in those patients in whom the procedure could potentially be of diagnostic benefit, e.g., lead to surgical intervention, the scope of this part of the study was, in effect, restricted to patients who were in an apneic, comatose state due to specific etiologies such as intracerebral trauma, including hematoma, cerebrovascular infarction, hemorrhage, and neoplasm. Although these criteria resulted in the exclusion of patients in whom cerebral angiography could not be justified—such as those with metabolic disorders, cardiorespiratory arrest, and drug intoxication— results from previous studies by us and others [35] allowed the assumption that the results from this group were applicable to apneic, comatose patients whose condition was due to other causes.

For patients to be entered into this validation study, it was a prerequisite that (a) he or she meet all clinical criteria for entry into the study; (b) his or her 30-minute EEG be isoelectric, i.e., demonstrate electrocerebral silence (ECS) or that repeated EEGs be probably isoelectric with artefacts or be persistently technically unsatisfactory; and (c) the following bolus study show no clear head bolus. There was one case that did not fully meet the last condition which was, nevertheless, included in the validation study; this will be discussed under the heading of results. A bolus study and EEG examination were repeated prior to and following angiography. Neuropathologic validation was also obtainable on the brains of a number of patients who met specified criteria.[36] Details of this pathologic study are also discussed elsewhere in the proceedings.[37]

FINDINGS

The initial ten pilot studies were done with limited controls, which included cerebral angiography and/or brain scanning. They yielded results that appeared to be all-or-none in nature, i.e., the presence of a bolus (FIGURE 3) suggesting the presence of cerebral blood flow (CBF) or the absence of a bolus (FIGURE 4) suggesting absent CBF or at least flow below a critical level. This gross qualitative measure, as indicated by such a step function, the presence or absence of a bolus, appeared to be even more desirable than a graded set of numbers, since there was less chance of overlap. This conclusion is based on the assumption that the critical level of CBF at which the bolus was absent is incompatible with cerebral viability.

All subsequent studies were performed employing the control probe and its simultaneous graphic readout. Such studies were only considered if the control tracing demonstrated an adequate bolus. In the absence of such an adequate control, no credence could be placed in the absence of a clear head bolus (FIGURE 5). In all but three patients, the femoral artery was used as a control. In these three, the femoral arteries were not available. A common carotid-artery control was used successfully in two (FIGURE 6). In the third precordial monitoring was not reliable enough to be considered technically satisfactory.[9]

As observed in the initial phase of the study, one type of tracing demonstrated a distinct bolus effect showing a relatively sharp rise and fall of activity, as noted in the patients illustrated in FIGURE 7. The sharp rise and fall of these tracings represent the bulk of intravenously injected bolus passing through the cerebral circulation and are essentially not distinguishable from tracings obtained in noncomatose individuals.[23, 24, 38–41] This will be referred to as a clearly

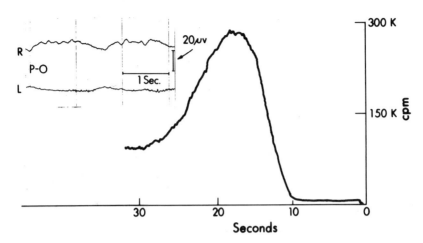

FIGURE 3. Patient was in deep coma because of episode of cerebral anoxia. Clinically, patient was never considered cerebrally dead according to Harvard criteria.[7] Although abnormal, EEG shows activity. EEG (right and left parietal occipital leads, R, L, P-O) is shown in inset. Probe tracing on patient clearly indicates bolus effect of intracranial flow. Tracing is essentially indistinguishable from tracings obtained on normal noncomatose patients. Patient expired two days after study. Autopsy showed bronchopneumonia and purulent peritonitis; in brain there was evidence of localized brain infarction only.

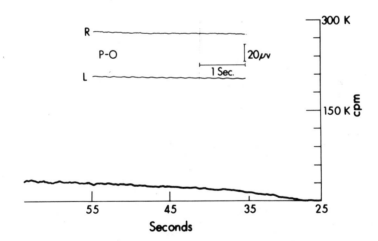

FIGURE 4. Patient was in coma secondary to transient cardiac arrest. EEG leads shown in inset are similar to those in FIGURE 3. EEG was isoelectric, and patient was considered to have been cerebrally dead according to Harvard criteria. Probe tracing on same patient reveals no bolus effect. Gradual rise of radioactivity starting 25 seconds after injection was regarded as due to extracerebral circulation. Note dramatic difference when compared to FIGURE 3. Patient expired with spontaneous and permanent cardiac arrest on the day after above study. Autopsy showed evidence of prior general brain death.

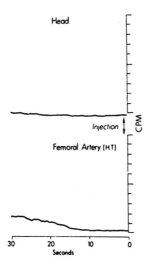

FIGURE 5. This study, as a whole, is considered inadequate because of failure to demonstrate a clear bolus effect in the femoral-artery tracing. Without this finding, the absence of a head bolus cannot be accepted as significant. In practice, the study can be repeated at any time.

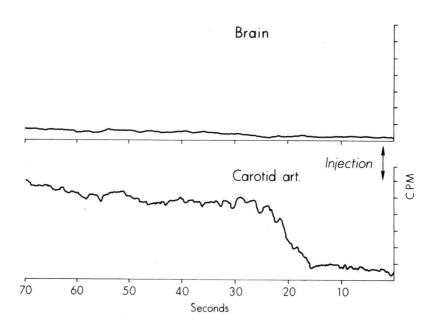

FIGURE 6. Training in a patient in whom the common carotid artery was used as a control is illustrated (*bottom*). Note that in the carotid artery there is not quite a "bolus" effect but a very large step-function phenomenon. This patient had no evidence of a head bolus by this technique (*top*).

normal head bolus. The appearance of the radioisotopic bolus in the femoral-artery area in the lower parts of the figure is similar but often slightly delayed when compared to the head tracing. These representative tracings were presumed to reflect sufficient CBF for maintenance of a viable, but not necessarily normal, cerebrum. The femoral controls indicate that the injection was satisfactory and that sufficient peripheral blood flow was present.

In sharp contrast to this, the second type of head tracing displayed a gradual, low magnitude, linear, graded increase in radioisotopic activity with no bolus effect from the head but with a normal femoral control. This is illustrated in FIGURE 8.

There was no distinct peak during the period of monitoring, which was

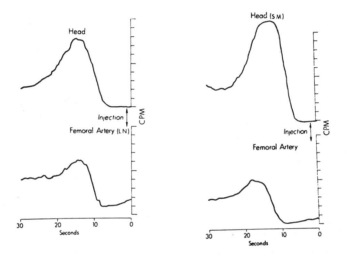

FIGURE 7. This illustrates the findings in two apneic, comatose patients in whom there was a "clear" head bolus (*top*) and normal femoral control (*bottom*). Note that the head bolus is usually greater in height than that from the femoral artery, that it occurs somewhat more rapidly, and that there is a distinct maximum. CPM refers to counts/minute; however, this measure should be considered entirely qualitative. The tracings were often run for more than one minute. Both of these patients had EEG activity.

continued for at least one minute following injection. This type of head time/activity tracing contrasts sharply with the passage of a distinct bolus through the femoral artery (FIGURES 7 and 8; lower portions of tracings). The lack of bolus effect in the head tracing was considered to be evidence of gross cerebral circulatory deficit. The relatively delayed, low-level, and gradual build-up in activity seen in the head tracings was presumably a reflection of the radionuclide activity in the extracerebral circulation. The evidence for this assumption will be further evaluated in the CONCLUSIONS AND DISCUSSION section.

One other type of result was found in a number of cases (FIGURE 9). This pattern showed a tracing from the head that was clearly different from the above two (FIGURES 7 and 8) in that it showed a minimal, very small rise in activity

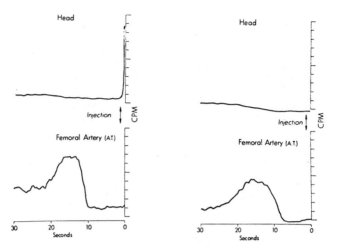

FIGURE 8. This illustrates tracings in two apneic, comatose patients with no evidence of significant CBF, as indicated by the absence of the head bolus (top) and by the presence of an appropriate femoral control (*bottom*). Both patients were brain-dead.

concomitant with a normal femoral-artery bolus response. This type of tracing was termed "intermediate." In some patients this was found in studies prior to or after an absent head bolus study was obtained. The significance of the "intermediate" tracing will also be analyzed in the CONCLUSIONS AND DISCUSSION section.

Finally, two patients showed a clear, but unusually small, head bolus (FIGURE 10). These cases will also be discussed below.

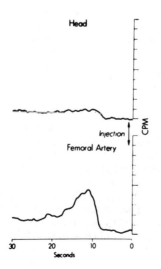

FIGURE 9. "Intermediate" tracing on patient with brain death. This shows a minimal, though not bolus, response (*top*) concomitant with normal femoral-artery bolus response (*bottom*). Compare with FIGURES 7 and 8.

RESULTS

The evidence used to assess the significance of the radioisotopic bolus study was basically of three different kinds:

1. The results were correlated and re-evaluated in the light of all clinical and laboratory evidence, including EEGs, following final disposition of each patient. This was done in 100 patients. No technically satisfactory or reliable bolus study could be obtained on 12 of these 100 patients, including three subjects in the initial pilot phase of the study in whom no reliable control to document adequate injection was available.

Every patient who did not finally have a clearly normal head bolus died, in the traditional sense of the word. There were 56 patients in this category. All

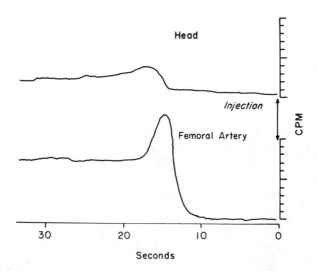

FIGURE 10. Single-head probe tracing illustrating the presence of a "small" head bolus. Contrast this with the usual tracing of a head bolus in FIGURE 7 and the intermediate tracing in FIGURE 9. Amplification is unchanged (see FIGURE 11).

other evidence in these patients also indicated the presence of brain death. The concomitant EEGs on all these patients showed ECS or were in some way persistently and technically unsatisfactory. One of these patients had had cerebral activity the day before the bolus study but had had spontaneous cessation of the heartbeat before the EEG could be repeated following the procedure. All nine patients with final "intermediate" tracings fell into the above category. The two patients with a minimal "small" head bolus, although not included in this category, met the criteria of brain death and also died.

Ten of 30 of the deeply comatose, apneic patients with a clearly normal head bolus survived. Significant cerebral blood flow (CBF) through the cerebral hemispheres was demonstrated by a variety of techniques used in 14 of these 30 patients in whom a head bolus was present. In the remaining patients evidence of cerebral circulation was indirect, i.e., patients had evidence of cerebral function, such as recovery, EEG activity, or transient improvement. Confirmation of CBF was made by utilizing cerebral angiography, brain scanning by sequential gamma-camera flow imaging, and/or by utilization of quantitative measures of CBF by means of the Kety technique.

2. Validation of the absence of a clear head bolus against four-vessel cerebral angiography in 20 appropriate patients was performed. The details of this study are given elsewhere in this volume. Suffice it to say here that in all 20 patients, the presence of cerebral death was confirmed angiographically in that none showed evidence of circulation through the cerebrum. Two of these

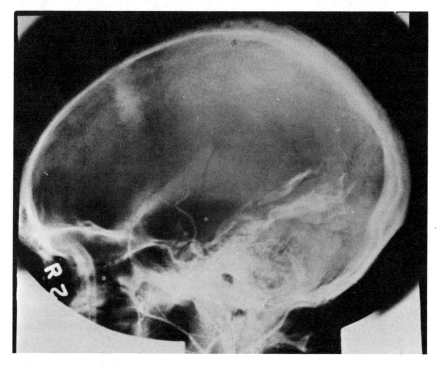

FIGURE 11. Lateral view of left common carotid angiogram of patient whose tracing was shown in FIGURE 10. Note extravasated contrast material in vicinity of right posterior cerebral artery and free tentorial edge. This extravasation persisted throughout the series. There was never evidence of venous opacification.

patients did, however, at the same time have angiographic evidence of flow through structures in the posterior fossa, albeit markedly abnormal, distorted and slow. Both of these patients, in addition to an absent head bolus, had ECS and were in unresponsive coma with no spontaneous respiration or cephalic reflexes. This phenomenon will be discussed below.

One of the two patients with a persistently "small" head bolus had cerebral angiography which showed bizarre supratentorial extraversation of contrast material and stasis (FIGURE 11); he was also felt to be cerebrally dead by angiographic criteria.

3. Pathologic examination of available brains from patients meeting the set criteria in this study also correlated with the absence of head bolus. Details of this validation are dealt with elsewhere in this volume.

In an attempt to determine a transitional level of CBF at which the appearance of the bolus changes, four patients were studied for quantitative CBF by Hass and his coworkers, using a modified Kety technique with argon. These studies indicated that an entirely normal bolus tracing was obtained on patients whose CBF was reduced to 24 percent of normal. Significantly lower levels of CBF could not be measured by this method.

THEORETICAL CONSIDERATIONS

The limitations of measuring CBF by means of external detection of diffusable radioisotopes have been previously considered and stressed in the literature.[27, 42, 43] Major problems have been encountered in distinguishing cerebral from extracerebral blood flow using multiple small probes. Furthermore, marked differences of regional circulation, for example, of the grey and white matter, have been well documented.[41, 44-46] These and other factors have led various investigators to conclude that the absence of intracranial blood flow, only as demonstrated by four-vessel angiography, is the sine qua non of brain death.[15, 42]

The results of the present study, in using the bolus technique as a qualitative indicator of cerebral circulatory deficit, suggest that under the special circumstances of arrested CBF, the extracranial circulation does not pose a significant problem. The reason for this apparent discrepancy with the results of previous investigators may be clarified if one considers that the head-flow tracings represent the passage of the radioisotopic bolus through two fundamentally different kinds of circulation.

First, the cerebral circulation involves a rapid transit of a large amount of blood flowing through a relatively small vascular reservoir. It has been calculated that the CBF normally is at least 750 cc/minute [47-49] and that it passes through a blood-pool reservoir of about 130 cc.[43] This very rapid transit through the relatively small cerebral blood reservoir causes a distinct registering of the arrival and departure of an intravenously injected bolus, which remains reasonably coherent after emergence from the left ventricle.

The appearance of such a tracing is essentially comparable to that which might be obtained over any large artery, such as the femoral. Such a clear bolus effect appears to be absent in the dispersed peripheral type of extracerebral circulation. In contrast, in this second type of circulation, the extracerebral blood flow involves a relatively small amount of blood with a very slow transit through a larger vascular reservoir in the scalp and skull.[47] This may be further illustrated by the studies of Ueda *et al.*[50] and Obrist *et al.*[41, 51, 52] In FIGURE 12 the differences in the clearance curves of the internal and the external carotid-artery injections of radioisotope illustrate the slow extracerebral flow in contrast to the more rapid flow through cerebral circulation. The cerebral circulation in turn may be separated into two compartments, but both appear to be more rapid than the extracerebral component.

The model developed by Obrist *et al.* (FIGURE 13, TABLE 2), which considers a three-compartment analysis of extracerebral and cerebral grey and white matter, confirms the major difference between the cerebral and extracerebral circulation. In the situation of arrested cerebral circulation, such as may be

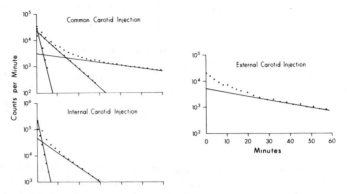

FIGURE 12. Clearance curves of tracer injection of ⁸⁵Kr directly into the common internal and external carotid arteries illustrating the partition of flow compartments of grey matter, white matter, and extracerebral circulation. (From Ueda *et al.*[50] Reproduced by permission.)

found in cases of brain death, the differences between white and grey matter are no longer significant; and the resultant flow tracing represents only extracerebral circulation, i.e., a tracing with an absent head bolus. To further test this hypothesis, a bolus study was performed with one probe over the femoral artery and another over the foot (FIGURE 14). The results confirm the similarity in the rapid transit of blood through a large artery, the femoral, which may be compared to the usual transit of CBF (which is not critically diminished). In contrast, the peripheral blood flow through the foot is similar to that of the extracerebral structures when the blood flow through the cerebrum is absent or critically impaired.

As stated above, levels of CBF in comatose patients, which are correlated with the presence of a clear bolus and EEG activity, have been found to be as low as 24 percent of normal. Studies of patients in deep coma associated with vascular disease who are not brain-dead have shown CBF values of about 50 percent of normal, while patients in deep barbiturate coma were found to have CBF values higher than 40 percent of normal.[53] Evidence indicates that

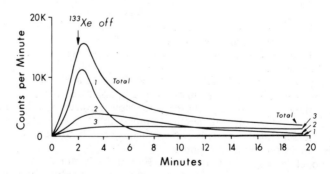

FIGURE 13. Three-compartment computerized model and results of ¹³³Xe washout curves: 1=grey matter, 2=white matter, 3=extracerebral circulation. The large curve represents the total circulation (see also TABLE 2). (Adapted from Obrist *et al.*[51])

TABLE 2 *

CEREBRAL AND EXTRACEREBRAL CIRCULATION †

Series	Method ¹³³Xe Clearance	Grey Fast Cerebral Component	White Slow Cerebral Component (ml/100 g/min)	Mean CBF
Ingvar *et al.* (1965)	Internal carotid injection	80	21	50
Obrist *et al.* (1967)	Inhalation, three-compartment analysis	75	25	55
Veall and Mallett (1966)	Inhalation, two-compartment analysis	53	10	32
Obrist *et al.* (1967)	Inhalation, two-compartment analysis	52	10	30

* Adapted from Obrist *et al.*[51]
† Extracerebral blood flow on this basis approximately 25 cc/100 g/min derived from mean CBF values above (maximal).

in situations where the clinical and electroencephalographic picture may simulate brain death but where the individual is in a reversible state, there should be sufficient CBF to produce a clearly "normal" bolus, as previously defined.[42, 54] In contrast, studies using a variety of techniques on patients who are brain-dead often show markedly reduced CBF. However, it should be understood that the reliability of some of these techniques is limited in situations in which there

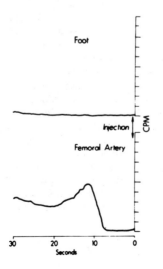

FIGURE 14. After the intravenous injection of isotope (⁹⁹ᵐTcO₄), note comparison of foot tracing (*top*) with collimator over the femoral artery (*bottom*) revealing two types of circulation—the slow, dispersed peripheral type of circulation is similar to the head tracings with no bolus. This suggests that in the absence of significant cerebral circulation, the blood flow detected by this technique is due to circulation through the skull and skin.

is marked reduction of CBF. Most investigators report CBF values of less than 10 percent in such patients.[30, 55-57] There appears to be a lower limit of CBF which is incompatible with cerebral viability and represents a threshold of irreversibility. Evidence suggests that this value is approximately 20 percent of normal CBF.[53, 56, 57]

Infrequently, patients who are brain-dead have been reported to have CBF higher than this and which presumably could have resulted in a false-positive, i.e., a bolus; but as noted, such an error is diagnostically acceptable.[56, 58] For example, Bès et al.[53] describe a patient who is brain-dead with a CBF of 22 percent of normal as measured by the intracarotid injection of ^{133}Xe (a diffusable tracer); but they note that there was no angiographic filling of vessels in the head. They consider the possibility that this figure represents either a more sensitive indicator of cerebral circulation or is due to extracerebral contamination or both. Since no normal bolus was ever seen by us in brain-dead patients who showed no intracranial circulation and who did show angiographic or clinical evidence of significant extracerebral circulation, this suggests that the maximal contribution of that extracerebral circulation would be equivalent to that seen in an intermediate tracing. The value of 22 percent of normal CBF in the brain-dead patient, as noted above, suggests, therefore, a significant component of extracerebral contamination.

The results of studies on another specific subset of patients in prolonged (months to years) irreversible coma should be further explored. Although terminology varies, one may unify this group under the term "persistent vegetative states," as suggested by Jennett and Plum.[59] This group of patients may have a variety in etiologies and localization of lesions. For example, there are reports describing patients as being in apallic states or as having "neocortical death."[11, 60, 61] The majority of patients in persistent vegetative states have complex patterns of brain-stem function without apnea and do not pose a problem in the differential diagnosis of brain death.[32] Of the two patients described as having neocortical death by Brierly et al.,[11] both had prolonged periods of ECS in their EEGs and one was apneic, requiring a respirator for 20 days. It is clinically significant that both of these patients always had pupillary reaction to light until the time of their death. Although no CBF studies were performed on these patients, the pathologic findings of marked bilateral, cortical, and basal ganglia atrophy and destruction suggest that the levels of the residual CBF would be related primarily to the remaining viable portion of the cerebrum, e.g., the thalamus. The reduction of CBF in such cases could be below 20 percent of normal, as was found by Ingvar[60] in one of his patients.|| Again, it is not known whether such patients would have a bolus tracing. Investigation evaluating the CBF and the bolus study in such patients would be of value. Despite these problems, all of the patients described above would not have met the criteria for brain death on clinical grounds, since they had cephalic reflexes, i.e., at least pupillary reaction to light, regardless of ECS in the EEG and regardless of the results of a bolus study.

Excluding such syndromes in which there are limited portions of supratentorial structures which are viable, it may be assumed that given the appropriate clinical criteria, CBF of less than 20 percent of normal is incompatible with survival of the cerebral hemispheres and will be reflected by the absence of a

---

|| See also the paper by Ingvar et al. in this volume.—J. K.

bolus on radioisotopic examinations during about a one-hour period, regardless of alterations in the extracerebral circulation.

An objection that may be raised against the bolus technique or against any method that evaluates CBF only may be the oft-stated proposition that it is not the CBF per se that is of concern in the problem of brain death, but rather the metabolism of neuronal cells, such as that reflected by the cerebral metabolic rate of oxygen consumption ($CMRO_2$). It is, in fact, the case that the fundamental living process is related to the metabolic activity and energy utilization in these cells.[41, 62, 63] Changes in $CMRO_2$ often parallel changes in CBF.[41] However, in many situations, especially in relation to hypothermia and drug-induced anesthetic states, the decrease of $CMRO_2$ is significantly greater than the relative decrease of CBF.[54, 64] Since such states are often reversible, we believe it is clinically feasible and more practical to consider the critical deficit in CBF rather than the critical deficit of $CMRO_2$ to determine irreversibility of destruction of the neuronal structures of the brain. Studies in the literature indicate that cerebral circulatory arrest of sufficient duration will lead to irreversible changes incompatible with cerebral viability. Miller and Myers[65] have described an upper limit of 20 minutes for this period. In the adult, if there is a demonstrable critical deficit in cerebral circulation, as measured by separate studies during a one-hour period, irreversibility can be considered virtually unequivocal regardless of etiology.

CONCLUSIONS AND DISCUSSION

It should be clear from what has been said above that the bolus technique does not evaluate for critical deficit of blood flow through the whole brain, only the supratentorial part. Indeed, two of our patients were shown to have some blood flow through the posterior fossa. If lack of viability of the posterior-fossa structures is also felt to be a significant consideration, the bolus technique may still be used in evaluation of the critical deficit of cerebral (supratentorial) blood flow. Other techniques or clinical evaluations could be used to determine the irreversibility of structures in the posterior fossa.[29, 66, 67] It is noteworthy that according to Von Bucheler *et al.*[68] in their angiographic studies of 21 patients with brain death, they commonly observed a temporal progression of lack of vascular filling of the cerebral arteries with subsequent involvement of the arteries in the posterior fossa. This was presumed to be usually related to progressively increasing pressure as the edematous cerebral hemispheres compressed and distorted the contents of the posterior fossa, thus leading to total brain death.

The two patients who did show flow in the posterior fossa were presumably in the later, though not final, stages of such a progression, since there was no evidence of function attributable to posterior-fossa structures.

Earlier in the study we felt that an "intermediate" study might represent a transitional stage between a head bolus and no head bolus and thus possibly reflect some CBF. We now feel its significance is the same as that of a no-head-bolus study, i.e., representing a critical deficit of CBF. This conclusion was drawn for the following reasons:

1. "Intermediate" and no-bolus studies were occasionally found following each other, in any order, on successive examinations. Neither type was ever followed by a clear head-bolus flow study.

2. All evidence outlined above for confirming or validating the presence of brain death, including angiography, was always positive in cases with "intermediate" results, including cases with only "intermediate" radioisotopic flow studies. The word "intermediate" is, therefore, not entirely appropriate for this finding.

The actual cause of an "intermediate" result may be the presence of some blood reaching into and again exiting via some major intracranial arteries supratentorially. There was some evidence to suggest this might occasionally be the cause in the angiographic validation study.[21] This will be further detailed elsewhere in this volume.[34]

There was, of course, never evidence of circulation through the cerebrum, as indicated by venous opacification. Reviewing all the studies, it was clear that an intermediate finding was significantly more likely when the examination was performed with two head probes, each placed laterally, than with a single-head probe placed at the forehead.[21] This occurred even when there was absolutely no angiographic evidence of intracranial filling.

Since major extracerebral vessels are located on the surface in the temporal area, it seems likely that extracranial arterial flow in larger vessels, especially near the detector, may cause an "intermediate" type of tracing. For this reason as well as for considerations of cost and ease of use, the authors find twin-probe (single-head probe) equipment preferable to triple-probe equipment.

The exact cause of the repeatedly abnormally small, but clear, head bolus in the two patients, one of which demonstrated contrast extravasation on angiography, is not clear. This small head bolus is like a clearly normal type of head bolus, except that it has a relatively lower amplitude when each kind of head bolus is judged in relation to the femoral bolus of the same study. It is clearly distinguishable from an intermediate tracing (FIGURE 9). In any case, the authors feel such a finding in itself has to be interpreted as not demonstrating a critical deficit of CBF. This would then in itself lead to a mistaken indication of cerebral viability. This underlines the axiom that such a mistake, not occurring frequently, is totally acceptable; whereas a mistaken indication of brain death in a confirmatory test is totally unacceptable. The latter mistake never occurred at any time in our studies. In such cases, as in all ambiguous situations, the clinician must use his judgment. For example, he may at this time consider four-vessel angiography if there is still doubt.

The passage of an intravenously injected radioactive bolus of $^{99m}TcO_4$ through the brain can also be imaged by a dynamic flow sequence with a gamma camera.[69] Since portable cameras are now becoming widely available and are used for many other purposes in hospitals, it has been suggested that this method of demonstrating the lack of passage of the bolus through the head is the method of choice.[70, 71] Before this pictorial display can be relied upon, a much more thorough and comprehensive investigation of its sensitivity would have to be undertaken. The flow images have a lower statistical basis in terms of the number of useful counts on which to base a finding. It must be proven that the level of nonvisualization of cerebral flow by dynamic images is below the level of critical deficit in CBF. Furthermore, these images require fine judgment and reproducible technique in order to decide that there is no cerebral flow. Such judgments leave room for potentially unacceptable types of error. In addition, the image studies can only be attempted once over a period of many hours.

Ten to 20 mCi of ^{99m}Tc must be used per study; this dose, in the form of ^{99m}Tc SC, especially if repeated, gives unacceptable radiation to the liver. The other agents available present too much residual background activity to allow for early repetition of the image examination. This means that if the initial bolus injection or other factors are inadequate, no early repetition is possible. Furthermore, routine confirmation in, say, one hour is also not possible. We disagree with Goodman *et al.*[70] that a single isotopic study, without EEG monitoring, is of itself adequate to make the crucial determination of the presence of brain death. In the presence of unequivocal EEG activity, a CBF study is irrelevant. Moreover, the total absence of blood flow for a period of less than one minute is not necessarily associated with nonviability of the brain. It should be pointed out that by using the probes and the associated time/activity curve method, any residual background activity can be negated simply by setting the pen at zero at the start of the examination.

We have discussed above, on theoretical grounds, the reasons why, with the possible exception of certain "persistent vegetative states," it should be anticipated that patients who do not have brain death, but who are in deep unresponsive coma with ECS, should demonstrate the presence of a head bolus. Although we did not have the opportunity to study any such patients, three such cases have been reported.[32, 72]

Two of these cases were in a study by Ashwal *et al.*,[72] using a modified application of the bolus technique in 15 infants and children, as described by those authors. In this study there were also two instances of an absent head bolus in newborn infants who did not have brain death. Ashwal *et al.* conclude that the absence of a head bolus over a short interval in infants under the age of one year is not as reliable as in more mature individuals.

The brains of neonatal infants are capable of tolerating greater degrees of ischemia and hypoxia, and currently this age limitation on the application of the bolus technique should be considered. One of the infants in the Ashwal study, who did survive, had a head bolus in the presence of ECS on a repeat examination. This underscores our firm belief that a radioisotope study showing an absent head bolus must be repeated at a suitable interval before reliance can be placed upon it. In our 100 adult cases (and in Ashwal and coworkers' 13 other childhood cases), there were no instances of an absent bolus that were not associated with cerebral death (the patients were also brain-dead).

The modification in technique used by Ashwal *et al.* was to place the control probe over the heart. In some early studies we used such a control but found that detection of the bolus in this circulation, which is not a peripheral arterial one, was not a reliable indicator of an adequate bolus injection.[9] So while we offer this as an alternative explanation for possibly apparent absence of a head bolus in these two cases, we also agree that at present the bolus technique must be used more cautiously in infants under one year.

It is our conclusion that, possibly except in infants and in patients with certain "persistent vegetative states," bolus studies performed over a 30- to 60-minute interval, showing the absence of a head bolus, are confirmatory proof of cerebral death, and with other appropriate clinical and laboratory criteria can be used to diagnose brain-death. This technique is safe, simple, and reliable; the equipment needed should be relatively cheap; and we advocate its clinical application.

ACKNOWLEDGMENTS

We wish to acknowledge the aid, cooperation, and participation of numerous individuals in the Departments of Neurology, Neurosurgery, and Radiology and the Division of Nuclear Medicine during this study, especially Drs. C. T. Randt, J. Ransohoff, and N. Chase. The technical assistance of Mr. C. Pierno in performing the bolus studies and of Ms. M. Kalmijn, Ms. E. Falek, Ms. V. Chao, and Ms. L. Levidow for performance of the EEGs is especially appreciated. The manuscript was prepared by Ms. G. Murphy.

REFERENCES

1. BALDY-MOULINIER, M. & PH. FREREBEAU. 1969. Cerebral blood flow in cases of fallowing coma after severe head injury. *In* Cerebral Blood Flow: Clinical and Experimental Results. M. Brock, C. Fieschi, D. H. Ingvar, N. A. Lassen & K. Schürmann, Eds. : 216–218. Springer-Verlag. Berlin.
2. BEECHER, H. K. 1970. Definitions of "life" and "death" for medical science and practice. Ann. N. Y. Acad. Sci. **169:** 471–474.
3. BENTAL, E. & U. LEIBOWITZ. 1961. Flat electroencephalograms during 28 days in a case of "encephalitis." Electroenceph. Clin. Neurophysiol. **13:** 457–460.
4. BICKFORD, R. G., B. DAWSON & H. TAKESHITA. 1965. EEG evidence of neurologic death. Electroenceph. Clin. Neurophysiol. **18:** 513–514.
5. BIRD, T. D. & F. PLUM. 1968. Recovery from barbiturate overdose coma with a prolonged isoelectric electroencephalogram. Neurology **18:** 456–460.
6. TENTLER, R. L., M. SADOVE, D. R. BECKA & R. C. TAYLOR. 1957. Electroencephalographic evidence of cortical "death" followed by full recovery: Protective action of hypothermia. JAMA **164:** 1667–1670.
7. BEECHER, H. K. 1968. A definition of irreversible coma: Report of the Ad Hoc Committee of the Harvard Medical School to examine the definition of brain death. JAMA **205**(6): 85–88.
8. BRAUNSTEIN, P., J. KOREIN, I. KRICHEFF, K. COREY & N. CHASE. 1973. A simple bedside evaluation for cerebral blood flow in the study of cerebral death: A prospective study on 34 deeply comatose patients. Am. J. Roentgen. **118**(4): 757–767.
9. KOREIN, J., P. BRAUNSTEIN, I. KRICHEFF, A. LIEBERMAN & N. CHASE. 1975. Radioisotopic bolus technique as a test to detect circulatory deficit associated with cerebral death: 142 studies on 80 patients demonstrating the bedside use of an innocuous IV procedure as an adjunct in the diagnosis of cerebral death. Circulation **51:** 924–939.
10. CLAR, H. E., A. AGNOLI & L. MAGNUS. 1972. Angiographische befunde bei intracraniellem kreislaufstillstand infolge erhhohten hirnducks. Acta Radiol. Vol. 13, Part 1, 9th Symposium, Neuroradiollogicum, Gothenberg, August 24–29, **1970:** 312–317.
11. BRIERLEY, J. B., D. I. GRAHAM, J. H. ADAMS & J. A. SIMPSOM. 1971. Neurocortical death after cardiac arrest: A clinical, neurophysiological, and neuropathological report of two cases. Lancet **2:** 560–565.
12. BROCK, M., K. SCHÜRMANN & A. HADJIDIMOS. 1969. Cerebral blood flow and cerebral death. Acta Neurochir. **20:** 195–209.
13. HUNT, W. E., J. N. MEAGHER, A. FREIMANIS & C. W. ROSSEL. 1962. Angiographic studies of experimental intracranial hypertension. J. Neurosurg. **19:** 1023–1032.
14. MITCHELL, O. C., E. DE LA TORRE, E. ALEXANDER, JR. & C. H. DAVIS, JR. 1962. The nonfilling phenomenon during angiography in acute intracranial hypertension. J. Neurosurg. **19:** 766–774.

15. HADJIDIMOS, A. A., M. BROCK, P. BAUM & K. SCHÜRMANN. 1969. Cessation of cerebral blood flow in total irreversible loss of brain function. *In* Cerebral Blood Flow: Clinical and Experimental Results. M. Brock, C. Fieschi, D. H. Ingvar, N. A. Lassen & K. Schürmann, Eds. : 209–212. Springer-Verlag. Berlin.
16. HASS, W. K., F. P. SIEW & D-J. YEE. 1968. Progress in adaptation of mass spectrometer to study of human cerebral blood flow. Circulation 38(Suppl. 6): 96.
17. WALD, A., W. K. HASS & J. RANSOHOFF. 1971. Tutorial: Experience with a mass spectrometer system for blood gas analysis in humans. J. Assoc. Advanc. Med. Instrument. 5: 325–342.
18. KRAMER, W. & J. A. TUYNMAN. 1967. Acute intracranial hypertension: An experimental investigation. Brain Res. 6: 686–705.
19. NIMMANNITYA, J. & A. E. WALKER. 1969. Significance of electroencephalogram in comatose respirator cases. Curr. Med. Digest 36: 189–200.
20. Final Report. 1977. An appraisal of the criteria of cerebral death: A summary statement. Collaborative Study of Cerebral Survival. HEW, NIH, NINDS, Contract 1–NS–1–2316. Bethesda, Md., April, 1974. JAMA 237: 982–986.
21. KOREIN J., P. BRAUNSTEIN, A. GEORGE, M. WICHTER, I. KRICHEFF, A. LIEBERMAN & J. PEARSON. 1977. Brain death: I. Angiographic correlation with the radioisotopic bolus technique for evaluation of critical deficit of cerebral blood flow. Ann. Neurol. 2(3): 195–205.
22. BRAUNSTEIN, P., I. KRICHEFF, J. KOREIN & K. COREY. 1973. Cerebral death: A rapid and reliable diagnostic adjunct using radioisotopes. J. Nucl. Med. 14(2): 122–124.
23. OLDENDORF, W. H. 1962. Measurement of the mean transit time of cerebral circulation by external detection of an intravenously injected radioisotope. J. Nucl. Med. 3: 382–398.
24. OLDENDORF, W. H. 1963. Measuring brain blood flow with radioisotopes. Nucleonics 21(4): 87–90.
25. MAYNARD, C. D., R. L. WITCOFSKI, R. JANEWAY & R. J. COWAN. 1969. "Radioisotope arteriography" as an adjunct to the brain scan. Radiology 92: 908–912.
26. BURKE, G. & A. HALKO. 1968. Cerebral blood flow studies with sodium-pertechnetate Tc 99m and the scintillation camera. JAMA 204: 109–114.
27. WELCH, T. J. C., E. J. POTCHEN & M. J. WELCH. 1972. Fundamentals of the Tracer Method. W. B. Saunders. Philadelphia, Pa.
28. ALLEN, N., J. D. BURKHOLDER, J. COMISCIONI & G. F. MOLINARI. 1976. Predictive value of clinical criteria in cerebral death (abstract). Neurology 26: 356–357.
29. PLUM, F. & J. B. POSNER. 1972. The Diagnosis of Stupor and Coma, 2nd Ed. F. A. Davis. Philadelphia, Pa.
30. SILVERMAN, D., M. G. SAUNDERS, R. S. SCHWAB & R. L. MASLAND. 1969. Cerebral death and the electroencephalogram: Report of the Ad Hoc Committee of the American Electroencephalographic Society of EEG criteria for determination of cerebral death. JAMA 209: 1505–1510.
31. SILVERMAN, D., R. L. MASLAND, M. G. SAUNDERS & R. S. SCHWAB. 1970. Irreversible coma associated with electrocerebral silence. Neurology 20: 525–533.
32. BENNETT, D., J. HUGHES, J. KOREIN, J. MERLIS & C. SUTER. 1976. Atlas of Electroencephalography in Coma and Cerebral Death. Raven Press. New York, N.Y.
33. AMERICAN ELECTROENCEPHALOGRAPHIC SOCIETY. 1976. Guidelines in EEG. : 21–28. Willoughby, Ohio.
34. KRICHEFF, I. et al. This volume.
35. KRICHEFF, I., P. BRAUNSTEIN, J. KOREIN, A. E. GEORGE & A. J. KUMAR. 1975. Isotopic and angiographic determination of cerebral blood flow: A correlation in patients with cerebral death. Acta Radiol. (Suppl. 347): 119–129.
36. PEARSON, J., J. KOREIN, J. H. HARRIS, M. WICHTER & P. BRAUNSTEIN. 1977.

Brain death: II. Neuropathological correlation with the radioisotopic bolus technique for evaluation of critical deficit of cerebral blood flow. Ann. Neurol. 2(3): 206–210.

37. PEARSON, J. This volume.

38. OLDENDORF, W. H. & M. KITANO. 1965. The symmetry of I^{131} 4-iodoantipyrine uptake by brain after intravenous injection. Neurology 15: 994–999.

39. OLDENDORF, W. H. & M. KITANO. 1965. Isotope study of brain blood turnover in vascular disease. Arch. Neurol. 12: 30–38.

40. OLDENDORF, W. H. & M. KITANO. 1967. Radioisotope measurement of brain blood turnover time as a clinical index of brain circulation. J. Nucl. Med. 8: 570–587.

41. PURVES, M. J. 1972. The Physiology of Cerebral Circulation. Cambridge University Press. Cambridge, England.

42. BROCK, M., C. FIESCHI, D. H. INGVAR, N. A. LASSEN & K. SCHÜRMANN, Eds. 1969. Cerebral Blood Flow: Clinical and Experimental Results. Springer-Verlag. Berlin.

43. OLDENDORF, W. H. 1969. Absolute measurement of brain blood flow using non-diffusible isotopes. In Cerebral Blood Flow: Clinical and Experimental Results. M. Brock, C. Fieschi, D. H. Ingvar, N. A. Lassen & K. Schürmann, Eds. : 53–55. Springer-Verlag. Berlin.

44. HOEDT-RASMUSSEN, K. 1967. Regional cerebral blood flow: The intra-arterial injection method. Acta Neurol. Scand. 43 (Suppl. 27).

45. INGVAR, D. H., N. A. LASSEN, B. K. SIESJO & E. SKINHOJ. 1968. Cerebral blood flow & cerebro-spinal fluid. Scand. J. Clin. Lab. Invest. 22 (Suppl. 102).

46. REIVICH, M., R. SLATER & N. SANO. 1969. Further studies on exponential models of cerebral clearance curves. In Cerebral Blood Flow: Clinical and Experimental Results. M. Brock, C. Fieschi, D. H. Ingvar, N. A. Lassen & K. Schürmann, Eds. : 8–10. Springer-Verlag. Berlin.

47. FOLKOW B. & E. NEIL. 1971. Circulation. Oxford University Press. New York, N.Y.

48. WRIGHT, S. 1971. Applied Physiology. : 143. Oxford University Press. London England.

49. BLINKOV, S. M. & I. I. GLEZER. 1968. The Human Brain in Figures and Tables. Basic Books. New York, N.Y.

50. UEDA, H., S. HATANO, T. MOLDE & T. GONDAIRA. 1965. Discussion II on: Compartmental analysis of the human brain blood flow. In Regional Cerebral Blood Flow. Acta Neurol. Scand. (Suppl. 14): 88–91.

51. OBRIST, W. D., H. K. THOMPSON, H. S. WANG & S. CRONQUIST. 1971. A simplified procedure for determining fast compartment CBF's by ^{133}Xenon inhalation. In Brain and Blood Flow. R. W. R. Russell, Ed. : 11–15. Pitman. London.

52. OBRIST, W. D., H. K. THOMPSON, C. H. KING & H. S. WANG. 1967. Determination of regional cerebral blood flow by inhalation of 133-Xenon. Circ. Res. 20: 124–135.

53. BÈS, A., L. ARBUS, Y. LAZORTHES, M. ESCANDE, M. DELPLA & J. P. M. VERGNE. 1969. Hemodynamic and metabolic studies in "coma depasse": A search for a biological test of death of the brain. In Cerebral Blood Flow: Clinical and Experimental Results. M. Brock, C. Fieschi, D. H. Ingvar, N. A. Lassen & K. Schürmann, Eds. : 213–215. Springer-Verlag. Berlin.

54. TABADDOR, K., T. J. GARDNER & A. E. WALKER. 1972. Cerebral circulation and metabolism at deep hypothermia. Neurology 22: 1065–1070.

55. GROS, C., B. VLAHOVITCH, P. FREREBEAU, A. KUHNER, M. BILLET, G. SAHUT & G. GAVAND. 1969. Criteres arteriographiques des comas depasses en neuro-chirurgie. Neuro-Chir. 15: 477–486.

56. HOYER, S. & J. WAWERSIK. 1968. Untersuchungen der hirndurchblutung und des hirnstoffwechsels beim decerbrationssyndrom. Langenbecks Arch. Chir. 322: 602–605.

57. BRODERSON, P., P. HEILBRUN, O. PAULSON, J. OLESON, E. SKINHOJE & N. A.

LASSEN. 1972. Cerebral blood flow and oxygen consumption in coma and brain death. *In* Diagnosis of Stupor and Coma, 2nd Ed. F. Plum & J. B. Posner, Eds. : 235. F. A. Davis. Philadelphia, Pa.

58. SHALIT, M. N., A. J. BELLER, M. FEINSOD, A. J. DRAPKIN & S. COTEV. 1970. The blood flow and oxygen consumption of the dying brain. Neurology **20:** 740–748.

59. JENNETT, B. & F. PLUM. 1972. Persistent vegatative state after brain damage: A syndrome in search of a name. Lancet **1:** 734–737.

60. INGVAR, D. H. 1971. EEG and cerebral circulation in the apallic syndrome and akinetic mutism. Electroenceph. Clin. Neurophysiol. **30:** 272–273.

61. INGVAR, D. H. & A. BRUN. 1972. Das complette apallisch syndrom. Arch. Psychiat. Nervenkr. **215:** 219–239.

62. GASTAUT, H. & J. S. MEYER, Eds. 1961. Cerebral Anoxia and the Electroencephalogram: The Proceedings of the Marseilles Colloquium. Charles C Thomas. Springfield, Ill.

63. KOREIN, J. 1966. Towards a general theory of living systems. *In* The 3rd International Conference on Cybernetic Medicine, 1964. A. Masturzo, Ed. : 232–248. Francesco, Giannino, and Figli. Naples.

64. WOLLMAN, H., A. L. SMITH & S. C. ALEXANDER. 1969. Effects of general anesthetics in man on the ratio of cerebral blood flow to cerebral oxygen consumption. *In* Cerebral Blood Flow: Clinical and Experimental Results. M. Brock, C. Fieschi, D. H. Ingvar, N. A. Lassen & K. Schürmann, Eds. : 242–243. Springer-Verlag. Berlin.

65. MILLER, J R. & R. E. MYERS. 1970. Neurological effects of systemic circulatory arrest in the monkey. Neurology **20:** 715–724.

66. KOREIN, J. & M. MACCARIO. 1971. On the diagnosis of cerebral death: A prospective study on 55 patients to define irreversible coma. Clin. Electroencephal. **2:** 178–199.

67. STARR, A. & L. J. ACHOR. 1975. Auditory brain stem responses in neurological disease. Arch. Neurol. **32:** 761–768.

68. VON BUCHELER, E., C. KAUFER & A. DUX. 1970. Zerebrale angiographie zur bestimmung des hirntodes. Fortschr. Roentgenstr. **113:** 278–296.

69. GOODMAN, J. M., F. S. MISHKIN & M. DYKEN. 1969. Determination of brain death by isotope angiography. JAMA. **209:** 1869–1872.

70. GOODMAN, J. M. & L. L. HECK. 1977. Confirmation of brain death at bedside by isotope angiography. JAMA **238**(9): 966–968.

71. NORDLANDER, S., P. E. WIKLUND & P. E. ASARD. 1973. Cerebral angioscintigraphy in brain death and in coma due to drug intoxication. J. Nucl. Med. **14:** 856–857.

72. ASHWAL, S., A. SMITH, F. TORRES, M. LOKEN & S. N. CHOU. 1977. Radionuclide bolus angiography: A technique for verification of brain death in infants and children. J. Pedat. **91**(5): 722–728.

ANGIOGRAPHIC FINDINGS IN BRAIN DEATH *

I. I. Kricheff, R. S. Pinto, A. E. George, P. Braunstein,
and J. Korein

Departments of Radiology and Neurology
New York University Medical Center
New York, New York 10016

INTRODUCTION

With advances in medical techniques, "life" may be supported even though irreversible brain † damage has occurred. To avoid prolonged efforts to maintain a brain-dead patient until systemic death occurs and to conserve organs for transplantations, it is necessary to rely on a diagnostic test that would aid in conclusively determining the irreversibility and scope of the cerebral insult. Although isotopic determination of a cerebral blood-flow deficit is a rapid and reliable diagnostic adjunct to determine cerebral † death,[3-5, 16, 17] there are times that in the clinical judgment of the examining neurologist, angiography is required before it can be stated with certainty that brain death has occurred.

Angiography may thus be necessary when the isotopic bolus study demonstrates an "intermediate" or small bolus pattern or is technically unsatisfactory, or when the EEG is not unequivocally isoelectric. Furthermore because of technical considerations the bolus technique is primarily limited to use in adults.[15] Therefore intracranial angiography may be necessary to document brain death in infants and small children.

Many European authors maintain that the *sine qua non* of brain death rests with the demonstration of absence of intracranial circulation by angiography.[2, 8, 23] Though serving a limited role in the diagnosis of brain death, the findings at angiography are recorded so that when this diagnostic test is used as the final confirmation of the determination of death, no confusion will result. It is our belief that when the advocates of angiography become familiar with the results obtained by the bolus technique, they will rarely resort to angiography.

METHOD

The angiographic studies in our series were done to evaluate and validate the critical deficit of cerebral blood flow that was found when the radioisotopic bolus technique was utilized. Intracranial angiography was performed only in those patients in whom it could be expected to yield some potential benefit. Twenty patients were studied by selective bilateral internal carotid artery and vertebral artery injections through a femoral arterial catheter. Eight cc of con-

---

* This work was supported in part by NINCDS Contracts Nos. 71–2319 and 1–NS–2307 from the National Institutes of Health and by Neurology Research Fund No. 8–0168–708 from New York University Medical Center.

† The words "brain death" and "cerebral death" are *not* used interchangeably in this paper.—*J. K.*

0077–8923/78/0315–0168 $01.75/0 © 1978, NYAS

trast medium was injected for each angiographic series. Several patients had repeated injections of 10 cc of contrast medium into the common carotid artery. Nineteen of our twenty patients met clinical and electroencephalographic criteria of brain death. The twentieth patient had a technically unsatisfactory EEG. These 20 patients included 14 with intracranial hemorrhage, four with intracranial trauma, and two with massive cerebral infarction presenting as a rapidly increasing space-occupying lesion.

The angiographic series was routinely prolonged for 30 seconds. Attempts were made to overcome increased vascular resistance secondary to increased intracranial pressure by increasing the pressure of the injection of the contrast medium.

In all cases where filling of intracranial vessels occurred the onset of filling and the duration of persistence of the contrast material were noted. In patients who demonstrated some intracranial circulation the time course of the circulation was measured. In patients in whom retrograde flow occurred, the time course and pathway of either the reflux or shunt was noted. The term "shunt" was used to indicate the flow of contrast material that made an abnormal exit from the cranial cavity via another artery without traversing into the venous sinuses. The term "reflux" was used to describe back flow when the contrast material entered and exited through the same artery. The time course of filling of the extracranial vessels was also noted. These included the superficial temporal artery, the middle meningeal artery, and the occipital arteries.

The angiographic findings were correlated with the findings obtained by the radioisotope bolus technique and electroencephalography.

RESULTS

The angiographic findings in the 20 brain-dead patients are classified into five groups which are summarized in TABLE 1.

Group I consisted of those patients with complete *absence* of intracranial flow or filling (FIGURES 1, 2 and 3). There were 10 patients in this group; all had EEGs with electrocortical silence, and bolus studies were performed both before and after the angiogram. Six of these patients had an absent bolus tracing prior to and after angiography and two had intermediate bolus tracings. There was one patient with an initial intermediate bolus tracing and the postangiographic study showed no bolus. One other patient had no bolus prior to angiography, and the repeat bolus tracing after angiography demonstrated an intermediate tracing.

Group II included three patients with absent intracranial circulation (i.e., no transit of contrast material from arterial to venous circulation), but in whom prolonged *stasis* filling of basal subarachnoid intracranial arteries was seen (FIGURE 4).

The arteries involved in such stasis filling were usually at the base, and included only first-order branches of the middle cerebral arteries, the Circle of Willis, and the basilar artery, as well as intracranial portions of the internal carotid artery. All patients demonstrated absent initial and postangiographic bolus tracings, except for one patient who had an intermediate tracing on a second postangiogram radioisotope study.

Group III consisted of four patients in whom a variety of *reflux* and *shunting* phenomena was observed (FIGURES 5 and 6). Although all these patients

TABLE 1

SUMMARY OF RESULTS IN 20 PATIENTS UNDERGOING ANGIOGRAPHY TO CONFIRM CEREBRAL DEATH

Patient No.	Etiology *	Angiography	EEG †	Bolus Study ‡		Head Probe
				Before Angiography	After Angiography	
Group I (10 patients)						
1	H		Iso	1	O	1
3	T		Iso	O	1	1
4	H		Iso	O	O	1
5	H		Iso	O	O	1
8	T	No intracranial filling	Iso	O	O	2
9	In		Iso	O	O	2
13	H		Iso	O	O	1
17	H		Iso	O	O	2
19	H		Iso	1	1	2
20	H		Iso	1	1	2
Group II (3 patients)						
6	H		Iso	O	O	1
11	H	Stasis	Iso	O	O	2
15	T		Iso	O	O,I	2

Group	No.	Cause*	Finding	EEG†	‡	‡	
Group III (4 patients)	7	T	Retrograde emptying	TU	I	I	1
	10	H		Iso	I	O	2
	12	H		Iso (artefact)	O	I	1
	16	H		Iso		O	2
Group IV (2 patients)	2	T	Posterior fossa flow	Iso	O	O	1
	18	H		Iso	O	O	2
Group V (1 patient)	14	In	Extravasation	Iso (artefact)	Small bolus	Small bolus	1

* H=hemorrhage, T=trauma, In=infarction.

† Iso=isoelectric or electrocerebral silences, TU=technically unsatisfactory.

‡ I=intermediate tracing, O=absent bolus.

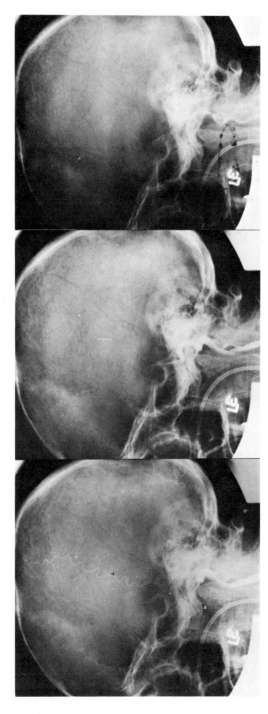

FIGURE 1. Left common carotid angiogram via femoral catheter demonstrating no intracranial filling of cerebral vessels (Group 1). (*Left*) lateral projection at 6 seconds shows good visualization of the external carotid artery and its branches including the middle meningeal, superficial temporal and occipital arteries. The internal carotid artery is opacified only as far as its precavernous segment. (*Center*) lateral projection at 10 seconds shows stasis filling of the internal carotid artery without antegrade progression of contrast medium further than the precavernous segment of the internal carotid artery. (*Right*) lateral projection at 29 seconds demonstrates persistent opacification of the extracranial internal carotid artery.

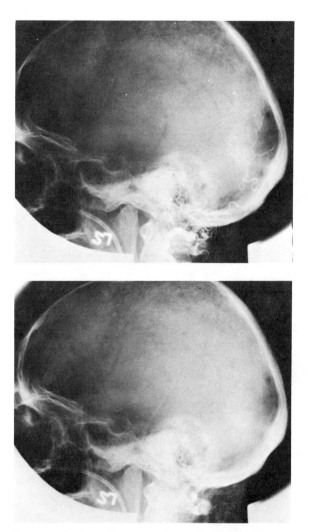

FIGURE 2. Left vertebral angiogram via femoral catheter in same patient as in FIGURE 1. (*Top*) lateral projection at 6 seconds shows good visualization of extracranial muscular and scalp vessels arising from the vertebral artery. The vertebral artery is opacified only to the level of C1. (*Bottom*) lateral projection at 12 seconds demonstrates persistent opacification of the cervical portion of the left vertebral artery without antegrade progression of contrast medium intracranially.

had electrocerebral silence on EEG, three demonstrated an intermediate tracing on the bolus radioisotope study. The phenomenon of retrograde flow was occasionally associated with stasis. As in Group II, there was no passage of contrast medium into the venous circulation.

Group IV included two patients in whom there was circulation in the *posterior fossa* vasculature only (FIGURE 7). Circulation was markedly prolonged (8 to 22 seconds), and one patient had stasis in the middle cerebral artery as well. Both patients had no evidence of bolus prior to or after angiography. Observation of transtentorial hippocampal herniation was noted with anterior

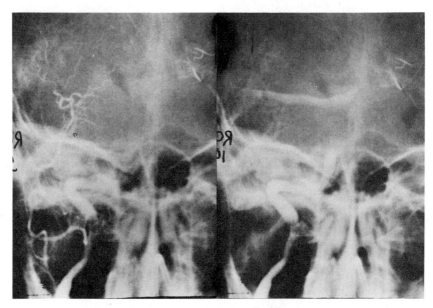

FIGURE 3. Right common carotid angiogram via femoral catheter (Group I). (*Left*) frontal projection at 5 seconds reveals opacification of the internal carotid artery only as far as its precavernous portion. Note excellent filling of the external carotid artery, particularly the occipital branch. (*Right*) frontal projection at 10 seconds fails to demonstrate cerebral filling. Opacification of the right transverse sinus is observed, filling presumably via an emissary vein.

displacement of the basilar artery, downward displacement of the superior cerebellar arteries, and posterior dislocation of the superior vermian branches of the superior cerebellar arteries. The contrast medium did reach the venous system on the posterior fossa study. It should be noted that at the time of angiography both patients had fixed and dilated pupils, with no evidence of brain-stem function and absence of spontaneous respiration. Therefore, these patients met all the nonangiographic criteria of brain death.

Group V comprises one patient with an unusual angiographic pattern of perivascular *extravasation* of contrast medium within the posterior cerebral

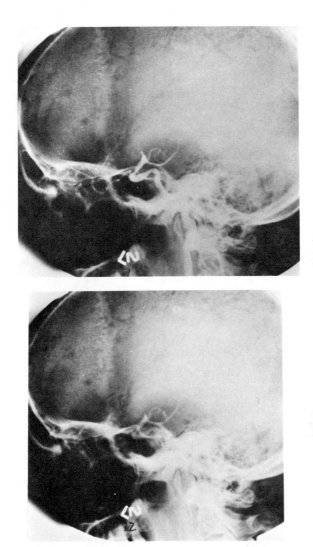

FIGURE 4. Left internal carotid angiogram via femoral catheter (Group II). (*Top*) lateral projection at 7 seconds reveals opacification of the ophthalmic artery, anterior choroidal artery, the posterior communicating artery, and the proximal portions of the left posterior cerebral artery. Miniscule filling of the proximal portions of the middle cerebral arteries bilaterally was observed in the frontal projections. (*Bottom*) lateral projection at 12 seconds demonstrates faint opacification of the ophthalmic anterior choroidal and posterior communicating arteries, as well as the proximal portions of the posterior cerebral arteries. The internal carotid artery is no longer opacified. This most likely represents retrograde washout.

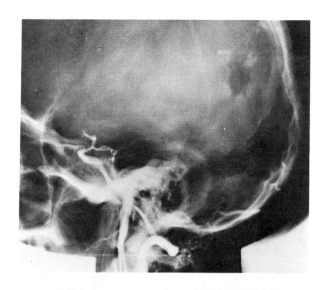

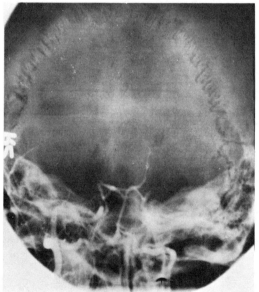

FIGURE 5. Right vertebral angiogram via femoral catheter (Group III). (*Top*) lateral projection demonstrates opacification of the right vertebral artery, the basilar artery, the proximal portions of both posterior cerebral arteries, both posterior communicating arteries, and both internal carotid arteries up to and just beyond the level of the anterior clinoids in antegrade flow. Retrograde opacification of the cavernous, precavernous, petrous and cervical portions of the internal carotid arteries, and reflux down the left vertebral artery are also observed. At no time was intracranial circulation noted. Excellent visualization of muscular branches arising from the vertebral artery as well as scalp branches apparently arising from the external carotid artery is noted. It is unclear whether these scalp vessels fill in antegrade or retrograde fashion. (*Bottom*) frontal projection demonstrates the shunting of contrast medium into the right internal carotid artery and left vertebral artery with stasis in the proximal posterior cerebral arteries, posterior communicating arteries, and basilar artery for several seconds.

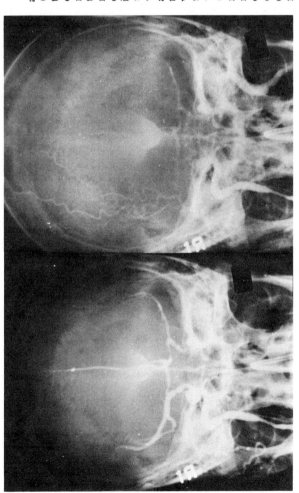

FIGURE 6. Right common carotid angiogram via femoral catheter (Group III). (*Left*) frontal projection at 2 seconds shows opacification of the right internal carotid artery, the right middle cerebral artery as far as the insula, the anterior cerebral arteries proximally, and the left middle cerebral artery up to the level of the insula. The most distal segments of the left internal carotid artery are also visualized. (*Right*) frontal projection at 4 seconds demonstrates opacification of external carotid branches, without further progression of contrast medium in the major intracranial vessels that was observed in FIGURE 6 (*left*). The intracranial vessels are more faintly opacified. The contrast material, however, has now clearly opacified the proximal (petrosal and cervical) segments of the left internal carotid artery indicating retrograde flow.

artery distribution on internal carotid artery injection (FIGURE 8). This region of extravasation persisted indefinitely and there was no posterior fossa filling from the vertebral artery. This patient had an EEG which was technically unsatisfactory, but which was probably isoelectric with artefacts. Radioisotopic bolus study revealed a small bolus prior to and after angiography.

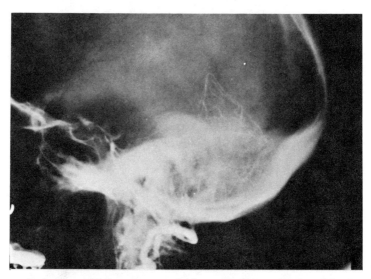

FIGURE 7. Left vertebral angiogram via femoral catheter (Group IV). Posterior fossa circulation, though prolonged, is demonstrated with a well-opacified arterial phase (intermediate and venous phase are not shown). Note the striking depression of the proximal portions of the superior cerebellar arteries and the compression of the vermis as a result of massive transtentorial herniation. The basilar artery is also anteriorly displaced and the tonsillar loop of the posterior inferior cerebellar artery is anteroinferiorly displaced, which is indicative of tonsillar herniation.

DISCUSSION

The clinical judgment of a physician in evaluating a patient who is diagnosed as brain-dead is to be considered paramount, and it must not be construed that angiography, more or less than any laboratory test, supersedes clinical judgment.[24] Nevertheless, demonstration of a cerebral circulatory deficit is the most direct corroborative study available for the documentation of such an awesome diagnosis. The results of this study show the intravenous radioisotope bolus technique to be the equivalent of angiography for this purpose.[15]

The bolus technique must be limited to adults, for infants and small children have not been included in this investigation. Therefore angiography may be considered a confirmatory diagnostic test in the diagnosis of brain death in infants and children.

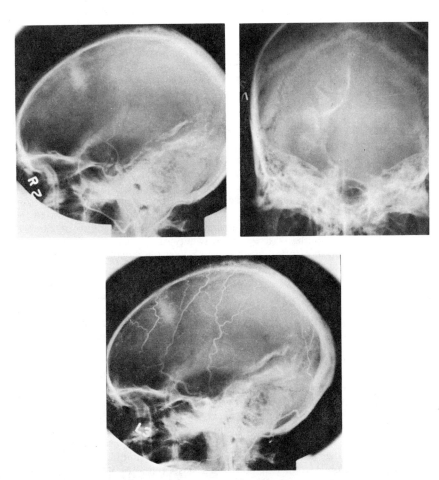

FIGURE 8. Right common carotid angiogram (Group V). (*Top left*) lateral projection reveals an opacified right internal carotid artery with numerous filling defects. The right posterior communicating artery is inferiorly displaced as a result of transtentorial herniation. Only the proximal portion of the right posterior cerebral artery is visualized. A large amount of contrast medium extravasates into the right posterior cerebral artery distribution. (*Top right*) frontal projection demonstrates the extravasated contrast medium to be within the distribution of the right posterior cerebral artery and free edge of the tentorium. (*Bottom*) left common carotid angiogram, lateral projection, done several minutes later than the two angiogram above shows persistence of the extravasated contrast medium, which remains unchanged in appearance. The left internal carotid artery and left ophthalmic artery are partially opacified. The external carotid artery branches are excellently visualized.

While electrocerebral silence on EEG has been reported in reversible coma states, such as those due to drug intoxication, hypothermia, metabolic disease and encephalitis, absent circulation has not been demonstrated.[21]

The conclusions from our earlier studies—that absence of a bolus, or an intermediate tracing in two successive tests performed approximately one hour apart, is incompatible with cerebral viability—have been confirmed by angiography.[3-5, 14, 16] It must be stressed that the bolus technique assists in the diagnosis of *cerebral death*. *Brain death* is the diagnosis that may be made in conjunction with other clinical and laboratory tests, especially those that test for brain-stem function. The reader is referred to previous papers that explicitly define these terms [14, 15, 17] and to other papers in this volume. Currently in the United States there is no uniform legal definition of death. The legal aspects of defining the irreversibility of brain function must consider the relationships and differences between cerebral and brain death, since this will possibly affect the significance of the confirmatory laboratory method that is used to determine the inviability of cerebral tissue.[14]

The angiographic findings of absence of contrast medium traversing from cerebral arteries to venous sinuses reflect absence of cerebral blood flow to the parenchyma of the brain and are incompatible with the viability of cerebral tissue.[12, 18, 20] This finding was seen in all twenty of our patients (FIGURE 1–8).

The mechanism most often presumed to reflect the angiographic demonstration of a cerebral circulatory deficit is that intracranial pressure has risen above the mean systemic arterial pressure or, more appropriately, the critical perfusion pressure, which therefore precludes perfusion of cerebral parenchyma.[6, 22] ‡ Most investigators report cerebral blood flow values of less than 10 percent in cerebrally dead patients.[7, 12, 13, 22] These appears to be a lower limit of cerebral blood flow that is incompatible with cerebral viability and represents a threshold of irreversibility. Evidence suggests that this value is in the range of 20 percent of normal cerebral blood flow with few exceptions.[2, 7, 13] §

The complete absence of cerebral and posterior fossa circulation at angiography (Group I) correlates with the absence of a head bolus on radioisotopic bolus study (FIGURES 1 and 2).

The presence of an intermediate tracing in two patients in Group I is probably related to the use of the now-abandoned dual-head probe which is excessively sensitive to the extracerebral circulation.[15] The dual-probe technique was used briefly and then dropped at the insistence of the funding agency.

On patient from Group I demonstrated stasis filling of the right transverse sinus, which fills via an emissary vein opacified by contrast material from the external carotid circulation (FIGURE 3). This adds further credence to the absence of intracranial venous filling. The emissary veins are a balance system receiving blood from both intracranial and extracranial structures. With lack of intracranial venous flow a low pressure system exists within the transverse sinus, allowing preferential flow from the extracranial circulation via emissary veins into the venous sinus.[9] Stasis filling of cerebral arteries as observed in Group II patients did not cause an intermediate tracing (FIGURE 4). Retrograde flow of contrast medium via reflux or shunting pathways (Group III) (FIGURES

---

‡ Other mechanisms are conceivable; e.g., see the paper by Pearson *et al.* in this volume.—*J. K.*

§ See also the paper by Ingvar *et al.* in this volume.—*J. K.*

5 and 6) from the supratentorial cerebral vasculature resulted in a persistent intermediate tracing even with a single-head probe. Such retrograde arterial emptying is considered incompatible with cerebral viability.[8, 17] Lin *et al.*[19] have shown that pressure injection of contrast material produces a transient elevation of intra-arterial pressure followed by a prolonged period of lower pressure, presumably due to a vasodilatory effect of the injected contrast medium. It is felt that in the brain-dead patient contrast material is mechanically forced into cerebral vessels, and that the reflux or shunting phenomena may be due to the proximal vasodilatation of extracerebral vessels that is known to occur with intra-arterial contrast medium injection.

The two patients listed in Group IV who had no angiographically demonstrated cerebral circulation, but had posterior fossa circulation (although it was abnormally slow), both demonstrated transtentorial herniation of supratentorial structures as a result of increased intracranial pressure (FIGURE 7). This posterior fossa circulation was undetected by the radioisotopic technique. Both patients had absence of spontaneous respiration and absent cephalic reflexes, with fixed and dilated pupils. The probability of potential return of brain-stem function in such instances is miniscule, and should not alter the clinical or angiographic diagnosis of cerebral and/or brain death. Buchler *et al.*[8] in their angiographic studies of 21 patients with brain death observed a temporal progression of lack of filling of cerebral arteries with subsequent involvement of arteries of the posterior fossa. This was presumed to be related to progressively increasing intracranial pressure, as the edematous cerebral hemispheres compressed and distorted the contents of the posterior fossa, and finally lead to total brain death.

The sole patient in Group V had angiographic evidence of perivascular extravasation of contrast medium in the posterior cerebral distribution (FIGURE 8). The radioisotopic study demonstrated a small bolus which presumably is related to repeated extravasation of radioisotope. Here the bolus study might be considered as giving a false indication of cerebral circulation, which would result in an error of diagnosing a patient with a dead brain as being alive. This mistake is acceptable, but the error that must never be made is quite the reverse.[4, 5]

The possible mechanism for perivascular extravasation of contrast medium rests in the complex physiology that separates the intravascular from the extravascular space of the brain. Suffice it to say that anoxic changes within brain parenchyma may lead to autolysis which effectively breaks down the blood-tissue barrier and allows transvascular diffusion of contrast media extravascularly.[10, 11]

CONCLUSIONS

The absence of intracranial circulation as demonstrated by angiography is considered incompatible with viability of neuronal tissue and therefore the *sine qua non* of brain death. Correlative studies with the radioisotopic bolus technique indicate that no bolus and intermediate bolus tracings represent a deficit of cerebral blood flow and confirmatory evidence of cerebral death.

The indications for four-vessel angiography to document brain death are relegated primarily to those ambigious situations when the EEG and bolus studies are nondiagnostic. Such angiography may be required in the diagnosis of brain death in infants and small children due to limitations of the radio-isotopic bolus technique. In terms of the medicolegal aspects of cerebral death, a distinction must be made between cerebral and total brain death, since the former is easily confirmed utilizing the bolus technique, whereas the latter necessitates appropriate testing of the brain-stem function.

SUMMARY

Intracranial angiographic investigation was undertaken to document the validity of the intravenous radioisotope bolus technique. Patients who met clinical and EEG criteria of brain death, showing flat or intermediate bolus tracings, were selected for angiography. All patients included in the study underwent bilateral carotid and vertebral basilar angiography performed by the femoral catheter technique. The angiographic series was prolonged so that the films covered a period of at least 30 seconds. All 20 patients who were investigated failed to demonstrate any supratentorial cerebral circulation. In 10 patients there was no intracranial circulation whatsoever. In three patients some stasis filling was noted in cerebral arteries, while in four patients arterial filling with retrograde emptying was noted. In these latter seven patients, there was never evidence of venous filling, indicating absence of cerebral viability. Two patients demonstrated abnormal slow posterior fossa circulation only. A final patient revealed only extravasation of radio-opaque material which persisted for many minutes. All but one patient met the clinical and EEG criteria of brain death. The exception was due to a technically unsatisfactory EEG. There were no instances where cerebral blood flow could be demonstrated by angiographic means where bolus technique indicated its absence. This angiographic study adds further credence to the efficacy of the bolus technique in the assessment of brain death.

REFERENCES

1. BENNETT, D., J. HUGHES, J. KOREIN, J. MERLIS, & C. SUTER. 1976. An Atlas of EEG in Coma and Cerebral Death. Raven Press. New York, N.Y.
2. BES, A., L. ARBUS, Y. LAZORTHES, M. ESCANDE, M. DELPLA & J. P. M. VERGNE. 1969. Hemodynamic and metabolic studies in "coma dépassé. A search for a biologic test of death of the brain. In Cerebral Blood Flow. M. Brock, et al., Eds. : 213–215. Springer-Verlag. Berlin.
3. BRAUNSTEIN, P., J. KOREIN & I. KRICHEFF. 1972. Bedside assessment of cerebral circulation. Lancet 1: 1291–1292.
4. BRAUNSTEIN, P., J. KOREIN, I. KRICHEFF, K. COREY & N. CHASE. 1973. A simple bedside evaluation of cerebral blood flow in the study of cerebral death: A prospective study on 34 deeply comatose patients. Am. J. Roentgenol. Radium Ther. Nucl. Med. 18: 757–767.
5. BRAUNSTEIN, P., I. KRICHEFF, J. KOREIN & K. COREY. 1973. Cerebral death: A rapid and reliable diagnostic adjunct using radioisotopes. Nucl. Med. 14: 122–124.
6. BRIERLY, J. B., D. I. GRAHAM, J. H. ADAMS & J. A. SIMPSON. 1971. Neocortical death after cardiac arrest—A clinical, neurophysiological and neuropathological report of two cases. Lancet 2: 560–565.
7. BRODERSON, P., P. HEILBRUN, O. PAULSON, J. OLESON, E. SKINHOJE & N. A. LASSEN. Quoted in Plum, F. & J. B. Posner. Diagnosis of Stupor and Coma. F. A. Davis Co. Philadelphia, Pa.

8. BUCHELER, VON E., C. KAUFER & A. DUX. 1970. Zerebrale Angiographie zur Bestimmung des Hirntodes. Fortschr. Geb. Roentgenstr. **113**: 278–296.

9. CHYNN, D. Y. 1963. Occipital emissary vein enlargement. Radiology **81**: 242–247.

10. GADO, M. H., M. E. PHELPS & R. E. COLEMAN. 1975. An extravascular component of contrast enhancement in cranial computed tomography. Part 1. The tissue-blood ratio of contrast enhancement. Radiology **117**: 589–593.

11. GADO, M. H., M. E. PHELPS & R. E. COLEMAN. 1975. An extravascular component of contrast enhancement in cranial computed tomography. Part II. Contrast enhancement and the blood-tissue barrier. Radiology **117**: 595–597.

12. GROS, C., B. VLAHOVITCH, P. FREREBEAU, A. KUHNER, M. BILLET, G. SAHUT & G. GAVAND. 1969. Critères arteriographiques des comas dépassés en neuro-chirurgie. Neuro-Chir. **15**: 477–486.

13. HOYER, S. & J. WAWERSIK. 1968. Untersuchungen der Hirndurchblutung und des Hirnstoffwechsels beim Decerbration syndrome. (Studies of cerebral blood flow and cerebral metabolism in the decerebration syndrome.) Langenbecks Arch. Chir. **322**: 602–605.

14. KOREIN, J. 1973. On cerebral, brain and systemic death. Current concepts of cerebrovascular disease. Stroke **8**: 9–14.

15. KOREIN, J., P. BRAUNSTEIN, A. GEORGE, M. WICHTER, I. KRICHEFF, A. LIEBERMAN & J. PEARSON. 1977. Brain death: I. Angiographic correlation with the radioisotopic bolus technique for evaluation of critical deficit of cerebral blood flow. Ann. Neurol. **2**: 195–205.

16. KOREIN, J., P. BRAUNSTEIN, I. KRICHEFF, A. LIEBERMAN & N. CHASE. 1975. Measurement of cerebral blood flow by the bolus technique as an adjunct in the diagnosis of cerebral death. 142 Studies on 80 patients of an innocuous IV procedure as an adjunct in the diagnosis of cerebral death. Circulation **51**: 929–939.

17. KRICHEFF, I., P. BRAUNSTEIN, J. KOREIN, A. E. GEORGE & A. J. KUMAR. 1975. Isotopic and angiographic determination of cerebral blood flow. Correlation in patients with cerebral death. Acta Radiol. Suppl. **347**: 119–129.

18. LANGFITT, T. W. & N. F. KASSELL. 1966. Nonfilling of cerebral vessels during angiography. Correlation with intracranial pressure. Acta Neurochir. **14**: 96–104.

19. LIN, J. P., I. I. KRICHEFF & N. E. CHASE. 1968. Blood pressure changes during retrograde brachial angiography. Radiology **83**: 640–646.

20. MITCHELL, O. C., E. DE LA TORRE, E, ALEXANDER & C. H. DAVIS. 1962. The non-filling phenomenon during angiography in acute intracranial hypertension. Report of 5 cases and experimental study. J. Neurosurg. **19**: 766–774.

21. SILVERMAN, D., M. G. SAUNDERS, R. S. SCHWAB & R. I. MASLAND. 1969. Cerebral death and electroencephalogram: Report of Ad Hoc Committee of American Electroencephalographic Society on EEG Criteria for Determination of Cerebral Death. JAMA **209**: 1505–1510.

22. SMITH, A. J. K. & A. E. WALTERS. 1973. Cerebral blood flow and brain metabolism as indicators of cerebral death: A review. Johns Hopkins Med. J. **133**: 107–109.

23. VLAHOVITCH, B., P. FREREBEAU, A. KUHNER, B. STOPEK, B. ALLAIS & C. GROS. 1972. Arrêt circulatoire intracranien dans la mort du cerveau. Acta Radiol. **13**: 334–349.

24. WALKER, A. E. *et al.* 1977. An appraisal of the criteria of cerebral death. A summary statement. A collaborative study. JAMA **237**: 982–986.

SURVIVAL AFTER SEVERE CEREBRAL ANOXIA WITH DESTRUCTION OF THE CEREBRAL CORTEX: THE APALLIC SYNDROME *

David H. Ingvar, Arne Brun, Lars Johansson, and
Sven Mårten Samuelsson

*Departments of Clinical Neurophysiology and Neuropathology
University Hospital, S-221 85 Lund; and the
Chronic Ward
Malmö General Hospital
S-111 45 Malmö, Sweden*

INTRODUCTION

In the present paper eight deceased patients are described who had all been exposed to severe cerebral anoxia and survived for varying periods of time (one week to 17 years). All showed a uniform clinical symptomatology with complete loss of higher functions (speech, voluntary motor activity, emotional reactions, signs of memory), but with good retention of brain-stem functions, including spontaneous respiration. These patients could be aroused by afferent stimulation, responding by primitive motor reactions, chewing, swallowing, respiratory changes, etc. The EEG was in all cases highly depressed, and in some cases isoelectric. The supratentorial cerebral blood flow was very low in the most chronic cases, and less so in a case with shorter duration. Neuropathologic studies showed a uniform picture with severe anoxic changes and an almost total destruction and disappearance of the telencephalic neurons. The neuron loss was especially marked in the patients who survived for several years, in whom the cortex had been replaced by a thin gliotic and fibrous tissue.

We have advocated the term "apallic syndrome" for states of the type described.[1] This term implies a loss of the "pallium," the cortical grey mantle that covers the telencephalon. It was introduced by Kretschmer[2] in 1940 to denote states with loss of telencephalic functions after severe anoxic, traumatic, infectious, degenerative, or cerebrovascular disorders. Gerstenbrand[3] also included acute, and to some extent transient, states following trauma with failing respiration and systemic circulation, epileptic symptoms, tonic cerebral seizures, etc. His definition was therefore somewhat difficult to outline, and this might have been why the diagnosis "apallic syndrome" has been used very little in the English literature. Instead, a number of terms have been employed such as "prolonged unconsciousness," "decorticate" or "decerebrate states," or simply "severe stuporous dementia."[4] In the French literature terms like "coma prolongé" or sometimes "coma vigile" have been advocated.[5] Some years ago Jennet and Plum suggested the term "persistent vegetative state" for similar types of patients.[6] Finally, Korein has introduced the term "cerebral death"

* This work was supported by grants from the Swedish Medical Research Council (Project No. B77–14X–84–13B and 12X–2037), from the Wallenberg and Thuring Foundations in Stockholm.

for patients with destruction of the major part of supratentorial structures [7] in contrast to "brain death," when the whole brain is destroyed.

The many diagnostic terms enumerated above have caused confusion, a fact to be regretted since the current discussion on brain death and related states puts great demands on clarity of nomenclature. Traditionally, one may label states of the type discussed in the present paper by emphasizing the functional and behavioral loss, by terms such as "permanent comatose states," "irreversible coma" and "persistent vegetative state." Another principle, preferred by us, stresses the pathoanatomic basis of the syndrome in question.[1, 6, 8] The term apallic syndrome has the advantage that it implies a severe total or almost total irreversible destruction of the cerebral cortex. This may serve to differentiate it from instances of transient disturbances of higher functions, as well as from states of permanent coma and unresponsiveness due to brain-stem lesions, in which there is severe dementia or global aphasia, and severe cortical lesions, sometimes in combination with brain stem-lesions.[3, 7-9]

TABLE 1

BASIC CLINICAL DATA ON THE EIGHT PATIENTS WITH APALLIC SYNDROMES

Case No.	Age at Death (yr)	Duration	Brain Weight (g)	Mean CBF (ml/100 g/min)	CMRO₂
1 (Ja. Fr.)	40	7 D	1250	. . .	. . .
2 (Ar. Ek.)	67	20 D	1370	. . .	. . .
3 (Ja. Br.)	53	30 D	. . .	28	. . .
4 (To. Ny.)	30	6 M	1345	13–16	0.34
5 (Ma. Lu.)	79	7 M	870	8	0.50
6 (El. He.)	55	12 M	1170	7	. . .
7 (Ag. Jo.)	43	8 Y	595	11	0.95
8 (Th. Sv.)	41	17 Y	315	9	. . .

Four of the present cases (numbers 3, 4, 6 and 7) have been discussed previously in another publication.[1] At that time, two of the patients (cases 6 and 7) were still alive. These two cases probably represent the longest survival ever reported—8 and 17 years, respectively—following complete loss of telencephalic functions. Due to the varying survival periods of the present patients it is possible to illustrate the progressive pathoanatomic changes that take place in the brain after severe anoxia (TABLE 1).

METHODS

Apart from routine clinical and neuroradiologic studies, as well as EEG examinations, measurements of regional cerebral blood flow (rCBF) were also carried out in six of the patients with the ¹³³Xe clearance technique (isotope injection in the internal carotid artery; 8 or 32 detectors) according to the method of Lassen and Ingvar.[10] The measurements were made without premedication and with controls of the arterial carbon dioxide tension. From the clearance curves various flow parameters were calculated. The main conclusions were based upon either so-called f_{init} values, calculated from the initial part of the clearance curve, or on f_{10} values, calculated from 10-minute clearance curves.

In three patients, cerebral venous samples were obtained via a cannula in the jugular bulb, introduced via a neck puncture of the internal jugular vein. From the arteriovenous oxygen difference, multiplied by the mean hemisphere flow, the supratentorial cerebral oxygen uptake was then calculated.

Neuropathologic examination was made on coronal sections of the brain which had been fixed in 10 percent formaldehyde. Representative sections were selected to cover all lobes and major circulatory territories, including the brain stem and cerebellum. After embedding in paraffin, whole brain sections, 6–8 microns thick, were obtained. The stains used included hematoxylin and eosin, luxol fast blue (for myelin), and cresyl violet. Some sections were also stained according to the method of Naoumenko for axons and with Sudan black B for lipids.

CASE MATERIAL

Case 1. The patient (Ja. Fr.) was a 40-year-old man who had had diabetes diagnosed at the age of 19. He had signs of retinal and peripheral neuropathy and had had angina pectoris for a year. The patient was observed to fall suddenly to the ground unconscious. He was admitted to the hospital within two hours in a deeply comatose state with ventricular fibrillation. After resuscitation pulmonary edema developed. And the deeply comatose state continued. Electroencephalography showed a severe general slowing and an amplitude depression that progressed. Much EMG activity was observed in all records. The patient developed spontaneous but irregular respiration after three days and he died in one week.

Autopsy showed an extensive myocardial infarction and bilateral bronchopneumonia. The brain weighed 1250 grams and was grossly unremarkable, apart from slight atherosclerosis of the larger vessels. Microscopically, however, there were signs of widespread severe ischemic neuronopathy with shrunken and retracted eosinophilic neurons with pale and pyknotic nuclei as well as diffuse glial hypertrophy and proliferation. These changes were mainly distributed within the cortical grey matter and basal ganglia. Some cortical areas in the unci and on the tops of the gyri were better preserved. There were also ischemic changes in the cerebellum. The brain stem was largely spared, the majority of the neurons there showing an entirely normal morphologic configuration.

Case 2. The patient (Ar. Ek.) was a 67-year-old man who had suffered from hypertension since the age of 30 years of age and from angina pectoris for the previous three years. His chest pains suddenly increased at home, and he lost consciousness. Immediate resuscitative measures were attempted and admission to the hospital followed 45 minutes later. An electrocardiogram showed ventricular fibrillation. Resuscitation regularized the heart activity and spontaneous respiration returned. Seizures were observed during the first 24 hours. The patient remained deeply comatose. Repeated EEG recordings showed initially continuous alpha wave activity also in frontal regions, unaffected by afferent stimulation, and much EMG activity in temporal regions. The frontal alpha wave then disappeared and the EEG showed a highly depressed low-voltage activity with a mean amplitude of less than 10 microvolts. The patient died after three weeks.

Autopsy showed an extensive myocardial infarction of the posterior and anterior wall of the left ventricle. The brain weighed 1370 grams and showed a general swelling without signs of herniation. Both hemispheres were softer than normal. Microscopic examination showed a widespread, severe, and in some places laminar, loss of neurons of the grey matter. The border zones between the middle cerebral and the anterior cerebral arteries showed especially marked changes. The occipital part showed the most severe damage which included the calcarine and pericalcarine cortical regions. Less pronounced changes were observed in basal parts. In general, the brain stem showed less pronounced changes. The cerebellar cortex showed an extensive loss of Purkinje cells. In places where the neuron loss was marked, astrocytic gliosis was observed.

Case 3. The patient (Ja. Br.) at the age of 53 years suffered a severe coronary thrombosis with ventricular fibrillation. He was brought deeply comatose to the hospital, where he was resuscitated. Eighteen days after the initial anoxic period the patient was still deeply comatose without any signs of higher cortical functions. His color was greyish and systolic pressure was 60–90 mm Hg. Respiration was irregular and there were slow but clear-cut motor reactions to afferent stimulation. The patient was, however, clearly arousable. The pupillary reactions were slow. Pain stimulation elicited a weak pupillary dilatation and weak withdrawal symptoms. The corneal reflexes varied. The spinal reflexes could not be elicited, and muscle tone was generally decreased. The Babinski sign was present on both sides. The EEG on the third day showed a very flat curve on the right side, and severely depressed slow activity on the left. Four days later no signs of remaining cortical electrical activity could be recorded. The EMG activity was, however, increased from muscles innervated by the trigeminal and facial nerves. The cerebral blood flow on the left side was highly reduced (28 ml/100 g/min; normal value 49.8 ± 5.4).[10] The patient died 40 days after the initial anoxic episode.

At autopsy a massive almost complete necrosis of the grey matter was found including extensive necrotic lesions of the putamina and globi pallidi. In basal cortical regions the necrosis was less evident. Unfortunately the brain stem was not examined. The microscopic examination of telencephalic structures showed many similarities to cases 1 and 2, reviewed above.

Case 4. The patient (To. Ny.), a 43-year-old man, had been diabetic for five years. He had increasing abstinence seizures related to alcoholism. The patient was found deeply unconscious at home with aspiration pneumonia. After resuscitation he remained in deep permanent coma with complete loss of all higher functions. Electroencephalography showed severe amplitude depression and general slowing. Brainstem reflexes were retained, including spontaneous respiration and vasomotor regulation. The corneal and pupillary reflexes were normal. There were active spinal reflexes and bilateral Babinski signs. On stimulation, primitive movements and altered respiration was observed. rCBF, measured five months after the anoxic injury, showed severe general reduction (14 ml/100 g/min; mean of four determinations) with an abnormal distribution, the highest values being recorded over structures representing the basal cortex and the upper brain stem. Verbal activation and cutaneous electrical stimulation did not change the flow pattern (FIGURE 1).

The patient died two weeks after the flow study, i.e., six months after the anoxic injury. Autopsy showed signs of juvenile diabetes with diabetic glomerulosclerosis. General atherosclerosis was also seen with bilateral necrosis and hemorrhage of the adrenal glands. There were also signs of bronchopneumonia and bronchitis.

At autopsy the brain weighed 1345 grams and appeared well preserved with only some atrophy of the frontal lobes and slight softening in the temporal regions. The basal vessels were smooth. Microscopic examination showed an extensive cell loss in the cortex, particularly in the depth of the sulci together with a brown and yellow discoloration of remaining cortical tissue. The cell loss and atrophy was particularly pronounced within the angular gyrus and temporal lobe, particularly on the right side, where a small cavity was seen. The corpus callosum was thinner than normal and the basal ganglia were well preserved. The brain stem and cerebellar hemispheres had a slight yellow discoloration. The pyramidal tracts appeared slender and greyish. The cortical destruction showed some regional variations. The crowns of the gyri were better preserved than the depths. The most severe involvement was found in the temporal lobes in parts of the insulae and adjacent parts of the operculae and parasagittal

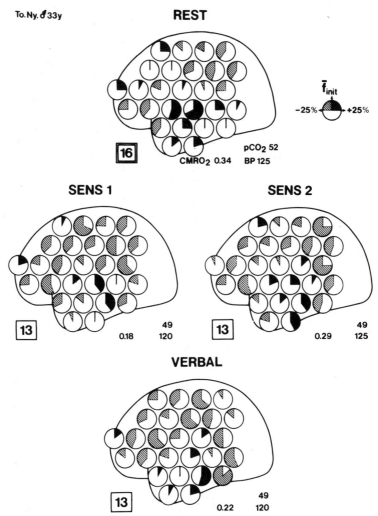

FIGURE 1. Case 4 (apallic syndrome following asphyxiation). Measurement of regional cerebral blood flow and oxygen uptake ($CMRO_2$) five months after cerebral anoxia. The values of rCBF measured by the different detectors have been plotted on an outline of the hemisphere drawn on a lateral skull x-ray. The clock symbols should be compared with the small figure in the upper right corner: the mark corresponding to 12 o'clock refers to the mean hemisphere flow values (16 ml/100 g/min) recorded at rest. *Black fields* to the right indicate values *above* the hemisphere mean and *shaded fields* indicate values *below* the mean. The three o'clock position indicates +25 percent and the nine o'clock −25 percent. The $CMRO_2$ values in the different situations are given in milliliters of oxygen per 100 grams per minute. Arterial pCO_2 and systolic blood pressure are given in mm Hg. Note the low resting mean hemisphere flow (16) with a concentration of the highest values of the basal detector fields, probably corresponding to the upper brain stem. Note that touch (sens 1) and pain stimulation (sens 2) as well as verbal arousal did not change the distribution of the flow. A moderate decrease was seen, possibly caused by a lowering of the pCO_2 due to increased respiration. (From Ingvar and Gadea Ciria.[8] Reproduced by permission.)

188

parts of the cortex, particularly frontally. Here the neurons had disappeared altogether and there was an intense gliosis and vascular proliferation. The white matter inside the gyri was demyelinated and gliotic. The striate body and the thalamus showed similar changes, but they were much less pronounced. The hypothalamus and the unci were well preserved. In the cerebellar cortex some Purkinje cells remained, although the majority had vanished together with parts of the granular layer. On the whole, the cerebellar lesions appeared less pronounced than those in the telencephalic cortex. The brain stem was best preserved, but here also some loss of neurons and some gliosis was seen.

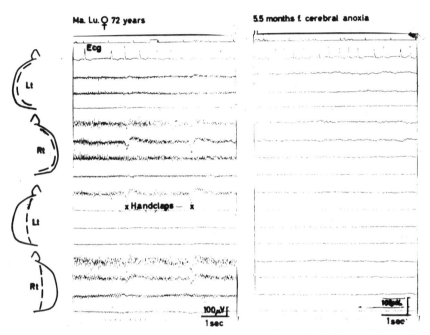

Figure 2A. EEG findings in Case 5. (*Left*) Tracing taken before administration of Selocurine. Note the tonic EMG activity and the blinking eye movements upon acoustic stimulation (x). (*Right*) Tracing taken after administration of selocurine shows absence of EMG activity. Note low-voltage EEG activity over right hemisphere.

Case 5. This patient (Ma. Lu.) at the age of 79 suffered severe coronary thrombosis, probably accompanied by cardiac arrest for an unknown period. On admission she was deeply comatose. Resuscitative measures re-established heart activity as well as spontaneous respiration. The patient remained deeply comatose without any sign of higher functions. Blood pressure was 150 mm Hg and there were no corneal reflexes. The pupils were initially contracted. Repeated EEG examination, (Figure 2A) (some done with the patient under "curarizing" or muscle-paralyzing agents) showed an almost isoelectric record on the left side, and some low-voltage EEG activity on the right with an amplitude not exceeding 10 microvolts. All EEG records showed massive artefacts from EMG activity in frontal and temporal regions, as well as from eye movements. A right-sided carotid angiogram was normal. After the initial phase, the patient's condition remained stable. She was clearly arousable. Stimulation with touch and pain elicited primitive motor reactions and some slow, blinking movements. Respiration was slightly irregular, often accompanied by swallowing and chewing. Normal pupillary reflexes were established later. The arm reflexes were normal bilaterally. No abdominal, patellar or achilles reflexes could be elicited. The Babinski sign was present bilaterally. Measurements of rCBF showed very low values with a mean hemisphere f_{10} of 8 ml/100 g/min (normal value about 50) (FIGURE 2B). A calculation of the relative weight of the grey matter (rapidly perfused compartments) showed a value of 8 percent (normal 50 percent). The supratentorial cerebral arteriovenous oxygen difference was 6.2 volume percent, a normal value. The mean supratentorial $CMRO_2$ was 0.5 ml/100 g/min, about one-sixth of the normal value.

The patient died seven months after the anoxic episode. At autopsy the brain was highly atrophic and weighed 870 grams (FIGURE 2C). Extensive fibrous adherences

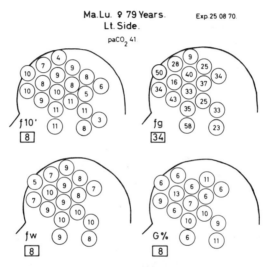

FIGURE 2B. Regional cerebral blood flow values in Case 5 calculated as so-called 10-minute values (f_{10}), grey flow (f_g), white flow (f_w) and G %. Note high reduction of all parameters (normal values f_{10}: 50, f_g: 80, f_w: 20 and G %: 50). The measurements were carried out four months following the initial anoxic episode caused by cardiac arrest.

were found between the brain and the meninges. Most gyri over the convexity were highly atrophic. The cingulate gyri and the unci were less damaged microscopically. The ventricles were highly dilated and in the atrophic cortical tissue small cavities could be seen. The thalamus and the hypothalamus were well retained. The hippocampi were sclerotic and atrophic. The white matter of the hemispheres was sclerotic and the peduncles were greyish. The cerebellum was also atrophic. There were no signs of herniation.

Microscopically, it was found that most of the telencephalic isocortex had been replaced by a severe gliosis which in some places had spared the second and third layers (FIGURE 2D). This was especially evident on the peaks on some gyri. There were many macrophages with iron pigments. In the white matter there was severe gliosis with fibrillary astrocytes and a loss of oligodendroglial cells, as well as fat inclusions in macrophages. The same picture was seen in the striatum and in the hip-

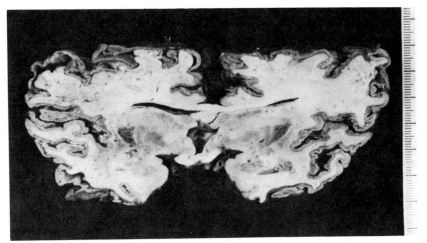

FIGURE 2C. Autopsy specimen (cm.) in Case 5. Note the extreme atrophy and shrivelled features of the cerebral cortex, upper brain stem.

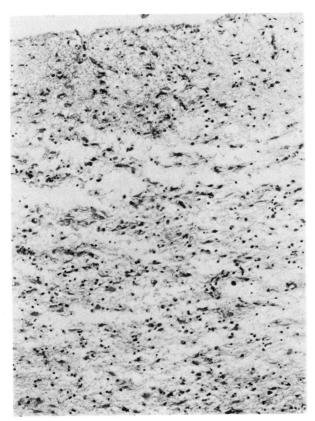

FIGURE 2D. Microscopic picture of the gliotic cortical tissue (cf. FIGURE 2C). Note the absence of neurons. Hematoxylin-eosin stain. (From Ingvar and Brun.[1] Reproduced by permission.)

pocampi. The cinguate gyri, the unci, the presubicular and entorhinal cortex were well preserved. Here the white matter was also well retained with normal oligodendroglial cells, retained myelin, and only a moderate giosis. The changes in the thalamus and hypothalamus were also relatively limited and most of the neurons appeared to be retained. The whole of the cerebellar cortex was completely atrophic in the depth of the sulci, some neurons were retained at the peaks of the folia. The brain stem showed normal findings in all nuclei, apart fom the substantia nigra, where minimal neuronal degeneration was seen. The reticular formation was well preserved. Here, however, a moderate diffuse astroglial proliferation was seen. The long corticospinal pathways showed a partial demyelination and some gliosis. The cerebellar pontine pathways were degenerated, and there was a severe gliosis in the inferior olives.

Case 6. The patient (El. He.), a 55-year-old man, had had alcohol problems for many years, having been admitted repeatedly to the hospital for gastric or duodenal ulcers, pancreatitis, methanol intoxication, etc. He had also been operated upon for rectal cancer, which showed no signs of recurrence. One year prior to his death the patient was admitted to a psychiatric ward. He had atrial fibrillation. One day he suddenly lost consciousness and was transferred to the intensive care unit, having cardiac arrest and no respiration. Routine resuscitation re-established heart activity. The patient remained deeply comatose, but after two days spontaneous respiration reappeared. Initially, the EEG showed suppression burst activity, but later no clear-cut signs of remaining cortical activity could be established. Much EMG activity was found from muscles innervated by the facial and trigeminal nerves. Movement artefacts from the eyes were also observed. Measurements of rCBF showed a low mean hemisphere flow of 7 ml/100 g/min (FIGURE 3). The highest values were found over the brain stem. No change in the flow was observed after intense sensory stimulation. The patient remained in a stable state of deep coma without signs of higher function for one year and then died.

Autopsy showed myocardial fibrosis. The brain weighed 1170 grams and was softened, particularly in parieto-occipital and temporal regions. There was an extreme cortical atrophy and disintegration of the underlying white matter. The unci were well retained and so was the brain stem. The cerebellum was atrophic and sclerotic. Microscopically, extensive damage of the whole of the neocortex was found. In some places the molecular layer was retained, with total destruction of the cortex underneath. In some places laminar necrosis was seen with a tendency to cavitation. In some regions there were smaller residues of the sixth laminar layer. The gliosis in the unci and the hypothalamus was only moderate. The optic chiasm, the optic tracts, and radiations were preserved. Otherwise the white matter showed severe general demyelination and gliosis. The cerebellum showed almost complete destruction of the

El. He. ♂ 55y

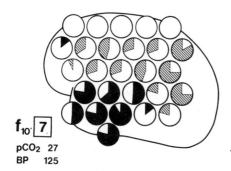

f_{10} ⎡7⎤

pCO₂ 27
BP   125

FIGURE 3. Case 6. Regional cerebral blood flow five months following the initial anoxic episode after cardiac arrest. Symbols are as in FIGURE 1: normal value $f_{10} = 50$ ml/100 g/min. Note the very low values over the periphery of the hemisphere and the high values over the brain stem (cf. FIGURE 1).

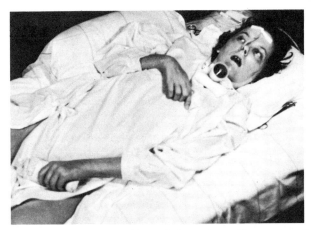

FIGURE 4A. Case 7. Habitual position of the patient. Photo taken four months after the initial anoxic episode.

Purkinje cells, partial destruction of the granular cell layer with demyelination, and gliosis of the white matter. The dentate nuclei were heavily damaged. The brain-stem nuclei were practically undamaged, and so was the reticular formation. In some places there was, however, some neuron loss and gliosis. The pyramidal tracts were demyelinated and shrunken.

Case 7. The patient (Ag. Jo.) was a 43-year-old woman (FIGURE 4A). For five years she had suffered from various transient, focal neurologic symptoms when, at the age of 35, she suffered a transitory left-sided hemiparesis. One year later she had a transitory right-sided hemiparesis and the following year weakness of the lower extremities and transient dysarthria. The diagnosis of multiple sclerosis was made. At the age of 35 she showed a moderate right-sided spastic hemiparesis, a slight dysarthria, and a sensory type of dysphasia. She then suffered acute severe cerebral anoxia caused by asphyxia due to dysphagia. There was no respiration for 15 minutes and the patient was admitted deeply comatose and cyanotic. Twenty-five minutes after onset of asphyxia no heart activity was observed. Resuscitation re-established heart activity and transient acute pulmonary edema followed two hours later. Artificial respiration was continued. Two days after asphyxia, weak pupillary reactions to light were observed. There were no Babinski signs, but weak patellar reflexes could be seen. EEG performed during this state (FIGURE 4B) did not show any signs of remaining cortical activity. A left-sided carotid angiogram (FIGURE 4C) three weeks after the initial anoxia showed normal findings. The patient had now regained spontaneous respration through a tracheal cannula. Two months later the patient developed a stationary condition which was confirmed in repeated clinical examinations.

When examined 13 months after the initial anoxic episode, she was lying down and had no movement unless stimulated. There were no signs of any higher functions. The eyes were kept open, the globes being somewhat divergent. Blinking movements were observed occasionally. The pupils reacted slowly to light and the corneal reflexes were weak. Audiopalpebral reflexes could easily be elicited. The spinal reflexes were normal on the left side and hyperactive on the right. Extension contractures had developed in both lower extremities. The Babinski sign was present bilateraly. The systolic blood pressure was 95 mm Hg, and heart activity was regular. All types of stimulation by touch, pain and noise elicited primitive stereotyped arousal reactions with rhythmic movements of the tongue and the cheek and some chewing and swallowing. The respiration also changed transiently. More intense pain stimulation elicited primitive withdrawal movements from other parts of the body. "Doll's eye" movements were produced, when the head was moved passively. When pressure was exerted on the carotid bifurcations, the heart rate slowed. Three months after the initial anoxic lesion a vertebral angiogram was taken and very slow passage of contrast medium was observed. Right-sided carotid angiography showed a slow passage of contrast and a marked filling of contrast in the choroid plexus. Angiography also showed signs of a moderate ventricular dilatation, but was otherwise unremarkable. Repeated EEG studies from the fourth day on did not give evidence of any remaining cortical activity.

Regional cerebral blood flow (FIGURE 4D) was measured twice, at three months and thirteen months, respectively, after the initial anoxic episode. Both studies

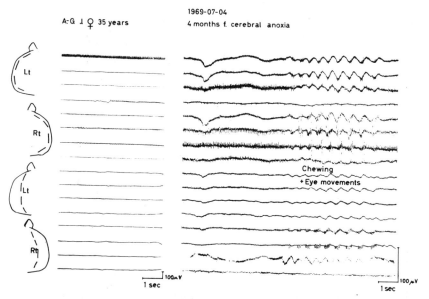

FIGURE 4B. EEG recording in Case 7 four months after the initial anoxic episode. Note extreme depression of the resting record with clearly visible EMG activity. On stimulation (right tracing) an increased EMG activity was seen including artefacts from eye movements and chewing.

showed similar results with a mean supratentorial CBF of 11 and 12 ml/100 g/min, respectively. The distribution of the flow values was highly abnormal in both studies, the highest flows being concentrated over the lower part of the detector field, over brain-stem structures. The second flow study was combined with jugular puncture. The arteriovenous oxygen difference was 8.5 volume percent, and the $CMRO_2$ was 0.95 ml/100 g/min. The patient remained in the above-described chronic state for eight years, when she died at the age of 43 after progressive deterioration.

Autopsy showed general atherosclerosis and bronchopneumonia. The brain weighed 595 grams and macroscopic examination showed very pronounced atrophy of the cerebral cortex. The brain stem and cerebellum appeared firm and shrunken. The medulla had a normal consistency. The ventricular system was widened and surrounded by only a 5-mm thick cerebral substance. The cortex and the basal ganglia were brown and yellow. Microscopically, the cortex was almost totally destroyed:

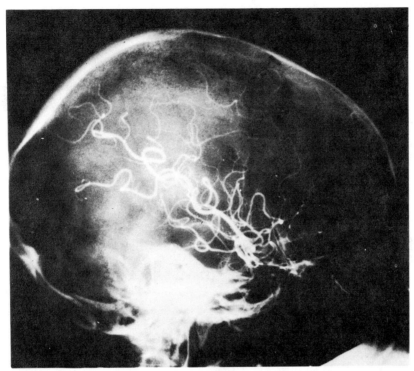

FIGURE 4C. Case 7. Internal carotid angiogram on the right side taken four months after the initial anoxic episode.

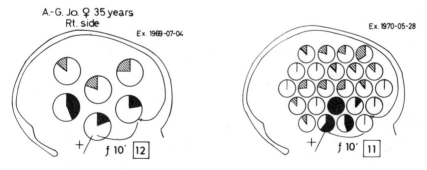

FIGURE 4D. Case 7. Regional cerebral blood flow four (*left*) and fifteen (*right*) months after the initial anoxic episode. Symbols are as in FIGURE 1. Please note the similarity between the two measurements carried out with seven and twenty-five detectors. Note also the same configuration of the rCBF distribution as in Case 4 (FIGURE 1) and in CASE 5 (FIGURE 3) with the highest values over the basal parts, probably corresponding to the brain stem. (Cf. Ingvar and Brun.[1])

There was a loss of most neurons and severe gliosis and spongiosis. However, the molecular layer was spared in some places, and there it also contained a few remaining neurons. The gliotic scar tissue contained macrophages with iron pigment. Groups of preserved neurons were seen, especially on the peaks of some gyri, but more consistently in the hypothalamus, the basal ganglia, and particularly in the unci, although with a loss of large portions of the neuronal population. The myelin was generally destroyed in the white matter, but remained to some extent preserved in the optic nerves and tracts and in areas containing neurons. In the cerebellum, the Purkinje cells had disappeared and were replaced by Bergman glial cells. The granular layer and the dentate nuclei were also heavily damaged. The brain stem showed gliosis and neuronal loss which, however, was much less pronounced than in the telencephalon. Some of the cranial nuclei were well preserved. Focal loss of myelin was seen in one of the cerebellar peduncles.

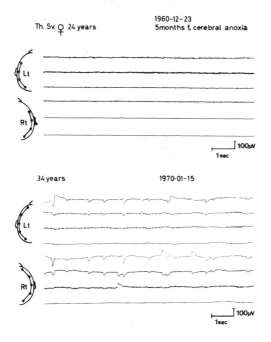

Th. Sv. ♀ 24 years

1960-12-23
5months f. cerebral anoxia

Lt

Rt

100μV
1sec

34 years

1970-01-15

Lt

Rt

100μV
1sec

FIGURE 5A. Case 8. EEG recordings five months (*top*) and ten years (*bottom*) after the initial anoxic episode. Note extreme depression and presence of artefacts from EMG and eye movements. In none of the records and in many others from this patient could it be established that any EEG activity remained.

Case 8. The patient (Th. Sv.) was a female who had been born in 1936. In July 1960, at the age of 24, she suffered severe eclampsia during pregnancy with serial epileptic attacks, followed by deep coma and transient respiratory and circulatory failure. In the acute phase, Babinski signs were present bilaterally and there was a transitory absence of pupillary, corneal and spinal reflexes. A left-sided carotid angiogram showed a slow passage of contrast medium and signs of brain edema. An EEG taken during the acute stage did not reveal any electrical cerebral activity (FIGURE 5A). The EEG remained isoelectric for the rest of the survival time (seventeen years). After the first three to four months the patient's state became stable with complete absence of all higher functions.

Examination ten years after the initial anoxic episode showed the patient lying supine, motionless, and with closed eys (FIGURE 5B). Respiration was spontaneous, regular and slow through a tracheal cannula. The pulse was regular. The systolic blood pressure was 75–100 mm Hg. Severe flexion contractures had developed in all

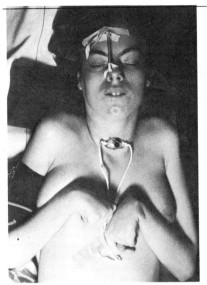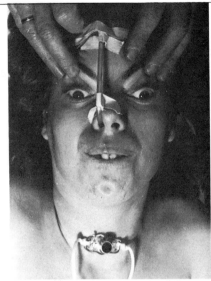

FIGURE 5B. Case 8. Habitual position of the patient ten years after the initial anoxic episode. There were flexion contractures and a divergent strabismus. The patient breathed spontaneously through a tracheal cannula.

extremities. Stimulation with acoustic signals, touch or pain gave rise to primitive arousal reactions including eye-opening, rhythmic movements of the extremities, chewing and swallowing, and withdrawal reflexes. The corneal reflex was present on the left side. When testing was done on the right side, transient horizontal nystagmus movements were elicited. Pupillary reflexes were present and normal on both sides. On passive movements of the head, typical vestibulo-ocular reflexes were elicited. The spinal reflexes were symmetrical and hyperactive. Patellar clonus was present bilaterally. Divergent strabismus was found when the eyes were opened. Measurement of the regional cerebral blood flow on the left side (ten years after the initial anoxic episode) showed a very low mean hemisphere flow of 9 ml/100 g/min (FIGURE 5C). The distribution of the flow was also abnormal, high values being found over the brain stem. The patient's condition remained essentially unchanged for seven more

Ty.Sv. ♀ 34 years
Lt. side

FIGURE 5C. Regional cerebral blood flow in Case 8. Symbols are as in FIGURE 1. The measurement was taken with the detectors placed close to the vertex. Note the same low flow value as in other cases in the series.

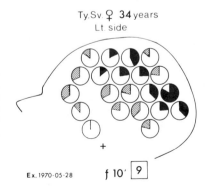

Ex. 1970-05-28   f 10' 9

years and she died seventeen years after the anoxic episode after repeated periods of pulmonary edema.

Autopsy showed a highly atrophic brain weighing only 315 grams (FIGURE 5D-H). The hemispheres was especially atrophied and they were in general transformed into thin-walled yellow-brown bags. The brain stem and cerebellum were sclerotic and shrunken. On the basal aspect some smaller parts of preserved cortex could be seen, mainly in the region of the unci. Microscopically the cerebral cortex was almost totally destroyed with some remnants of a thin gliotic molecular layer and underneath a microcystic spongy tissue with macrophages containing iron pigment. The white matter was completely demyelinated and rebuilt into gliotic scar tissue, and there were also scattered macrophages containing iron pigment. The basal ganglia were severely destroyed, whereas less advanced destruction was found in the subfrontal basal cortex, the subcallosal gyrus, the unci, the thalamus and hypothalamus, and in the subicular and entorhinal areas. In the cerebellum the Purkinje cells had almost

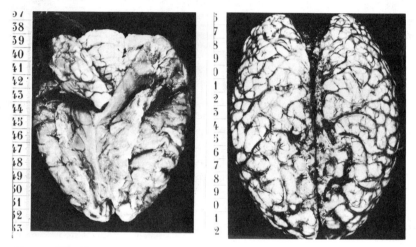

FIGURE 5D. Case 8. Upper view of atrophic brain weighing 370 grams. To the right a normal brain is shown for comparison. Note preservation of the cerebellum and islands of remaining telencephalic cortex in the apallic brain.

completely disappeared and were replaced by glial cells. The granular layer was partly destroyed. The cerebellar white matter was partly demyelinated. In the brain stem some neurons had disappeared and a diffuse gliosis was found. Several cranial nerve nuclei remained spared. The long sensory and motor tracts were completely demyelinated and gliotic, whereas transverse pontine tracts remained well myelinated.

DISCUSSION

It should be evident from the case material presented that all eight patients showed a similar clinical picture of deep permanent coma with total loss of higher functions and pathoanatomic findings dominated by very severe neocortical ischemic lesions. These lesions varied from extensive cortical neuronal damage in the cases of short duration to an almost complete loss of cortical cells in the patients who survived for years. This series of cases thus depicts the

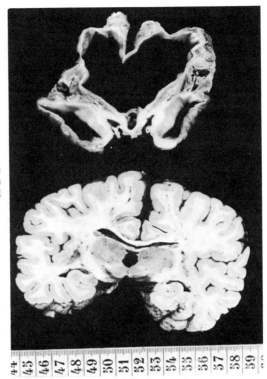

FIGURE 5E. Gross appearance of frontal brain slices in the apallic (Case 8) (*above*) and normal brain (*below*).

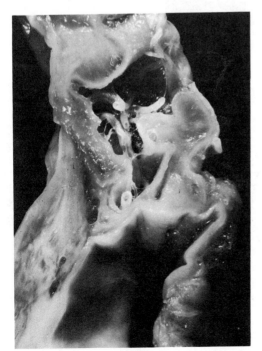

FIGURE 5F. Perisylvian area with white and temporal horn at the bottom and the lateral ventricle to the left. Underneath the solid white ribbon of the meninges and the molecular aganglionic layer, the cortex and white matter appear gelatinous and spongy.

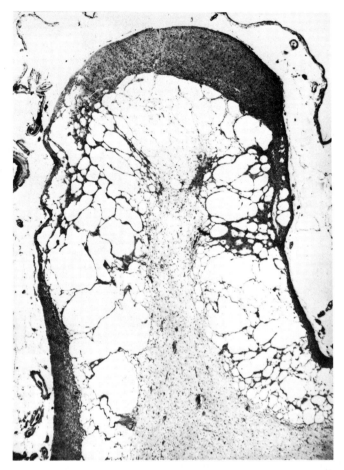

FIGURE 5G. Atrophic cortical gyrus from Case 8 with a mushy core of scarred cortex and white matter with small caps of partly preserved supragranular layers. (Magnification ×15. Hematoxylin and eosin stains.)

clinical and pathoanatomic course of survival after severe brain anoxia for periods varying from one week up to 17 years.

Patients surviving severe cerebral anoxia have been discussed previously by several authors.[2-8, 11-15] Brierley et al.[16] described two cases very similar to the present ones which were termed "neocortical death." Korein [17] has introduced the term "cerebral death" for patients suffering from loss of supratentorial structures. He stressed the difference between such states and the classical brain death in which there is complete destruction of all central nervous tissue down to the first cervical segment (C-1). Korein's term "cerebral death" appears to us authors less well chosen due to its linguistic similarity with the term brain death. Laymen and indeed many doctors do not always appreciate the difference between the *brain* (all structures from the cortex to segment C-1) and the *cerebrum* (the telencephalon). Criticism may also be raised against the term "neocortical death" of Brierly *et al.* Although it emphasizes the main patho-anatomic feature of the apallic syndrome, the inclusion of the word "death" tends to create some confusion with total brain infarction, i.e., brain death.[17]

The main additional information provided by the present series is the mea-surement of the cerebral blood flow (six patients) and of the cerebral metabolic rate (three patients). In addition, the autopsy findings picture the progressive nature of a severe anoxic lesion involving mainly the telencephalic cortex.

The main features of the eight cases presented are the following:

1. All patients had an episode of severe cerebral anoxia as the main etiologic factor. In six patients this was caused by cardiac arrest due to myocardial infarction, and in two by asphyxiation.

2. After resuscitation a deep comatose state developed with complete and permanent absence of all higher functions such as speech, voluntary movements, emotional reactions, and signs of memory functions.

3. Within the first few days brain-stem reflexes did come back in most of the patients as did spontaneous respiration. Thus, pupillary, corneal and spinal reflexes returned as well as an intense, often tonic EMG activity in muscles innervated by the trigeminal and facial nerves. Ocular movements were also observed which, however, were irregular and not of the roving or orienting type.

4. In the patients who survived the longest, i.e., more than a few months,

FIGURE 5H. Microscopic view of brain stem at the mesencephalic level showing well-preserved midline structures with retained neurons. (Magnification ×70. Hema-toxylin and eosin stains.)

thermoregulation was preserved and the electrolyte and water balance appeared normal.

5. All patients were clearly arousable, exhibiting primitive avoidance movements, chewing, and respiratory alterations on stimulation with touch or pain.

6. In some of the patients the EEG initially showed paroxysmal discharges of varying type, frontal alpha, as well as a severe depression. In all cases a very marked depression then developed in the EEG record which often had to be made with the patient under curare due to the intense EMG activity and the ocular movements. In some cases no electrical cortical activity could be recorded, and the EEG in these cases was diagnosed as isoelectric. No alterations of the EEG record were seen on afferent stimulation, i.e., there was an absence of EEG arousal.

7. The cerebral blood flow, measured in six of the patients, showed very low values (around 20 percent of normal). In one case of shorter duration the flow depression was less marked. In three cases in which the cerebral oxygen uptake was measured, extremely low values were seen. The distribution of the flow values over the hemisphere was highly abnormal, the highest flows being recorded over the brain stem. In addition, no flow changes could be elicited in two of the patients during sensory stimulation.

8. Pathoanatomic examination showed severe anoxic ischemic lesions of neurons of the cortex and a well-retained brain stem. In the patients who survived only a short time widespread acute severe ischemic neuronal changes were observed in the neocortex. In the cases with long-lasting survival, almost all of the cortex had been replaced by gliotic scar tissue except in the cingulate gyri and in the unci.

We have chosen to denote patients of the type described here as having an *apallic syndrome* since the main factor, confirmed at autopsy, responsible for the clinical picture was the loss of the cortical grey mantle, the pallium. Admittedly, some of the patients showed remnants of cortical tissue in isolated islands, mostly in basal parts of the telencephalon, in the cingulate gyri and the unci. However, the clinical observations did not reveal in any of the patients that functions remained that are localized to the neocortex. From the functional point of view all patients may therefore be considered as having a total apallic syndrome.

In his monograph, Gerstenbrand [3] uses the term "das apallisches Syndrome" less strictly. He includes within it many types of patients, as well as those suffering from decerebrate rigidity after brain trauma, and chronic stuporous state with severe dementia. According to the detailed descriptions given, a number of telencephalic functions could still be demonstrated in several of his patients and in some the symptoms were only transient. Many patients showed grasp reflexes and primitive, possibly purposeful voluntary movements, as well as complex, primitive emotional reactions including vocalization. Most patients were severely aphasic and several of them had a retained but highly pathologic EEG recording of higher voltage. Elsewhere [8] it has been suggested that such patients, who clearly differ from those described in the present series, might represent ""dyspallic" or "incomplete apallic" syndromes.

The differential diagnosis in patients with apallic syndromes and those with *brain death* does not present any problems.[7, 8, 12, 17, 18] Brain death, which implies a total brain infarction,[17] results in a complete loss of all cerebral *and* brain-stem functions, including respiration. Furthermore, it should be stressed that the state of brain death does not last more than three to five days in the majority of cases, apart from that seen in children, in which cardiac activity may continue for two or three weeks at the most. As pointed out by Korein and others,[7, 17, 19, 20] brain death is accompanied by absence of cerebral circulation, which can be demonstrated by four-vessel angiography and often by isotope encephalography. In the present cases of apallic syndrome intracranial (including supratentorial) blood flow was clearly demonstrated with the ^{133}Xe isotope technique as well as with cerebral angiography in three cases.

When comparing apallic syndromes with other *comatose states* it should be stressed that apallic patients with a still functioning brain stem all show an arousability to a greater or lesser extent, reacting with primitive movements, chewing and swallowing, and withdrawal reactions on afferent stimulation. Some autonomic responses (heart rate changes) could also be elicited, most clearly in the long-surviving chronic patients described above. It should be noted, however, that these primitive arousal reactions did not include any EEG if such activity could be recorded.

States of coma (in a more narrow sense) caused by lesions of mesial brain-stem structures, including the reticular formation, differ principally from apallic syndromes by the patient's being *nonarousable*.[9, 18, 21, 22] One case of a selective lesion of the reticular core is of special interest in the present discussion. This patient had a mesencephalic cerebrovascular lesion with almost complete destruction of the periaqueductal reticular formation, which resulted in a comatose state lasting three years. His EEG was very slow and there was a complete absence of all higher functions as well as a lack of arousability and no arousal reactions on the EEG. Remarkably enough autopsy examination showed that the atrophic-degenerative changes in the cerebral cortex were very limited. If this case and similar ones[4] are compared to the eight cases presented above, they illustrate the advantage of using the term arousability in the clinical analysis of patients in coma who lack all higher functions. This term may contribute to an operational definition of coma, and one may thus avoid the difficult decision of whether a given patient is conscious or not.

Patients with so-called *coma vigile*[5, 18] should also be recalled here. They show a reactionless state with complete loss of higher functions, spontaneous movements and speech. Some such patients are diagnosed as suffering from *akinetic mutism*[6, 18] caused by lesions of efferent pathways and/or upper brain-stem structures. Such patients may have a normal EEG and they also have a high cerebral blood flow and metabolism.[8] Related cases may have retained eye-movement control and clear-cut signs of mental activity (*locked-in syndromes*).[6, 8] †

The Pathogenesis

It is not possible at present to explain the selective massive anoxic destruction of the telencephalon in the patients summarized above. In none of the cases was there evidence at autopsy of a tentorial herniation that could have explained the extensive supratentorial brain lesions. However transient such herniation and indeed brain edema might be in the acute phase, it might com-

† See the paper by Posner in this volume—*J. K.*

promise the carotid flow, including the flow in the posterior cerebral artery, while leaving the circulation to the upper and lower brain stem, including the thalamus and the hypothalamus, essentially intact.[23]

It is natural here to recall that the present apallic cases illustrate the classical principle of selective vulnerability, which implies that the telencephalic cortex and the cerebellar cortex are more vulnerable to anoxia than are the brain stem and spinal cord.[14, 24] However, hemodynamic factors should not be excluded. They could play a role in the preservation of basal cortical parts in the cingulate gyri and in the unci. In some of the cases of shorter duration there was also evidence that the watershed areas between the territories of the larger cerebral arteries showed more pronounced changes than did the cortical fields in between.[25, 26]

In several brain specimens, islands of cortical neurons, mainly in the molecular layer, were seen, especially on the peaks of the gyri. The mechanism responsible for this distribution of the lesions is unknown. Possibly, acute brain edema, exerting its most profound influence along the walls of the sulci, could have played a role. A persistent nutrient flow in superficial vessels could have saved some neurons at the cortical surface in this situation. But, to judge from the clinical symptoms and the EEG, these remaining neurons did not retain any function at all.

Another etiologic factors responsible for the severe cortical neuron loss could have been the epileptic seizures taking place in the acute phase once cerebral blood flow had been re-established. Such activity was observed in two of the patients before severe EEG depression developed. It is well known that the metabolic demands in an epileptic cortex are highly increased.[26] Such an increased demand in the postanoxic state with a failing systemic circulation and blood pressure could have been deleterious, and further increased the anoxia of the brain tissue, causing edema and further compromising the tissue perfusion. Epileptic seizures could thus have contributed to the vicious circle that resulted in the enormous destruction of the cortical neurons.

The neuropathologic findings in the brains of the eight patients indicate that the degenerative changes in the apallic syndrome develop progressively. In the initial stages widespread ischemic changes are seen in the cortical neurons of varying intensity with pale or pyknotic cell bodies, eosinophilic neurons, small, dense nuclei, etc.[14, 24] Slowly the neurons disappear, being substituted by a shrunken gliotic scar. Later, the axons also disappear, resulting in a secondary severe atrophy and vacuolization of the white matter. Finally, the whole of the telencephalic cortex is transformed into a shrunken mass. In many cases in the present series only the cingulate gyri and the unci were saved. The cerebellum appeared less consistently and less completely involved, but a main feature was the loss of Purkinje cells. Here it should be recalled that morphologic changes of the type described are also seen around an infarction. Fresh infarcts show retained neuronal elements with anoxic changes of varying intensity, while in later stages the neurons disappear and a gliotic scar develops.

The Cerebral Circulation in Apallic Syndromes

As shown in six of our cases, the supratentorial blood flow was highly reduced. In three patients this was also demonstrated by cerebral angiography, even after months of apallism. It appears that the gliotic supratentorial tissue may retain a normal configuration for a long time, allowing for a normal vascular pattern to appear in the angiographic picture.

The intra-arterial ^{133}Xe studies demonstrated clearly that the blood flow in the long-surviving cases was reduced to extremely low values (to about 10–20 percent of the normal level). This is even below the normal flow for the white matter of the brain, which is usually about 20 ml/100 g/min.[10] The low supratentorial flow illustrates the reduced metabolic demand of the gliotic scar tissue, a conclusion that is supported by the determination of $CMRO_2$ in three of the cases, in which values of 0.34, 0.50 and 0.95 ml/100 g/min were found. The low flow and metabolism apparently represent the basic requirements for the gliotic tissue lacking neurons which are responsible for the high oxygen consumption and blood flow of the normal cortex. One should, however, introduce a word of caution here. The findings with cerebral venous sampling in apallic patients, in whom the cerebral circulation is reduced, appear uncertain since such samples may be contaminated by venous blood from nonsupratentorial cerebral structures. Therefore the accuracy of the arteriovenous oxygen differences obtained is open to question.

One feature of the rCBF pattern should be emphasized. Many patients showed a distinctly abnormal distribution of rCBF with very low values, or no recordable flow over hemisphere structures, and the highest flows, in some cases around 20–30 ml/100 g/min, over the upper brain stem in the lower part of the detector field. This pattern appears pathognomonic for apallic cases and might be of diagnostic value in chronic comatose cases. In the shorter-surviving cases higher blood flow values were seen. Such high flows could have been caused by a remaining postanoxic lactacidosis of the brain tissue, which becomes hyperemic when the systemic circulation is restored and vasoparalysis in the brain still prevails.

The Electroencephalogram

Concerning the EEG the main finding in the present series of cases was the severe amplitude depression which developed once the clinical state had stabilized and become permanent. In some patients no certain EEG activity could be recorded and these records were hence labeled isoelectric. This appears natural in view of the massive destruction of the cerebral cortex. However, some low-amplitude EEG activity was recorded in some cases, which was probably generated by remaining basal cortical or brain stem tissue. Possibly, isolated denervated cortical islands could also have given rise to bursts of electrical activity with a low amplitude. In apallic cases it would appear necessary to use depth electrodes in order to show fully whether electrical activity is present or not in supratentorial structures. It should also be emphasized that EEG recordings in apallic cases often have to be carried out with the patient under a muscle paralysant drug in order to eliminate artefacts from the increased tonic EMG activity and the eye movements induced from the active brain stem. However, both the EMG activity and the ocular movement potentials have diagnostic importance since they prove the survival of the oculomotor, trigeminal, and facial neurons in the brain stem.

Concluding Remarks

Finally, the existence of the apallic syndrome demands a consideration of the ethical issues involved. This syndrome represents a tragic example of the possible results of modern resuscitative measures. Similar conditions will most likely continue to be produced when facilities for acute treatment of cerebral anoxia are better developed. Furthermore, with increasing quality of care of comatose patients their life expectancy will most likely also increase. Although apallic syndromes of long duration do not appear to be numerous, their existence merits special consideration since, as shown above, survival time may be extremely long (being as long as 17 years in one of our cases). There is no need to discuss here the psychological effects upon the relatives of these patients in whom all signs of higher functions (i.e., all types of mental activity) are lacking. Nor will we discuss here the enormous economic cost of chronic intensive care.

The fundamentally important question might, however, be raised as to whether apallic patients with a destroyed telencephalon have any form of brain activity, which we normally consider a prerequisite for mental activity and consciousness. Indeed, the primitive arousal reactions seen in all our patients cannot, as such, be taken as a proof of remaining mental activity, only as a sign of persisting brain-stem functions. However, as a basis for further discussion of ethical aspects of resuscitative measures, and of the clinical handling of so-called noncognitive states, it appears that we need several additional detailed clinical analyses of chronic comatose patients studied by neuroradiologic techniques, EEG (with the patient under curare), measurements of the cerebral blood flow and oxygen uptake at rest and during activity, computerized tomography, and the like in order to reach a certain diagnosis. Such clinical studies may then form the basis for judging the patient's prognosis and for informing his or her family. Furthermore, such information may be useful in forthcoming discussions if limitations should be introduced in the care of permanently comatose patients who for months and years lack all signs of mental activity, and in whom it has been proved that the prerequisite for mental activity, the cerebral cortex, is permanently lost.‡

Addendum

During the preparation of this paper, the proceedings from a symposium held in 1973 in Florence, Italy have been published.§ This volume is of great significance to the current discussion on the outcome and sequelae of anoxic, traumatic, metabolic, and other severe generalized brain injuries. In the 36 contributions the clinical features, etiology, and the pathologic anatomy of various types of apallic syndromes are discussed. Under the heading "Apallic Syndrome" many of the authors include acute transient states of defective neocortical functions, as well as combined injuries of the brain stem and the cortex, as outlined previously by Gerstenbrand.[3] Many such patients might be

---

‡ This discussion may also be applied to anencephalic infants.—*J. K.*

§ ORE, G. D., F. GERSTENBRAND, C. H. LÜCKING, G. PETERS, & U. H. PETERS, Eds. 1977. The Apallic Syndrome. Springer Verlag. Berlin and New York.

considered as having "functional transient apallism," since they (in contrast to the present patients with total apallism) in their subsequent course often showed clear-cut signs of recovery with remaining neocortical functions ("dyspallism"; see above) and high-voltage pathologic EEG activity. Of special interest is the contribution by Heiss, who reports a reduction of the cerebral blood flow in 30 patients with symptoms of apallism. From the clinical history and the (relatively high) flow values reported, it is evident that his series, like others in the volume, includes many patients with acute head injuries with short survival time, as well as other less severe cases, even including some who "recovered completely." It may therefore be concluded that the present eight cases, as emphasized above, constitute a group of "pure" apallic syndromes in which the persistent and stable symptomatology was fully compatible with a total irreversible destruction of the neocortex and survival of the brain stem.

REFERENCES

1. INGVAR, D. H. & A. BRUN. 1972. Das komplette apallische syndrome. Arch. Psychiat. Nervenkr. **215:** 219–239.
2. KRETSCHMER, E. 1940. Das apallische Syndrom. Z. Gesamte. Neurol. Psychiat. **169:** 576–579.
3. GERSTENBRAND, F. 1967. Das Traumatische Apallische Syndrom. Springer Verlag. Berlin.
4. PLUM, F. & J. E. POSNER. 1966. Diagnosis of Stupor and Coma. : 86–101. Blackwell Scientific Publications. Oxford, England.
5. MOLLARET, P. & M. GOULON. 1959. Le coma dépassé.. Rev. Neurol. **101:** 3–15.
6. JENNET, B. & F. PLUM. 1972. Persistent vegetative state after brain damage. Lancet (April 1) : 734–737.
7. INGVAR, D. H. & P. SOURANDER. 1970. Destruction of the reticular core of the brain stem. Arch. Neurol. **23:** 1–8.
8. INGVAR, D. H. & M. GADEA CIRIA. 1975. Assessment of severe damage to the brain by multiregional measurements of cerebral blood flow. *In* Outcome of Severe Damage to the Central Nervous System. : 97–120. Elsevier. Amsterdam.
9. LASSEN, N. A. & D. H. INGVAR. 1972. Radioisotopic assessment of regional cerebral blood flow. Progr. Nucl. Med. **1.** S. Karger. Basel.
10. LINDSLEY, D. B., J. W. BOWDEN & H. W. MAGOUN. 1949. Effects upon the EEG of acute injury to brain stem activating system. Electroenceph. Clin. Neurophysiol. **1:** 475–481.
11. JEFFERSON, M. 1962. Altered consciousness associated with brain stem lesions. Brain **75:** 55–67.
12. BELL, J. A. & H. J. E. HODGSON. 1974. Coma after cardiac arrest. Brain **97:** 361–372.
13. OBRADOR, S. 1970. Damaged sub-responsive human brain. Acta Neurochir. **22:** 113–123.
14. SCHNEIDER, H., W. MASSHOFF & G. A. NEUHAUS. 1969. Klinische und morphologische Aspekte des Hirntodes. Klin. Wochenschr. **47:** 844–859.
15. SNYDER, B. D., M. RAMIREZ-LASSEPAS & D. LIPPERT. 1977. Neurologic status and prognosis after cardiopulmonary arrest: I. A retrospective study. Neurology **27:** 807–811.
16. BRIERLEY, J. B., J. H. ADAMS, D. I. GRAHAM & J. A. SIMPSON. 1976. Neocortical death after cardiac arrest. Lancet Sept. 11 : 560–565.
17. KOREIN, J., P. BRAUNSTEIN, A. GEORGE, M. WICHTER, I. KRICHEFF, A. LIEBERMAN & J. PEARSON. 1977. Brain death: I. Angiographic correlation with the radioisotopic bolus technique for evaluation of critical deficit of cerebral blood flow. Ann. Neurol. **2**(3)**:** 195–205.

18. PEARSON, J., J. KOREIN, J. H. HARRIS, M. WICHTER & P. BRAUNSTEIN. 1977. Brain death: II. Neuropathological correlation with the radioisotopic bolus technique for evaluation of critical deficit of cerebral blood flow. Ann. Neurol. 2: 206–210.
19. BRODERSON, P. & E. JØRGENSEN. Cerebral blood flow and metabolism in severe coma and brain death.
20. MATAKAS, F., J. CERVOS-NAVARRO & H. SCHNEIDER. 1973. Experimental brain death. I. Morphology and fine structure of the brain. J. Neurol. Neurosurg. Psychiat. 36: 497–508.
21. SIESJÖ, B. K., L. NILSSON, M. ROKEACH & N. N. ZWETNOW. 1971. Energy metabolism of the brain at reduced cerebral perfusion pressures and in arterial hypoxaemia. In Brain Hypoxia. : 79–93. William Heinemann Medical Books Ltd.
22. SCHOLZ, W. 1939. Histologische Untersuchungen über Form, Dynamik und pathologisch-anatomische Auswirkung funktioneller Durchblutungsstörungen des Hirngewebes. Z. Gesamte. Neurol. Psychiat. 167: 424–429.
23. LINDENBERG, R. 1963. Patterns of CNS vulnerability in acute hypoxaemia, including anaesthesia accidents. In Selective Vulnerability of the Brain in Hypoxaemia. J. P. Schadé & W. H. McMenemey, Eds. : 189–210. Blackwell. Oxford, England.
24. WEINBERGER, L. M., M. A. GIBBON & J. H. GIBBON. 1940. Temporary arrest of the circulation to the central nervous system. II. Pathologic effects. Arch. Neurol. Psychiat. 43: 961–986.
25. MILLER, J. R. & R. E. MYERS. 1970. Neurological effects of systemic circulatory arrest in the monkey. Neurology 20: 715–724.
26. LASSEN, N. A. 1966. The luxury-perfusion syndrome and its possible relation to acute metabolic acidosis localized within the brain. Lancet ii: 1113.

DISCUSSION

FEIN: I would like to point out that angiographic features are not necessarily static. Occasionally you will encounter patients, and we have had experience with three such patients in the last two years, who develop intracranial hypertension. An angiogram was performed which showed no intracranial flow. In these patients, we injected a bolus of mannitol and then repeated the angiogram, which revealed subsequent return of intracranial flow. These patients obviously had severe neurologic involvement but the status of their cerebral blood flow (CBF) is dynamic and may change.

PINTO: As I stated, CBF is based on a critical perfusion pressure. I believe that is why at one time you may see flow and another time you may see more or less flow using angiography.

FEIN: There is a current misconception that patients with total brain death can be maintained indefinitely or for a prolonged period of time by means of mechanical and other life-support measures. Dr. Ingvar has just alluded to the fact that this is not true. Eventually, these patients will deteriorate despite all supportive measures. The process may be delayed but not be prolonged indefinitely. Dr. Ingvar, would you comment on this?

INGVAR: Yes; it is our experience in Swedish hospitals that patients meeting the criteria of brain death, that is, unresponsive coma, apnea, absent cephalic reflexes, isoelectric EEG and nonfilling of all intracranial vessels on angiography, cannot be maintained for a significant period. The mean period of continuing activity of the heart is only three to five days. This appears to us to be a rather important fact.|| This should suffice to counteract the false notion that we are filling up our hospitals with brain-dead patients. This is not so. In contrast, what we may be doing is producing apallic patients by our resuscitative efforts, and to my mind this condition represents the state closest to brain death. But I certainly think it is important to point out that total brain death is not a prolonged state and of itself will never be a major medical or economic burden to society.

GOLDENSOHN: Although I don't have the exact figures, more than 200 of the 287 patients who met the criteria for brain death in the Collaborative Study had irreversible cardiac standstill after 48 hours. Therefore, the results from the Collaborative Study support Dr. Ingvar's statement.

M. NATHANSON (*State University of New York, Stony Brook, N.Y.*): In September 1977 in Amsterdam, Dr. T. Swick and I presented a paper reviewing 4 cases similar to those of Dr. Ingvar. These patients lived from 6 to 96 days after cerebral insult. The paper described these patients with persistent brain-stem reflexes and ECS. We were surprised when Dr. Ingvar stated in the discussion that he had a series of such patients who lived up to 17 years. Our findings were essentially corroborated by those of Dr. Ingvar and his colleagues. We believe these findings are very important. I agree with Dr. Ingvar that at this stage we should closely correlate the clinical and neurophysiologic findings underlying this marked dissociation between electrocerebral activity, decreased CBF, and persistence of brain-stem function.

In earlier studies on altered states of consciousness, I did work with caloric stimulation and oculovestibular stimulation. I was convinced that changes in ocular responses paralleled the depth of unconsciousness of the patient. For example, if the oculocephalic and the oculovestibular reflexes were absent, the patient was in a deep state of unconsciousness. I realize now that our conclusions were limited.

I believe that the term apallic syndrome is a good one because it tells us something. But I believe that the term coma as used in relation to some aspects of brain-stem activity should be confined to situations in which it is suspected that all the brain-stem functions are absent. For example, we had patients with brain-wave activity in whom there were no oculocephalic or caloric responses, and the pupils were fixed and dilated. These patients expired. In contrast, I will describe one case of a patient who survived for 96 days until cardiac asystole occurred. The patient had all pupillary reflexes and caloric responses were present. The EOG during caloric testing showed gross quick- and slow-phase activity, gritting of the jaw, and other stereotyped cephalic reflexes with absent EEG activity.

Pathologic examination of the brain revealed that the cortical mantle was gone and that lesions were present in the caudate and putamen. Microscopic examination of the cerebral cortex showed almost complete absence of neurons. In the cerebellar cortex, there were almost no Purkinje cells. In the brain stem, at the level of the third nerve nucleus, the neurons were intact, similar to the cases described by Dr. Ingvar.

|| In adults who are brain-dead, the maximal time to irreversible cardiac standstill does not appear to exceed one week; in children who are brain-dead, the maximal time to cardiac standstill may exceed two weeks with full life-support measures.—*J. K.*

One of the reasons for reporting these cases is that they are occurring more frequently, especially in patients with cardiopulmonary arrest. All of the four patients we described had cardiopulmonary arrest with subsequent resuscitation. If such patients have brain-stem reflexes, often a neurologist is not called and an EEG is not requested until four or five days later. Then, when a neurologist is consulted, we may be surprised to find that there is no brain-wave activity, even when the EEG is repeated.

MOLINARI: I have three questions, all for Dr. Ingvar and all directly related. First, how soon after the onset of cardiac arrest can one distinguish total cerebral infarction from an apallic syndrome?

Second, would you ever consider a patient in an apallic syndrome as a possible donor for organ transplantation?

Finally, is the norm in Scandinavia for determining total cerebral infarction still the clinically available angiogram or is it a sophisticated determination of blood flow?

INGVAR: To start with the last question, most places in Sweden still require four-vessel angiography to demonstrate the nonfilling phenomenon. This is to confirm the diagnosis of total brain infarction or brain death when the patient is being considered as an organ donor. I think I can say that is the official rule.

Your question as to whether we should consider patients in a complete apallic condition as potential donors raises a very important moral issue. As I tried to emphasize, these patients have permanently lost the prerequisites for mental activity. We can probably use the computerized tomography scan to see these atrophic brains, thus simplifying the diagnosis of the apallic syndrome. However, reviewing our own cases and those of Dr. Nathanson, it apparently takes some years before the white matter disappears. The apallic syndrome appears as a progressive pathologic picture when initiated by pronounced ischemic lesions of the neurons. Then, after a time, they disappear. After a longer period, the white matter is substituted by a glial scar.

As to your second question about whether such persons should be organ donors, I do not believe that we can answer that question currently. We still consider these patients to be "alive." At present, we do not have enough knowledge, nor have we sufficiently explored the moral and ethical issues in this type of case. But I think we will arrive at that point in the not too distant future with these patients.

As to your first question, I would say that in most of these patients spontaneous respiration returned within two to four days. However, most of the patients had cephalic reflexes at the onset, as well as EEG and CBF activity and therefore could easily be differentiated from patients with brain death. Then the course may often fluctuate dramatically. Respiratory, circulatory, and cardiac activity may show marked alterations. In order to clearly differentiate the apallic syndrome from other states, excluding brain death, I would like to observe the patient for a period of three to four months. In actuality, the pathologic substrate for the apallic state is present within the first to second week; to fully establish the clinical diagnosis would require several months, as I mentioned; the massive atrophy, however, clearly takes a longer time, probably many months to years.

PAMPIGLIONE: There is one point in relation to Dr. Ingvar's paper that I was not sure about. In the patient with the tremendously shrunken brain of less than 400 grams, there did not seem to be any thalamic system recognizable, at least at postmortem examination. I was wondering whether Dr. Ingvar has any comment on this particular point, since this would be more than just an apallic state.

I have further questions for those investigators who have done angiography and the bolus studies and have experience with these techniques. Did they find an absence of a bolus effect in patients with "inactive" EEG rather than ECS?

The other additional point in relation to the bolus is the question of the 30-second period. The 30-second period may be too short in situations involving obstruction of the superior vena cava, abnormal circulation due to multiple emboli, or severe cerebral edema. These factors may be responsible in part for the patient's comatose condition.

The last point that I want to make is about hypothermia. In general, the patients are warmed up to normal temperature before the EEG is performed, but even if the patients are hypothermic, we have found that the electric activity of the brain persists provided there is no hypothermia below 20° C of internal temperature. This does not refer to external temperature but to temperature measured from the rectum or the ear cavity. I think the general idea that ECS is the EEG might be due to hypothermia should be deleted from the general criteria.

INGVAR: Concerning the thalamus in the case you referred to, I presented the pathologist's report. The basal ganglia were severely destroyed. Less advanced destruction was found in the subfrontal cortex, the uncus, the thalamus, hypothalamus, and the subicular region. There was some thalamic tissue left, but this was present in a section anterior to the section illustrated in our paper. The hypothalamus was always retained in the patients. This is a prerequisite for the retention of thermoregulation, water and electrolyte balance.

BRAUNSTEIN: In reference to your question of the 30-second duration in studying CBF by means of the bolus technique and angiography, we often continued the procedure for well over a minute and even several minutes in many patients and there was no significant difference in our findings.

We were never able to study a patient with ECS who had a bolus. We did study some patients who had technically unsatisfactory EEGs, but there have been three case reports of patients with ECS. One of these patients who had a bolus survived.

PAMPIGLIONE: Have you seen patients with electrical activity but an absent bolus effect?

BRAUNSTEIN: No, never.**

J. GOODMAN (*Indiana University, Indianapolis, Ind.*): I would like to make a few comments about the gamma imaging technique of diagnosing brain death at the bedside. We first began to use isotope angiography for determining brain death at Indiana University in 1968, and in 1969 we wrote a paper in the

---

** In a more recent communication, S. Ashwal and S. Schneider (unpublished material) have reported seven children (age 0.25–30 months) with the clinical findings of brain death and absent cerebral circulation (four determined by bolus and three by angiography). In all these children, EEG activity was reported to have persisted throughout their course, which lasted from two to 32 days until cardiac standstill. Autopsy on one patient showed a respirator brain and CT scan on another also showed destruction of the brain. If this unusual finding is confirmed by others, it may represent another limitation of the use of EEG on young children and infants in the problem of diagnosing brain death.—*J. K.*

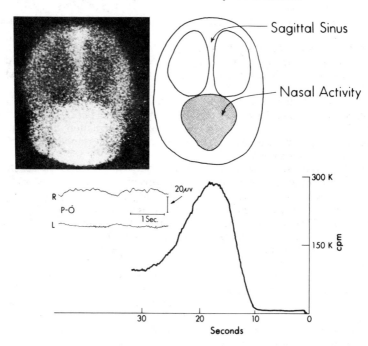

DISCUSSION FIGURE 1. Static gamma camera image, EEG tracing, and bolus study on apneic, comatose patient who is not brain-dead. Note presence of sagittal sinus.

Journal of the American Medical Association proposing that the absence of CBF on isotope angiography be considered a confirmatory test for brain death.

Dr. Braunstein and his group criticized the article, perhaps rightly so, by saying it involved taking a critically ill patient with all the respiratory equipment attached, to the x-ray department for this nuclear brain scan.†† Nevertheless, we continued to do it and, fortunately, we have had no mishaps so far and have done many such procedures.

In a typical isotope angiogram, a few seconds after injection one may, by using a tourniquet on the scalp to partially occlude the extracranial circulation and then by removing it, visualize the carotid arteries coming up the neck and stopping at the base of the skull.

Also, in diagnosing brain death by isotope angiography, we find absence of the intracranial sinuses. In our experience with brain scanning, it is rare to find absence of the intracranial sinuses unless the patient is brain-dead.

†† Dr. Goodman should be given full credit for his work using gamma imaging as an ancillary test in diagnosing brain death. In DISCUSSION FIGURES 1 and 2, there is a comparison between two patients, both of whom are in unresponsive coma and apneic. In DISCUSSION FIGURE 1, the gamma image, the bolus and the EEG are compared in a patient who is not brain-dead. In DISCUSSION FIGURE 2, these three tests are compared in a patient who is brain-dead. These studies were based on Dr. Goodman's original work and are referred to in the paper by Braunstein *et al.*—*J. K.*

About three years ago, a portable gamma camera became available and since that time, rather than using a bolus technique, we found it very useful to use the isotope angiogram with the portable equipment. There are now five companies making such portable equipment. The new portable machine can be used at the bedside and it has even greater resolution than those previously used. After we are sure that clinical brain death exists by all of the clinical criteria, we call the nuclear medicine department and they wheel up this machine. All the technicians in the department know how to use the apparatus. It is very simple and only a few minutes are needed to get a picture.

In the isotope angiography now performed with the portable equipment, a tourniquet is not required. Visualization of the subclavian vein allows us to determine that there is a good injection. The carotid arteries are also visualized in patients who are brain-dead, while there is no visualization of the anterior or middle cerebral arteries. We follow this procedure for a couple of minutes in order to obtain a scan with a higher count rate and increased resolution. The lateral and saggital sinuses are also not visualized.

We have used this technique for almost nine years and we believe that it is an extremely reliable adjunct in confirming the diagnosis of brain death. In fact, it has been so reliable in the last few years that we have not found it necessary

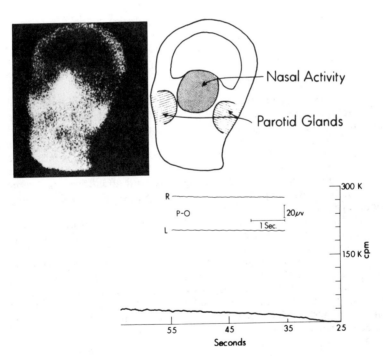

DISCUSSION FIGURE 2. Static gamma camera image, EEG tracing, and bolus study on a comatose, apneic patient who is brain-dead. Note absence of sagittal sinus and relatively empty appearance of brain area. Head is tilted because of tracheostomy in this patient. EEG and bolus show no activity or cerebral blood flow, respectively.

to do electroencephalography in most cases. The pictures derived from the test are very helpful; they can be shown to families and placed in the records.

BRAUNSTEIN: I will respond very briefly to Dr. Goodman's comments. Our main reservation about the gamma camera technique is that the background cannot be subtracted and it is important to be able to repeat the examination at short intervals in order to confirm the diagnosis of brain death. A single examination, we feel, is probably not enough. I know you can reproduce the static images later, but the flow study cannot be repeated in a short time.

GOODMAN: Nevertheless we believe that the pictures are good enough, and we prolong the test long enough in those patients in whom the diagnosis of brain death is being considered, so that we do not feel that a repeat study is required. We do not repeat most of our neuroradiologic studies.

PEARSON: I believe that Dr. Ingvar's figures showed between 18 and 22 percent of normal CBF in the patients that became apallic. In the bolus studies, the figure of 24 percent or normal CBF was mentioned as the threshold. This figure was presented in the context of studies indicating that above 24 percent of normal CBF a bolus would be present. The problem is that we do not know what the CBF values are when there is no bolus. We have assumed, on the basis of research performed by us and others, that no bolus would be present when the CBF is below 20 percent of normal. It could be anywhere between 0 and 20 percent. I wanted to mention this so that there is no confusion between the different types of CBF studies.

INGVAR: I agree with Dr. Pearson. This appears to be the range of decreased CBF where you might feel there is a limitation in reliability in using the bolus technique. In apallic patients, in whom the flow is very low, you may have a radioisotopic tracing similar to what you describe as a "small" bolus. I believe that the bolus test is qualitative and therefore may be unreliable in these circumstances.

BRAUNSTEIN: I agree that the results of the bolus technique are entirely qualitative, but in the large majority of the patients studied the transition from bolus to no-bolus state appears to be an all-or-none phenomenon related to a critical deficit of CBF below which cerebral neurons cannot survive. We believe that this is the 20 percent of normal CBF that Dr. Pearson referred to. The small bolus does not appear to be a transitional phase. One of the two patients with the small bolus, in fact, had angiography with absent cerebral circulation. The small bolus was apparently related to supratentorial extravasation of the radioisotope.

One of the exceptions that I pointed out was that in neocortical death or apallic states, we might not get a bolus, but these would be distinguished from brain death on clinical grounds.

HASS: To reiterate an obvious truism: I do not think that the bolus technique would be employed at our institution if the patient had intact cephalic reflexes; and I think that the diagnosis of brain death is not related to any particular test, however clear and absolute the result may seem, but is primarily a clinical diagnosis which may then be confirmed by a clinical EEG or other bedside technique.

COMA AND OTHER STATES OF CONSCIOUSNESS: THE DIFFERENTIAL DIAGNOSIS OF BRAIN DEATH

Jerome B. Posner

Department of Neurology
Memorial Sloan-Kettering Cancer Center
New York, New York 10021

The concept of brain death is now well established in the thinking of physicians and, to a lesser degree, in the thinking of the general population. As this Conference has demonstrated, there is also widespread agreement among the experts about both the concept and the definition of brain death. Although details of the criteria that define brain death have varied from committee to committee, the general principles of definition as outlined in TABLE 1 are all similar.[1-5] The first general criterion is that the nature of the process causing coma in the examined patient be understood, at least to the extent that one is certain that no endogenous or exogenous toxins or major metabolic or physiologic disturbance of the body's internal or external milieu be present. All criteria require that it be clearly established that the patient is not overdosed with sedative drugs, not hypothermic at the time the observations are made, and that the patient's acid-base balance and blood oxygenation are relatively normal when brain death is pronounced. In addition, some definitions incorporate into this section a set period of time over which the observations must be made so that one can be certain that metabolic abnormalities have not caused a state of apparent brain death.

The second general criterion is cerebral unresponsivity. Some define this simply by the neurologic examination;[2,4] others additionally require electroencephalography with one or often two isoelectric EEGs over a set period of time.[1,3] Korein and other investigators have shown that this criterion can also be met by demonstrating a critical deficit in cerebral blood flow, either by arteriography or by bolus injection of radioisotope.[6,7]

The third criterion is absence of brain-stem function, including nonreactive pupils, absent oculovestibular responses (tested by injection of ice water against the tympanic membrane), and failure of spontaneous respiration (tested by an adequate period off the respirator without evidence of respiratory movement). Some committees suggest that pupils be dilated rather than just unresponsive[3] since dilated pupils effectively rule out all sedative drugs except glutethimide. Others have suggested electrical tests of brain-stem function such as auditory evoked potentials as being confirmatory of the findings on neurologic examination.[8]

Whatever the criteria one uses to establish these three general principles, the results are much the same. The collaborative study headed by Walker has recently reported on 503 comatose and apneic patients using the above criteria; 187 patients appeared to have suffered brain death on the initial examination, and 185 of those patients died.[3] The two patients who did not die suffered from drug overdosage and thus, of course, "failed" the first criterion, i.e., that there be no toxic products causing coma. Thus, the evidence from this study and all of the other studies subsequently reported is that if strict attention is paid to the

0077-8923/78/0315-0215 $01.75/0 © 1978, NYAS

TABLE 1

GENERAL CRITERIA FOR THE DIAGNOSIS OF BRAIN DEATH

1. *Coma of established cause*
    No toxins
    Physiologic abnormalities corrected

2. *Cerebral unresponsivity*

3. *Absent brain-stem reflexes*
    Pupils
    Oculovestibular responses
    Respiration

criteria indicated above, diagnosis is 100 percent accurate, i.e., no patient who meets these criteria will recover consciousness, and in all these patients cardio-vascular function will cease within a matter of days. In the strictest sense, therefore, there is no differential diagnosis of brain death since the criteria have been so drawn that all patients whose brains are not dead are eliminated from consideration. One has only to attend scrupulously to the diagnostic criteria indicated at this symposium and one will not then include any comatose patients whose brains are, in fact, not dead.

There are, however, pitfalls in the diagnosis of brain death, particularly when coma occurs in hospitalized patients or those who have been chronically ill. Almost none of these will lead to serious error in diagnosis if the examining physician is aware of the potential pitfalls and if he attends to them when examining individual patients who are considered brain-dead. Some of the pitfalls that neurologists may encounter in attempting to make a diagnosis of brain death are outlined in TABLE 2.

In comatose patients, pupillary fixation does not always mean absence of brain-stem function. In rare instances, the pupils may have been fixed by pre-existing ocular or neurologic disease, but more commonly, particularly in a patient who has suffered cardiac arrest, atropine has been injected during the resuscitation process and widely dilated, fixed pupils may result from the atropine and not indicate the absence of brain-stem function. Neuromuscular blocking agents can also produce pupillary fixation, although in these instances the pupils are usually midposition or small rather than widely dilated.[9]

Similarly, the absence of oculovestibular responses does not necessarily indicate absence of brain-stem vestibular function. Like pupillary responses, oculo-vestibular reflexes may be absent if the end organ is either poisoned or damaged. Some patients otherwise neurologically normal suffer labyrinthine dysfunction from peripheral disease which pre-existed the onset of coma. Other patients with chronic illnesses have suffered ototoxicity from a variety of drugs, including antibiotics such as gentamicin.[10] In these patients, oculovestibular responses may be absent even though brain-stem processes are still functioning. Finally, a variety of drugs including sedatives, anticholinergics, anticonvulsants, and tricyclic antidepressants may suppress vestibular and/or oculomotor function to the point where oculovestibular reflexes disappear.[11]

Pitfalls also exist in the diagnosis of apnea in comatose patients who have been on respirators.[4, 12, 13] Many patients who are on respirators are hyper-ventilated, so that when the physician observes the patient after disconnection from the respirator, the patient begins with a low CO_2 tension. Since CO_2 production is often decreased in patients who are deeply comatose and since the threshold for respiratory drive in comatose patients may be raised, several minutes may have to elapse before the arterial pCO_2 rises to a level that will stimulate the respiratory center. Schaefer and Caronna [13] have estimated a rise of 3.2 mm of CO_2 tension per minute, so at least 10 minutes of apnea are required to be certain of a pCO_2 level that will stimulate respiration. If the patient is to be left off the respirator for 10 minutes, some method must be used to oxygenate him during that time.[4, 12, 13] The technique of apneic oxygenation allows one to disconnect the patient from a respirator for the requisite 10 minutes to be certain that there is no spontaneous respiration. To carry out this technique, the patient is first placed on 100 percent oxygen on the respirator for approximately 15 minutes until he is fully denitrogenated. Some have suggested that 5 percent CO_2 can be added to 95 percent O_2 to assure a relatively normal pCO_2 when the respirator is discontinued.[4] The patient is then disconnected from the respirator and a catheter is placed to deliver 100 percent oxygen, at about 6 liters per minute, to the endotracheal or tracheostomy tube. This technique allows for diffusion of oxygen across the alveolar membrane in sufficient quantities to keep the body fully oxygenated. One can then allow the pCO_2 to rise over a period of 10 minutes or more of apnea until it reaches 50–60 mm Hg to be certain that the patient has no spontaneous respiratory function.

The absence of motor activity also does not guarantee loss of brain-stem function. Neuromuscular blockers are often used early in the course of artificial respiration when the patient is resisting the respirator and, if suspected brain death subsequently occurs, there may still be enough circulating neuromuscular blocking agent to produce absence of motor function when the examination is carried out. A recent report has described the simulation of brain death by excessive

TABLE 2

SOME PITFALLS IN THE DIAGNOSIS OF BRAIN DEATH

Finding	Possible Cause
1. Pupils fixed	Anticholinergic drugs Neuromuscular blockers Pre-existing disease
2. No oculovestibular reflexes	Ototoxic agents Vestibular suppressants Pre-existing disease
3. No respiration	Posthyperventilation apnea Neuromuscular blockers
4. No motor activity	Neuromuscular blockers "Locked-in" state Sedative drugs
5. Isoelectric EEG	Sedative drugs Anoxia Hypothermia Encephalitis Trauma

sensitivity to succinylcholine.[9] In this case the EEG established cerebral viability.

Overdoses of sedative drugs likewise may abolish reflexes and motor responses to noxious stimuli. In patients with structural damage to the cortical spinal tracts sparing the reticular activating formation (the locked-in state), there may be absence of motor activity even though parts of the brain-stem subserving consciousness remain intact. On the other hand, the presence of some motor function does not guarantee that the brain-stem or brain are functioning. Multiple reports now exist of preserved spinal reflexes in patients whose brains are dead, and most committees no longer require total absence of motor function to reach a diagnosis of brain death.[14]

There are also pitfalls in using the EEG as an ancillary technique in the diagnosis of cerebral death. Isoelectric EEGs with subsequent recovery have been reported with sedative drug overdosage after anoxia, during hypothermia, following cerebral trauma, and after encephalitis.[3] Bennett *et al.* have carefully defined the artefacts that may appear in an attempt to establish an EEG diagnosis of brain death, and included in their atlas is a protocol for recording variables and placement of electrodes required to be certain that the EEG is isoelectric.[15]

Brain death is only one of the possible descriptions of brain function and the brain's relationship with the external milieu. How can one classify other states of consciousness? There are really four broad categories that describe brain function and its relationship with the world (TABLE 3): Those states in which cognitive functions are normal and the patient is fully responsive to appropriate stimuli (even though the patient may not be fully conscious at the time the examination begins); those states in which cognitive functions are diminished but in which the patient responds appropriately at least to some outside stimuli (states variously called delirium, dementia or stupor, depending on their clinical picture); those states in which cognitive functions are diminished and the patient is unresponsive to all outside stimuli (coma); and those states in which cognitive functions are normal or relatively normal but the patient is unresponsive on all or parts of the neurologic examination (pseudocoma).

In the first category in TABLE 3 (normal cognitive function/responsive), there are three possible states of brain function, i.e., wakefulness, slow-wave sleep, and REM sleep. These states differ markedly from each other in their clinical appearance but resemble each other metabolically. Only the first of these fits Cobb's definition of consciousness, i.e., awareness of environment and self.[16] However, in all three of these normal states the physician can easily

TABLE 3

CATEGORIES OF CONSCIOUSNESS

Category	Example
1. Cognitive function normal/patient responsive	Normal state
2. Cognitive function diminished/patient responsive	Delirium, dementia
3. Cognitive function diminished/patient unresponsive	Coma
4. Cognitive function normal/patient unresponsive	Pseudocoma

TABLE 4

DECREASED STATES OF CONSCIOUSNESS

Acute	Chronic
Delirium (clouding of consciousness)	Dementia
Stupor	Severe dementia
Hypersomnia	Hypersomnia
Coma	Coma
Sleep-like coma	Persistent vegetative state
Akinetic mutism	Akinetic mutism
Death	Apallic syndrome

arouse the patient to a state of full and sustained awareness which satisfies Cobb's definition. The first state is wakefulness; the degree of wakefulness may vary from extreme alertness to inattention and preoccupation, but in all instances in which wakefulness is normal, the patient can be made to attend to his environment and respond appropriately to tests of mental states. Sleep is also a normal state, which, at first examination, may resemble coma. Slow-wave sleep as defined electroencephalographically may vary from light to deep. There may be marked differences in the ease with which the patient can be aroused to attend to the mental status examination, but in all instances patients with normal sleep can be wakened. Cerebral blood flow and metabolism are normal.[17] The third normal state of consciousness is rapid eye movement (REM) sleep, from which the patient can likewise be awakened and after which he often reports the presence of dreams. All of these normal states have certain aspects in common. In each the patient can be brought relatively easily to a state in which his mental status examination is normal. In all, the EEG either reveals a normal waking record or can be made to become a normal waking record after attempts are made at arousal of the patient. Most importantly, in all these subjects the cerebral blood flow and oxygen uptake are either normal or significantly increased in REM sleep,[18] but in none is there diminution of either cerebral blood flow or oxygen uptake, as there is in most diminished states of consciousness.

The second two categories in TABLE 3 encompass the spectrum of diminished consciousness, which in man is wide (TABLE 4) and ranges from mild disorders of cognitive function called, depending on the setting, delirium or dementia, through stupor and coma to brain death. Even though in the milder states the patient is often aware of his environment and himself, all of these states have in common the inability of the patient to perform tests of cognitive function at his previously accustomed level no matter what the outside stimulus. These diminished states of consciousness are also usually characterized by a variety of abnormalities found on noncognitive neurologic examination (e.g., pupillary, respiratory, vestibulo-ocular, and motor abnormalities), by abnormal electrical activity of the brain (the EEG generally slows in direct proportion to the decreased state of consciousness, although there are exceptions, which include desynchronized EEGs in the acute delirium of drug withdrawal and normal alpha activity in the EEG of some patients unconscious after brain-stem infarction or cardiac arrest—alpha coma [19]). In addition, the cerebral metabolic rate is reduced in patients with diminished states of consciousness and the reduction in cerebral metabolic rate is in most instances proportional to the electroencephalographic slowing [20] and the patient's reduction of consciousness. Several different clinical pictures of stupor or coma have been described in the acute state: The common one is a sleep-like coma in which the patient lies unarousable with his eyes closed and demonstrates a variety of abnormal respiratory, pupillary, ocular and motor movements. A second state, hypersomnia, looks very much like normal sleep in that patients can often be transiently aroused to answer questions appropriately, only to fall off to sleep again. Findings on neurologic examination may otherwise be normal, although pupillary and oculomotor abnormalities are common. Such abnormalities have been described in lesions in the posterior hypothalamus and upper brain stem. A third comatose state is akinetic mutism,[21] a state of coma in which the individual's eyes are open and in which he appears to follow the examiner around the room, but from whom no speech and no movement can be elicited and in which the EEG is slow.

Sleep-like coma, which is the common form of coma in acutely developing states, does not occur in the chronic state. Nor is delirium or stupor a common finding in patients whose brains have been chronically damaged. Instead, patients with chronic brain damage may be demented, either mildly or severely, or, if comatose, they may have sleeping and waking cycles, often lying with eyes open and making some primitive responses to their environment, a state called by Jennett and Plum a "persistent vegetative state." [22] Akinetic mutism and hypersomnia, unlike sleep-like coma, may also occur in the chronic state.

As important as those states of decreased consciousness are the states in which the patient is unresponsive, but is in fact not unconscious. These states are classified in TABLE 5. The first is catatonia. Patients with catatonia are in fact awake, but may not respond to environmental stimuli, either verbal or noxious. Those with psychiatric catatonia may arouse themselves and usually remember and are able to report all the events of their supposed unconsciousness. Catatonia, however, is a symptom and not a disease, and symptoms similar to psychiatric catatonia occur with frontal lobe dysfunction and have been reported with drug-induced states.[23] Some patients with severe frontal lobe disease are so withdrawn that they appear to have decreased consciousness and may occasionally appear comatose. This state at times resembles akinetic mutism, but the patient is awake rather than comatose.[24] Finally, and most impor-

TABLE 5

STATES OF CONSCIOUSNESS MIMICKING COMA ("PSEUDOCOMA")

State	Cause
Catatonia	Psychiatric
	Frontal lobe disease
	Drug-induced
Abulia	
"Locked-in" state	Pontine lesions
	Polyneuritis
	Drugs (succinylcholine)

TABLE 6

ANATOMY OF ALTERED CONSCIOUSNESS

Site of Lesion	Symptom
Left hemisphere	Transient coma—aphasia
Frontal lobes	Abulia
Bilateral hemispheres	Coma—persistent vegetative state
Diencephalon	Akinetic mutism
Hypothalamus	Hypersomnia
Midbrain reticular formation	Coma
Basis pontis	"Locked-in" state

tantly, is the locked-in state.[2] Patients who are awake and reasonably alert may be unable to respond to their environment in any way because metabolic or structural disease of the nervous system has prevented the motor expression of cerebral function. Such patients are locked into their own bodies. The commonest cause are lesions of the basis pontis, in which all voluntary motor activity of lower cranial nerves and extremities may be absent. Some patients are able to move their eyes in an upward and downward direction or to blink their eyes, and some of these patients can use this eye movement as a method of communication. The EEG may be normal in these individuals, and in fact it may be the EEG that gives the only clue to the fact that the patient is not comatose. Similar locked-in states have been described in severe polyneuritis and with drugs, particularly neuromuscular blockers such as succinylcholine.

TABLE 6 is an attempt to classify altered states of consciousness anatomically. There is, in fact, so much overlap among these various states that it is impossible to do so with any certainty. In general, unilateral hemispheral lesions do not produce gross alterations in the state of consciousness. Left hemispheral lesions have been reported by some investigators to produce transient coma,[25] and grossly aphasic patients often appear lethargic and withdrawn and are less responsive to the environment than simply their language difficulty would warrant. With bilateral frontal lobe disease, there is a diminution of responsivity to the environment, and the patient becomes hypokinetic and at times mute. This state may become so profound that it may resemble stupor, but if patients can be urged or coaxed into responding, they are frequently in surprisingly good contact with their environment. With diffuse bilateral hemispheral disease, patients acutely enter sleep-like coma, and if the state remains chronically, they develop the persistent vegetative state in which eyes are opened and occasionally rove but in which the patients may make no more than primitive responses to noxious stimulation in their environment. Patients with lesions surrounding the third ventricle may develop a state called by Cairns akinetic mutism.[21] In this state the patient often appears awake, with eyes opened, and at times appears to follow the examiner. However, the patient does not move spontaneously, speak, or respond to noxious stimuli, although perioral reflexes, including swallowing, may be present. The EEG is invariably slow, and if the pathologic process can be reversed, when the patient wakes up he remembers nothing of the akinetic mute state. Hypersomnia,[26] a state in which the patient appears to be normally asleep and from which some degree of arousal can be elicited by noxious stimulation, has been described in patients with lesions in and around the hypothalamus. When these patients are aroused, they are often surprisingly in contact with their environment, but as soon as the noxious stimulus is eliminated, the patient often falls back into his hypersomnolent state. Lesions of the midbrain reticular formation produce in their early phase sleep-like coma and, if the patient survives into a chronic state, they yield a picture resembling the persistent vegetative state which is not clinically differentiatable from bilateral hemispheral diseases. Lesions of the lower pons and medulla do not produce coma, but lesions of the basis pontis may produce the locked-in state.

Since there are a variety of comatose or unresponsive states that may on first examination be confused with the state of brain death, a practical classification of the unresponsive states producing an unresponsive clinical picture is useful. These are included in TABLE 7. The first state is coma, which should be subdivided in the physician's mind into those comatose states that are reversible and those that are irreversible. Irreversible coma, however, is not brain

TABLE 7

CLASSIFICATION OF "COMATOSE" STATES

Coma	Reversible
	Irreversible
"Pseudocoma"	Psychogenic
	Structural
	Metabolic
Death	

death. Plum and his colleagues in this volume have presented criteria that often allow one to make a diagnosis of irreversible coma as opposed to brain death. A second unresponsive state is that of pseudocoma, which should be subdivided in the physician's mind into those that are psychogenic and can often be reversed by the use of "Amytal® interviews," those that are due to structural disease such as the locked-in state, and those that are drug-induced and due to metabolic disease. Finally, the third unresponsive state is that of brain death, the criteria for which have been listed in TABLE 1. Each time an unresponsive patient is approached by the physician, he should bear in mind four questions:

1. Is the patient comatose? Is the patient in fact unconscious or is the unresponsive state one of the pseudocomas?
2. What is the cause of coma? Is is due to structural or metabolic disease?
3. Is the coma reversible?
4. Does the patient meet the criteria for brain death?

All of these questions can be answered and a diagnosis of the particular unresponsive state from which the patient is suffering made by paying careful attention to the elements of the examination. All patients require a complete general physical and laboratory evaluation, particularly with respect to metabolic disorders which might be producing unresponsiveness. Neurologic examination should pay careful attention to both cerebral and brain-stem function. The EEG should be recorded. Radiologic tests, particularly the computerized tomography scan, are often necessary to find structural disease of the cerebral hemispheres or brain stem, and lumbar puncture is also often helpful in defining the nature of coma. Finally, in appropriate patients in whom the diagnosis is still unclear, regional blood flow and metabolic studies, as outlined in this volume by Dr. Ingvar, may be of great help in arriving at a diagnosis.

REFERENCES

1. BEECHER H. K. 1968. A definition of irreversible coma: Report of the Ad Hoc Committee of the Harvard Medical School to examine the definition of brain death. JAMA **205:** 85–88.
2. PLUM, F. & J. B. POSNER. 1972. The Diagnosis of Stupor and Coma, 2nd ed. F. A. Davis. Philadelphia, Pa.
3. 1977. An appraisal of the criteria of cerebral death. A summary statement. A collaborative study. JAMA **237:** 982–983.
4. 1976. Diagnosis of brain death. Statement issued by the honorary secretary of the Conference of Medical Royal Colleges and their Faculties in the United Kingdom on 11 October 1976. *Brit. Med. J.* November 13 : 1187–1188.
5. VEITH, F. J. *et al.* 1977. Brain death. I. A status report of medical and ethical considerations. JAMA **238:** 1651–1655; II. A status report of legal considerations. JAMA **238:** 1744–1748.
6. KOREIN, J. *et al.* 1977. Brain death. I. Angiographic correlation with the radioisotopic bolus technique for evaluation of critical deficit of cerebral blood flow. Ann. Neurol. **2:** 195–205.
7. PEARSON, J. *et al.* 1977. Brain death. II. Neuropathological correlation with the radioisotopic bolus technique for evaluation of critical deficit of cerebral blood flow. Ann. Neurol. **2:** 206–210.
8. STARR, A. 1976. Auditory brain-stem responses in brain death. Brain **99:** 543–554.
9. TYSON, R. N. 1974. Simulation of cerebral death by succinylcholine sensitivity. Arch. Neurol. **30:** 409–411.
10. JACKSON, G. G. & G. ARCIERI. 1971. Ototoxicity of gentamicin in man: A survey and controlled analysis of clinical experience in the United States. J. Infect. Dis. **124:** S130–137.
11. MLADINICH, E. K. & T. J. CARLOW. 1977. Total gaze paresis in amitriptyline overdose. Neurology **27:** 695.
12. SCHAEFER, J. & J. J. CARONNA. 1978. Duration of apnea needed to confirm brain death. Neurology **28:** 661.
13. BRANDFONBRENER, M., G. KROLL & C. BORDEN. 1969. Posthyperventilation apnea and the criteria of brain damage and death. Am. Heart J. **78:** 573–574.
14. JØRGENSEN, E. O. 1973. Spinal man after brain death. Acta Neurochir. **28:** 259–273.
15. BENNETT, D. R. *et al.* 1976. Atlas of Electroencephalography in Coma and Cerebral Death. EEG at the Bedside of in the Intensive Care Unit. Raven Press. New York, N.Y.
16. COBB, S. 1958. Foundations of Neuropsychiatry, 6th ed. Williams & Wilkins. Baltimore, Md.
17. MANGOLD, R. *et al.* 1955. The effect of sleep and lack of sleep on the cerebral circulation and metabolism of normal young man. J. Clin. Invest. **34:** 1092.
18. SEYLAZ, J. *et al.* 1975. Human cerebral blood flow during sleep. *In* Brain

Work, The Coupling of Function, Metabolism and Blood Flow in the Brain. Proceedings of the Alfred Benzon Symposium VIII, Copenhagen, May 26–30, 1974. D. H. Ingvar & N. A. Lassen, Eds. : 235–252. Munksgaard. Copenhagen.
19. GRINDAL, A. B., C. SUTER & A. J. MARTINEZ. 1977. Alpha-pattern coma: 24 cases with 9 survivors. Ann. Neurol. 1: 371–377.
20. INGVAR, D. H., B. SJÖLUND & A. ARD. 1976. Correlation between dominant EEG frequency, cerebral oxygen uptake and blood flow. EEG Clin. Neurophysiol. 41: 268–276.
21. CAIRNS, H. et al. 1941. Akinetic mutism with an epidermoid cyst of the 3rd ventricle (with a report on the associated disturbance of brain potentials). Brain 64: 273–290.
22. JENNETT, B. & F. PLUM. 1972. Persistent vegetative state after brain damage. A syndrome in search of a name. Lancet April 1: 734–737.
23. GELENBERG, A. J. 1976. The catatonic syndrome. Lancet June 19 : 1339–1341.
24. POECK, K. 1969. Pathophysiology of emotional disorders associated with brain damage. In Handbook of Clinical Neurology, Vol. 3: Disorders of Higher Nervous Activity. P. J. Vinken & G. W. Bruyn, Eds. : 343–367. North-Holland. Amsterdam.
25. ALBERT, M. L. et al. 1976. Cerebral dominance for consciousness. Arch. Neurol. 33: 453–454.
26. SEGARRA, J. M. 1970. Cerebral vascular disease and behavior. I. The syndrome of the mesencephalic artery (basilar artery bifurcation). Arch. Neurol. 22: 408–418.

DISCUSSION

INGVAR: I wish to discuss one expression. I know that my opinions may differ from those of Dr. Plum, and perhaps Dr. Posner, concerning the expression "persistent vegetative state." We have not discussed it in detail previously and I believe that we should expand on this now.

This expression seems a bit awkward to me because it does not tell very much about the patient other than he is vegetative. Since English is not my native tongue, it is not clear to me what "vegetative" means, although I know what "persistent" means. The expression may be unclear because it does not tell us the pathoanatomic basis of the problem.

PLUM: Dr. Ingvar, I believe that the only unfortunate part of the original term that Jennett and I used is the word "persistent." The description "vegetative state" is, I think, probably the least committal and yet most physiologically accurate term that we have to describe the clinical phenomenology in such patients since they undergo a variety of complex serial clinical changes following serious injury to the central nervous system.

The term was not taken from common lay usage. In fact, we were extremely sensitive to terminology which in some way may demean a sick human being. We found, however, that any set of terms that we considered were not those used by the friends or families involved. In fact, it was the families who most often implied that someone who had lost his higher mental functions, that is, was noncognitive, was a "vegetable."

The source of our terminology was derived from the studies of physiology initiated by the French in the early part of this century and expanded by Cannon to describe the vegetative or noncognitive components of the nervous system. Our description of patients who are vegetative includes those individuals who clinically have autonomic function. The term "persistent autonomic state" could have been employed almost equally well, except that the term is less flexible and would be less well understood by the patient's family. We were using the term, "vegetative" as a synonym for "autonomic" to imply loss of cognitive neurologic function.

A number of other terms have been used. "Akinetic mutism," for example, is a term I find confusing because its definitions vary so widely. These include patients who are catatonic, those who lack motivation, patients with frontal lobe disease, and patients with periaqueductal injury of the brain stem. The last mentioned are certainly mute. In many of these situations one cannot determine whether they are cognizant or not. Besides the fact that it helps to be a Greek scholar to understand its derivation, the term "apallic syndrome" implies that we have knowledge of the neuropathologic anatomy underlying the clinical symptoms—knowledge that, in fact, we do not yet possess. The anatomic distribution of injury to the central nervous system in patients who are functioning at a vegetative level varies enormously. This is particularly true among subjects who are passing through a reversible vegetative state in transition to a higher level of recovery, as discussed by Dr. Levy and his coworkers elsewhere in this volume.

Therefore, it appeared to Jennett and me at that time that "vegetative" was the most noncommittal word we could use in describing the clinical state of such patients, despite the fact that we knew of Dr. Ingvar's work on the apallic syndrome. Some of these patients do, in fact, have manifestations of brain-stem dysfunction which makes them more than apallic; it makes them hypomesencephalic. This is a nice illustration of use of terminology in which I may not necessarily agree with my colleagues. In the situation in which the patient has his eyes open and we wish to have an operational definition of coma, we must evaluate whether the patient is noncognitive. If the patient is noncognitive we use the term "vegetative state." Such forms of coma may be transient. Many patients recover to the point of awareness. The duration varies widely, but is apparently of no prognostic significance. In contrast, we consider patients with eyes closed and no evidence of self-awareness to be truly comatose. With the exception of this small difference of opinion, my views are identical to those of Dr. Posner.

BOSHES: Dr. Posner's paper raises a number of questions in my mind, particularly in relation to patients with various types of pontine lesions and the differential diagnosis of the so-called "locked-in syndrome." We may record our observations on examination and we may evaluate the patient's clinical motor response but can we evaluate what sensory stimuli the patient is capable of receiving?

In our earlier work in spinal man we developed a hierarchy of signals to which the isolated spinal cord will respond. For example, the spinal cord is most responsive to the application of ice cubes, which results in primitive spinal reflexes. There is a sequential increase in difficulty in obtaining the spinal reflex using stimuli such as a pinprick, a pinch, plucking of hair on the extremity, and finally, touch, in that order. With repetitive stimuli, reflexes are more complex and are related to serial inputs to the cord, which are summated.

Now if one uses similar peripheral stimuli in patients in the so-called "locked-in syndrome," what signals may be derived at the cortical level? For example, in some recent research in a patient with a pontine lesion, we were surprised that there was very little cortical response using auditory evoked potentials. However, application of ice to the soles of the foot, pinch, pinprick, and plucking of hairs on the extremity did give us definite alterations of cortical activity that we have not yet analyzed in detail. This particular patient has been in a totally locked-in "awake" state for more than three months. We have run her EEG as long as 10 or 12 hours. We have never recorded any sleep activity. One cannot communicate with this patient; her eyes move spontaneously with a suggestion of seeking movements, but cannot be used for communication. My question is: What sensory stimuli is she receiving? What impulses are being derived from sensory and other neural transmission systems?

POSNER: The problem with the neurologic examination is that one is only capable of examining the most distal loss of function. For example, a patient with no muscle function (if the muscles are destroyed), cannot be examined for peripheral nerve motor function or central motor function. You cannot examine brain-stem or cerebral function below the level of spinal cord destruction or transection.

In a patient with destruction of the brain stem, one cannot directly examine cortical function on neurologic examination. This can be done by means of electroencephalography, evoked potential work at times, and by Dr. Ingvar's very nice regional cerebral blood flow and metabolic studies, which indicate alterations produced by external stimuli. Dr. Becker has recently reported in the *Journal of Neurosurgery* the use of five modalities of evoked potentials to predict the outcome of head injuries. This does not necessarily apply to brain death since electroencephalographic and clinical criteria may clearly indicate that the brain is destroyed. It does apply to the differential diagnosis of comatose states, which can, at times, be very difficult.

GRENVIK: Spinal cord reflexes are sometimes confusing and include leg withdrawal and abdominal wall rigidity. An illustrative example of a case that has confused us was in a woman who met all criteria for brain death and demonstrated very bizarre arm movements. During the test for apnea, after two minutes she very slowly raised the left arm up to 90°, which was followed by supination of both hands, and finally she extended her left arm, hand and fingers at her side with flexion of the right elbow and extension of the right hand an fingers. We believe that this was initiated by neurochemical alterations with increased pCO_2, which was in the 50s in arterial blood and because of hypoxia. The arterial pO_2 at the time was also in the 50s. To date, we have seen only two patients of 175 who met the criteria of brain death but who had arm movements. Dr. Posner, can you explain the pattern of arm movements I have described to you?

POSNER: No.

PLUM: I suspect that most neurophysiologists would regard that kind of motor movement as requiring more than a spinal cord. They suggest a component of brain-stem reflexes. If that woman died, what were the autopsy findings?

GRENVIK: The patient had a large hematoma in the right cerebellar hemisphere and high intracranial pressure prior to death.

PLUM: What was the histologic findings in the brain-stem?

GRENVIK: Unfortunately we have no report on the pathologic examination of the brain stem.

PLUM: It is difficult to be positive, but I believe that most clinicians and physiologists would consider that kind of movement inconsistent with what has been observed from studies of spinal-cord reflexes in higher primates.

GRENVIK: Some of the pediatricians we consulted believe that it was possible that these reflexes could be of spinal cord origin.*

* The upper extremity reflexes described probably denote a component of brain stem function. Repetitive or additional studies should be considered prior to diagnosing such a patient as having total brain death.—*J. K.*

ANCILLARY STUDIES IN THE DIAGNOSIS OF BRAIN DEATH

A. Earl Walker

Department of Surgery
Division of Neurosurgery
University of New Mexico
School of Medicine
Albuquerque, New Mexico 87131

Introduction

In patients who meet the clinical criteria of cerebral * death, the usual confirmatory examination is an electroencephalogram (EEG). However, resuscitative equipment, nursing services, and labile cardiorespiratory states of the patient introduce artefactual material into these records. For this reason, the interpretation of electrocerebral silence (ECS) requires more than average experience in reading EEGs. Accordingly, if the clinical data are incomplete, or the EEG findings are equivocal, additional confirmatory tests are needed to substantiate the diagnosis of cerebral death.

These ancillary examinations are measurements of cerebral metabolism, cerebral blood flow or cerebral potentials, each of which provides an independent estimate of cerebral death.

In this presentation the discussion will be limited to the examination of tests which may confirm the diagnosis of a dead brain in a person who meets the basic clinical criteria of cerebral death—namely, apnea, unresponsivity, and absence of all cephalic reflexes. No attempt will be made to examine refinements of clinical determination of cerebral or brain-stem function such as the intravenous injection of atropine. Nor will the ancillary tests—such as electroencephalography (EEG), angiography, and bolus transit curves—that are discussed elsewhere in this volume be more than mentioned. Rather, those examinations of parameters of brain function that may provide absolute evidence of cerebral death will be surveyed in terms of accuracy, availability, and practical application. Such confirmatory evidence of a dead brain may be necessary only if a diagnosis is required within a few hours of an ictus or if other criteria are equivocal.

Metabolic Criteria of Cerebral Death

In the absence of neuronal and glial activity the brain utilizes no oxygen so that the cerebral metabolic rate of oxygen consumption ($CRMO_2$), which is measured in liters per 100 cc of brain tissue per minute, is practically zero. Similarly, the oxygen content of blood entering and leaving the brain ($AVDO_2$) is almost the same. And since in most cases some intracellular enzymes are still

---

* The term "cerebral death" as used in this paper is synonymous with "brain death"
—*J. K.*

0077–8923/78/0315–0228 $01.75/0 © 1978, NYAS

active after oxygen is depleted, their activity must be supported by the breakdown of intracellular stores of glycogen and protein, the end-product of which is lactic acid. Hence an acidosis must develop in the brain. Accordingly, the presence of cerebral death may be established by determination of the $CMRO_2$, $AVDO_2$ or lactic acid content of the brain.

Theoretically, a measurement of cerebral metabolism ($CMRO_2$) should be the ultimate technique for the establishment of cerebral death. It is calculated from estimates of cerebral blood flow (CBF) and the arteriovenous difference of the O_2 content across the brain ($AVDO_2$). If the cerebral hemispheres have not extracted any, or insignificant, amounts of O_2 from the blood passing through them, they may be considerel nonfunctional. The proof that the brain is dead requires evidence of $CMRO_2$ inactivity for a time variously estimated from five minutes to as long as an hour.

The determination of $CMRO_2$ requires the placement of needles or catheters in the jugular bulb and in an artery, so that blood may be withdrawn for analysis of O_2 and CO_2. This technique has two deficiencies: (1) the cerebral blood flow measurements cannot be obtained for the entire brain; and (2) in the event of little or no cerebral circulation, the blood obtained from the jugular bulb may not be representative of intracranial venous blood, but may be grossly contaminated by extracranial blood from vessels at the base of the skull. Hence, the $CMRO_2$ determinations in cerebral death suspects may show erroneously low values.

Because the determination of the cerebral metabolic rate requires multiple vascular punctures and complicated equipment such as the mass spectrometer for the assay of O_2 in arterial and venous blood, the technique is mainly used in large medical centers and usually on a research basis. For this reason, relatively few reports of $CMRO_2$ determinations in cases of cerebral death have appeared.

Pevsner et al.[29] found strikingly reduced levels of oxygen consumption in two comatose patients who had isoelectric EEGs; these levels were 0.6 and 0.0. cc O_2/100 gm brain/minute, respectively. These investigators recommended $CMRO_2$ as a reliable method of determining cerebral death. Held and Gottstein [14] measured the CBF and $CMRO_2$ in eight patients with irreversible coma who died within five days. The $CMRO_2$ levels were greatly reduced in three cases of cerebral death to the point where the O_2 consumption was not measurable. In other cases the CBF was only slightly decreased and the $CMRO_2$ was 2–3 ml/gm/min. They concluded that a $CMRO_2$ below 1 ml/gm/min may be taken as an indication of a dying or dead brain. Brodersen and Jørgensen [4] concurred in this conclusion and stated that such a low rate was incompatible with return of consciousness. Because of the disadvantages and limitations of $CMRO_2$ determinations, increased attention has been given to the measurements of factors that modulate O_2 consumption, namely, PvO_2 and differences in the O_2 content of arterial and venous blood.

Arteriovenous Oxygen Difference ($AVDO_2$)

Although in cerebral death the PvO_2 may be unusually high due to the failure of the brain to take up O_2, the estimates of the differences of the O_2 content of arterial and jugular bulb blood are of more value for the determination of cerebral death than is the level of O_2 tension. Theoretically, if, as assumed in cerebral death, there is no CBF, any difference in the O_2 content of arterial and jugular bulb blood should represent extracerebral metabolism which is low in comparison with the high rate of $CMRO_2$. Hence, the PvO_2 is high, and the arteriovenous difference is commonly less than 2 vol percent. Paulson et al.[28] have commented upon the high O_2 content of jugular blood in cerebral death. To show that this was due to the external circulation, Minami et al.[23] clamped the external carotid artery and found that the jugular PO_2 dropped to the level of that of mixed venous blood. Other metabolic substances—glucose, lactate, and pyruvate—are less predictive of brain death. Although in most cases of cerebral death the $AVDO_2$ is below 3 vol percent, some patients with dead brains have normal $AVDO_2$ values (6 vol percent). On the other hand, comatose patients with luxury perfusion may have $AVDO_2$ levels below 2 vol percent. For these reasons determination of the $AVDO_2$ is not a completely reliable test for cerebral death.

However, the $AVDO_2$ may differentiate drug-induced from other irreversible comas. In barbiturate intoxication, the $AVDO_2$ is normal or increased.[31] This is in line with Sokoloff's report [31] that in severe barbiturate intoxication, the $CMRO_2$ is more reduced than the CBF so that the cerebral O_2 supply is more than adequate.

Lactic Acid Content of the Cerebrospinal Fluid

Although lactate is somewhat increased in the CSF in all cases of coma except those caused by barbiturate intoxication, in cerebral death the lactic acid content is abnormally high (10–15 mEq/l). As expected, the lactate dehydrogenase level is also elevated. Yashon et al.[36] believe that there is a correlation between the elevated lactic acid levels, the presence of ECS and cerebral death, for at lactic acid levels of 3.77 mEq/l, the brain is capable of producing potentials above 6–7 Hz, whereas when the CSF lactic acid reaches 6.72 mEq/l, as it does in cerebral death, the cerebrum is unable to develop potentials demonstrable with conventional recording.

The biochemical syndrome of cerebral death consists of the triad of an archaic respiratory quotient, a marked drop in the arteriovenous O_2 difference to less than 2 vol percent, and an increase in CSF lactic acid to more than 3 mg percent.†

CEREBRAL BLOOD FLOW

The conclusions of Opitz and Schneider [27] that the critical level of oxygen tension for the maintenance of cerebral functions is approximately a venous pO_2 of 19 mm Hg have been generally accepted. At this point their animals lost consciousness and death ensued when the venous pO_2 reached the range of 12–14 mm Hg. Recently, however, MacMillan and Siesjö [19] have shown in rats that the ability of the brain to withstand anoxic insults is also dependent upon the cerebral perfusion. They found that lowering the venous pO_2 to 10 mm Hg

---

† In general metabolic studies are more of a research tool than a clinically viable technique to confirm the diagnosis of brain death.—J. K.

did not produce significant derangements of cerebral oxidative metabolism, provided that the arterial blood pressure and cerebral perfusion pressures were maintained in the normal range. Conversely Eklöf and Siesjö [7] demonstrated that serious metabolic derangements occurred if the cerebral perfusion was decreased, even though the venous pO_2 fell only to 33 mm Hg.

Further evidence that the brain has greater resistance to simple anoxia than was previously believed is derived from work by Olsson and Hossmann,[26] who showed that cats were able to withstand a long period of anoxia provided that the brain was perfused, even with a nonoxygenated electrolyte solution. The accumulation of toxic products of cerebral metabolism (such as lactic acid) may be the factor producing irreversible brain injury, rather than hypoxia per se. For this reason the estimation of cerebral blood flow has valuable prognostic implications. However, for the diagnosis of cerebral death, the presence of no flow is an adequate indicator.

Because the quantitative determination of cerebral blood flow (CBF) requires arterial and venous samples of blood, which are sometimes difficult to obtain, especially in persons with a failing vascular system, qualitative tests for CBF have been sought that would be less traumatizing and easier to interpret. Some investigators have used isotopic clearance tests, others have studied physical phenomena associated with cerebral blood flow, and still others have based their studies upon rheogenic electrical potentials.

DIRECT DEMONSTRATION OF CEREBRAL BLOOD FLOW

Angiography

Contrast angiography was originally used to demonstrate the intracranial perfusion of blood, but in patients suspected of cerebral death the stresses of the techniques used seemed to some physicians sufficient to weight adversely the balance in persons hovering between life and death. For this reason, other methods, not stressful to the individual have been sought. However, in many clinics, especially in Europe, cerebral angiography by femoral catheterization is routinely used.

Isotope Angiography

After the intravenous injection of a gamma-emitting isotope, the major cerebral arteries and the dural sinuses of normal individuals are clearly visualized by rectilinear scans or imaging cameras. However, if the CBF is absent, the cerebral scan shows an empty cranium.[24]

Bolus Transit Curve

An intravenous isotope bolus may be followed through the head by a collimated cephalic probe which is fed into a linear scanner recorder. A second probe over the femoral artery serves as a control of the systemic circulation of the bolus. In case of no cerebral blood flow, the usual bolus hump is missing. Korein et al.[14] report the details of this technique.

Intra-arterial Isotope Perfusion

Several investigators have used tracer clearance techniques to measure cerebral blood flow in patients with brain death. Baldy-Moulinier and Frèrebeau [2] concluded that a flat trace indicated the arrest of cerebral circulation and cerebral death.

Intracerebral Techniques

To eliminate the possibility of regurgitation to the external carotid circulation, Lazorthe and Bes [15] injected ^{133}Xe into the cerebral parenchyma and followed the clearance. They considered that a plateau indicated an absence of cerebral circulation and that two such curves at ten-minute intervals represented a dead brain. Zwetnow [37] injected ^{85}Kr intracerebrally through a burr hole in 40 cases and found by external detectors no clearance of the isotope in brains that had arrested circulation.

Inhalation Techniques

The nitrous oxide method of Kety and Schmidt is vitiated in patients with brain death by the incomplete uptake of nitrous oxide and the contamination of jugular blood from dilated extracranial venous channels. Hence the low values (9–15 ml/100 mg/min) reported by Hoyer and Wawersik [11] and Shalit et al.[30] are not necessarily accurate estimates of cerebral blood flow.

INDIRECT METHODS OF DETERMINING CEREBRAL BLOOD FLOW

Echoencephalography

The presence or absence of cerebral circulation may be determined by the echoencephalographic demonstration of intracranial vascular pulsations. Leksell[16] described a midline pulsatile echo synchronous with the heart beat, but pulsating echoes may be demonstrated throughout the brain substance. These pulsations in the brain can be depicted by gating any desired portion of the reflected echo. Such hemispheral pulsations are almost entirely due to carotid shock waves, whereas the midline pulsations are in part derived from basilar pulsations. Accordingly, the hemispheral pulsations may be absent while the midline pulsations persist. For this reason some investigators have used the absence of the hemispheral pulsations as evidence of cerebral death and others have recorded midline pulsations in the belief that they are more sensitive indicators of cerebral circulation. The proof that these pulsations are related to cerebral blood flow stems from both clinical and experimental studies. Lepetit et al.[17] and Marasasa [22] found that absence of the echo pulsations coincided with obstruction of cerebral circulation and nonfilling of the cerebral vessels in angiograms.

Arnold et al.[1] noted that midline echo pulsations, probably due to pulsations in the stems of the carotid and basilar arteries, may still be detected after cerebral circulation can no longer be demonstrated angiographically. Lepetit et al.,[17] who consider that an absence of hemispheral pulsatile echoes is evidence of arrest of carotid circulation and implies irreversible loss of cerebral function, admit vertebrobasilar echoes may be detected for some time after the cessation of hemispheral pulsatile echoes. They conclude that the presence of three criteria—stage IV coma, a flat EEG tracing, and immobile hemispheral echoes —is sufficient to prove death of the brain.

Uematsu and Walker[34] used an electronic switch controlled by a pulse generator to gate any desired time interval. The gated midline echo was converted to a sequence of pulses, each of which was proportional in amplitude to the appropriate echo pulse and could be recorded on any strip chart recorder, oscillograph or EEG pen writer. To ensure stability of the transducer, a head band was devised to hold the ultrasonic transducer so that it could be adjusted manually and maintained in an appropriate position.

Patients with normal cerebral blood flow invariably had pulsation of the midline echo. In a series of 45 comatose patients normal pulsatile midline echo was present in 3 obtunded patients, 15 unresponsive patients, and 2 of 27 patients suspected of cerebral death. In the remaining 25 cases of cerebral death the midline echoes did not pulsate. Four patients suspected of brain death in whom angiograms were done had absence of echo pulsation and non-filling of the intracranial blood vessels. The dissociated findings of an isoelectric encephalogram and a pulsating echo may be the result of an ischemic brain still being irrigated, of pulsations arising from the stump of an occluded carotid or basilar artery, or of a fall in perfusion pressure sufficient to abolish the electro-encephalogram, but not pulsations detectable by echography. It is well known that the biologic activity of the EEG may disappear as the blood pressure falls to subshock levels, then reappear when vasopressor agents elevate the blood pressure to near normal levels. In the patients having dissociated findings in this series, the arterial pressure fluctuated from imperceptible to shock levels. This severe hypotension apparently was inadequate to sustain neuronal activity, but sufficient to produce shock waves capable of distorting the walls of the third ventricle.

Ophthalmic Artery Blood Flow

Several investigators have attempted to assess the presence and/or direction of blood flow in the opthalmic arteries or their terminal branches as an index of flow in the intracranial portions of the internal carotid arteries. Direct observation of the retinal flow is possible by ophthalmoscopy, at least in the early stages of cerebral death. Later, the cornea may become milky and opaque as it dries out or is covered with ointments to prevent drying. However, at the initial examination, especially if the pupils are dilated and fixed, the retinal vessels may be seen to have a slow circulation with sludging of erythrocytes or complete cessation of circulation, in which event the clumped erythrocytes appear like strings of sausages in the vessels. Sludging is not common in the retinae of patients with a dead brain (it occurs in about 20 percent of such cases), but when present, would appear to indicate absence of cerebral blood flow and a dead brain.

Providing a corollary to clinical studies of retinal circulation, Vlahovitch and Boudet[35] examined the ophthalmic circulation by carotid angiography with compression. In half of 25 cases of deep coma, persistent opacification of the choroidal crescent and ophthalmic artery indicated circulatory arrest. Thus, although the ocular supply is derived in part at least from extracranial sources, in cerebral death it is often arrested.

Lobstein *et al.*[18] and Mantz *et al.*[21] have studied the arm-retinal circulation time using fluorescein injected by a catheter into the subclavian vein while the retinal vessels were being observed ophthalmoscopically. Because in two-thirds of 33 cases of coma dépassé, the circulation time was greatly increased from the normal rate of 8–14 seconds, they concluded that a circulation time greater than 30 seconds was a certain sign of coma dépassé. Using a Doppler directional flowmeter, Muller[25] and Despland and DeCrousaz[6] believe that they can diagnose cerebral death on the basis of a complex of rheographic findings, namely, (1) a high systolic flow in the carotid arteries with replacement of the continuous diastolic flow by a reversal of flow in part of diastole, and (2) a lack of (in the case of cerebral lesions) or an intermittent (in posterior fossa lesions) orthodromic flow in the ophthalmic artery. These techniques, although requiring special equipment and a certain expertise, are simple and harmless, and, if positive, give confirmatory evidence of the arrest of cerebral circulation.

Rheoencephalography

The rheoencephalogram, derived from intracranial electrodes, becomes flat at the same time as the EEG when the intracranial pressure approximates arterial tension; when the pressure is lowered, the rheoencephalogram returns to normal before the EEG does.[14] Under these circumstances rheoencephalography adds a refinement to the diagnosis of cerebral death, but depth impedance studies are not always desirable and surface records may not correspond to the depth findings. Hence, complete reliance cannot be placed on clinical rheoencephalograms.

ELECTRICAL ACTIVITY OF THE BRAIN

For many years it has been recognized that cerebral activity is accompanied by changing electrical activity. When the concept of a dead brain was introduced, it was suggested that an isoelectric electroencephalogram would indicate the loss of cerebral function. However, experience showed that a number of conditions—such as drug intoxication, hypothermia, or arterial hypotension—might produce an isoelectric record which, when the causative factor was remedied, might again show changing electrical potentials. The value and limitations of electroencephalography in the determination of cerebral death is discussed elsewhere. However, since certain ancillary techniques have been proposed for the confirmation of cerebral death, these procedures related to the electrical potentials of the brain are presented here.

Depth Recording

It is known that scalp electrodes may not detect changes in electrical potential in subcortical areas. For this reason, when an isoelectric EEG was proposed as a criterion of cerebral death, the question was raised as to the possibility of the persistence of electrical activity in basal ganglia, thalamus and brain stem in the presence of an isoelectric scalp record. Recording from the subcortical structures by means of depth electrodes is complicated by extraneous artefacts making their interpretation difficult. In the majority of cases, if the surface electrodes show ECS, the depth recording is also isoelectric, but in some cases, activity may be present in subcortical ganglia, such as the thalamus, when the scalp records show inactivity. Findji et al.[8] studied ten patients in deep and irreversible coma. In two of three patients no activity was found at any level; in the third patient, examined 24 hours after respiratory arrest, slow waves 1–2 per second about 10–20 microvolts in amplitude were seen. In the other 7 patients electrical activity was present at all levels, including the scalp. That scalp isoelectric records may be associated with depth activity has been confirmed by others.

EVOKED POTENTIALS

The ordinary scalp electroencephalogram is essentially a record of the resting brain. But physiologists have known for years that under conditions of narcosis and hypothermia the spontaneous activity of the brain might be depressed without eliminating the electrical activity associated with neuronal excitation. Thus, even in deep anesthesia, visual, auditory or somatosensory stimuli may induce cortical electrical responses. It may be necessary to summate these potentials in order to distinguish them from low-voltage background "noise." This is customarily done by "averaging" a series of responses in a computer. However, at times the individual evoked responses can be detected by the naked eye.

An attempt is made to evoke cortical potentials by auditory, visual and tactile stimulation when recording on any patient suspected of cerebral death. However, individual responses are difficult to differentiate from background activity without averaging techniques when biological activity is present; even when the tracing is flat, a cortical potential is rarely visible.

Trojaborg and Jørgensen[33] studied the evoked responses in 50 comatose patients being artificially ventilated. If the cranial nerve reflexes were present, visual and somatosensory cortical responses could be evoked, although the response was delayed and simple in form (without late components). In patients with no cephalic reflexes, induced somatosensory potentials and usually visual potentials could not be demonstrated. Starr[32] found that auditory evoked potentials from the brain stem have a long latency in patients with a dying brain. As the brain dies, the potentials are of lower amplitude and eventually with death, if a response is obtained at all, it is only an attenuated wave I of long latency.

Steady Potentials

The stationary potentials of the head, approximately 20 mV above the potential of the nose, are, according to Manaka and Sano,[20] in cerebral death are reduced to zero and in lesser degrees of brain hypoxia are decreased proportionally to the degree of brain damage. Bushart and Rittmeyer[5] also consider the DC negative shift to be a useful guide to cerebral death. They found that the usual response to hypoxia, a negative shift, was absent when cerebral circulation was abolished and the brain was dead.

INTRACRANIAL PRESSURE

Because the intracranial cavity is a relatively closed box, an increase in its contents will raise the pressure, at times, sufficiently to prevent blood from entering it. Under normal circumstances the arterial pressure is great enough to force blood through the intracranial contents. This force, referred to as the perfusion pressure, is defined as the difference between mean systemic arterial (SAP) and the cerebral venous pressures. Gros and his associates [9] showed that when the intracranial pressure (ICP), which corresponds to the cerebral venous pressure, was raised to more than 70 percent of the systolic blood pressure, cerebral blood flow ceased. This might occur either when the ICP was increased or the SAP was decreased. Experimentally, Brierley et al.[3] found that irreversible brain damage occurred when the SAP was lowered so that the perfusion pressure was less than 25 mm Hg, and Ingvar et al.[12] noted that increasing the intracranial pressure to such an extent that the perfusion pressure was less than 40 mm Hg also caused irreparable brain damage. In patients, as the ICP/SAP approaches unity, Jørgenson [13] states that the clinical state deteriorates, the intracranial pulsations decrease in amplitude and cease, and the EEG becomes isoelectric. However, in cerebral death the ICP/SAP ratio may vary from 0.7 to 1.17.

On the basis of these data, it would seem that although the CBF may be absent with an ICP/SAP ratio of 0.7, for a reliable conclusion of no CBF, the ratio should be at least unity.

How long must cerebral blood flow be absent to conclude that the brain is dead? Although a few minutes' absolute cessation of cerebral blood flow in animals will produce an irreparably damaged brain, in clinical practice the minimal time is variously estimated from 15 to 30 minutes. Hence, an intracranial pressure equal to the mean systolic arterial pressure for a period of 30 minutes should assure a dead brain.

MISCELLANEOUS TESTS

A number of confirmatory tests which may be used to establish cerebral death have been suggested but their value and limitations are not known.

Intrathecal Spinal Injection of RISA

As a means of demonstrating the absence of the craniospinal circulation, the lumbar injection of a gamma-emitting isotope has been proposed. In normal individuals, this isotope rapidly diffuses in the CSF to the head and may be detected by counters placed over the scalp. If there is a block at the foramen magnum such as usually occurs in cerebral death, the isotope cannot be detected over the cranium, and often not even over the cervical spine. No large series of such studies has been reported, so that the validation and limitations of the technique are not known.

Cerebral Temperature

A few reports of the brain temperature as determined by intracerebral thermocouples have indicated that in brain death the intracerebral temperature is lower than that of the body. However, since this test requires a burr hole and intracerebral penetration, it has not been generally accepted. No data are available regarding the minimal difference between brain and body temperature that is indicative of brain death.

Computerized Tomography

The increasing use of CT scans in comatose persons has suggested its usefulness in the confirmation of cerebral death. It may serve as an ancillary test for cerebral death by reason of its demonstration of (1) the primary cause of cerebral death, (2) the state of the cerebral blood flow, and (3) the pathologic changes that are associated with a dead brain.

Often the etiology of a coma is not apparent from clinical examination of an unresponsive patient. Yet if the diagnosis could be established as an irreparable lesion of the brain, other specialized examinations such as electroencephalography and angiography might not be required to establish brain death. The value and reliability of computerized tomography in the diagnosis of many intracranial lesions have been validated by its routine use in many of the larger hospitals. Although some irreversible conditions may not be demonstrable in the first day or two by this technique, many, especially hemorrhage, are quite apparent in the first few hours after an ictus. Certainly the reversible toxic states that may be confused with cerebral death would show a normal image of the brain that should lead the physician to initiate or continue appropriate therapy.

Another benefit of computerized tomography is the possibility that enhancement may indicate the presence or absence of CBF, for under normal conditions the internal carotid and middle cerebral arteries are visualized by this technique. If there is no CBF, these vessels would not be seen. However, the validity and limitations of this method for demonstrating the cerebral blood flow in normal patients and in those with cerebral death have not been established.

The third advantage of computerized tomography in cerebral death suspects may be the possibility of demonstrating pathologic alterations of the brain that are characteristic of cerebral death. This aspect has not been adequately explored as yet, but what little experience has accumulated suggests that the pathologic brain changes are too variable to be considered pathognomonic of cerebral death. Certainly the early diagnosis of cerebral death does not seem possible on the basis of computerized tomography. Later, when pathologic changes are well pronounced, the diagnosis may be possible, but by that time cerebral death is usually obvious on clinical or other laboratory examinations.

Hence the definitive role of computerized tomography in the diagnosis of cerebral death is not yet determined. At the present time, its main advantage would seem to be to establish the etiologic factor of the comatose state.

DISCUSSION

Ancillary tests for cerebral death are desirable when an early diagnosis of a dead brain is needed, for example, if organs are to be transplanted, or when findings on the usual clinical examinations are equivocal. The examinations that have been discussed have certain advantages and limitations that are presented in TABLE 1.

It is apparent that many of the techniques used for the determination of cerebral death require operative procedures and delicate and intricate manipulations by highly skilled personnel. Consequently it is almost impossible to perform them in addition to resuscitative and diagnostic examinations within six

TABLE 1

ADVANTAGES AND LIMITATIONS OF ANCILLARY TESTS

Test of:	Technique	Time Performed * 0–6–12–24	Invasive Arterial	Venous	Cranial	Validity (%)	Time Present (min)
Cerebral blood flow	Angiography (4-vessel)	√	√			99	30
	Angiography (isotope)	√			√	99	30
	Bolus	√			√	99	30
	Echoencephalography	√				99	30
	Rheoencephalography	√			√	Undetermined	—
	Intracranial pressure	√			√	Undetermined	—
	Quantitative	√	√	√		95	30
Metabolic function	ADVO₂	√		√	√	95	30
	PVO₂	√			√	Undetermined	—
	CMRO₂	√		√	√	99	Once
	CSF	√				99	Once

* Time after insult when tests can usually be performed, viz., 0–6=zero to 6 hours, etc.

hours of admission to an emergency room. Some of these tests might not be carried out for 12 or 24 hours.

In addition, many of these techniques required venous, arterial or cranial punctures, which, although of little risk in a normal person, may be hazardous in a seriously ill person.

REFERENCES

1. ARNOLD, H., P. ANSORG, P. VOIGTSBERGER, H. EGER, & H. RITTER. 1972. Beitrag der Pulsationsechoenzephalographie zur Todeszeitbestimmung. Acta Neurochir. **27**: 263–275.

2. BALDY-MOULINIER, M & P. FRÈREBEAU. 1969. Cerebral blood flow in cases of coma following severe head injury. *In* Cerebral Blood Flow: Clinical and Experimental Results. M. BROCK, *et al., Eds.* : 216–218.
3. BRIERLEY, J. B., J. H. ADAMS, D. I. GRAHAM, & J. A. SIMPSON. 1971. Neocortical death after cardiac arrest. A clinical, neurophysiological, and neuropathological report of two cases. Lancet **2:** 560–565.
4. BRODERSEN, P. & E. O. JØRGENSEN. 1974. Cerebral blood flow and oxygen uptake, and cerebrospinal fluid biochemistry in severe coma. J. Neurol. Neurosurg. Psychiat. **37:** 384–391.
5. BUSHART, W. & P. RITTMEYER. 1969. Kriterien der irreversiblen Hirnschaedigung bei Intensivbehandlung: Elektroenzephalographische und klinische Verlaufsueberwachung. Med. Klin. **64:** 184–193.
6. DESPLAND, P. A. & G. DECROUSAZ. 1974. L'apport de l'ultrasonographie Doppler au diagnostic de la mort cérébrale. Schweiz. Med. Wochensch. **104:** 1454–1459.
7. EKLÖF, B. & B. K. SIESJÖ. 1971. Cerebral blood flow and cerebral energy state. Acta Physiol. Scand. **82:** 409–411.
8. FINDJI, F., J. GACHES, J. P. HOUTTEVILLE, P. CREISSARD & A. CALISKAN. 1970. Enregistrements éléctroencéphalographiques corticaux, transcorticaux, et souscorticaux dans dix cas de coma profound ou dépassé (note préliminaire) Neurochirurgia **13:** 211–219.
9. GROS, C. 1972. Les critères circulatoires et biologiques de la mort, du cerveau (à l'éxclusion des problèmes cliniques et électro-encéphalographiques). Neuro-Chir. **18:** 9–48.
10. HELD, K. & U. GOTTSTEIN. 1972. Durchblutung und Stoffwechsel des menschlichen Gehirns nach akuter cerebraler Ischemie. Verh. Dtsch. Ges. Inn. Med. **78:** 665–668.
11. HOYER, S. & J. WAWERSIK. 1968. Untersuchungen der Hirndurchblutung und des Hirnstoffwechsels beim Decerebrationssyndrom. Langenbecks Arch. Chir. **322:** 602–605.
12. INGVAR, D. H., N. A. LASSEN, B. K. SIESJÖ, & E. SKINHOJ. 1968. Cerebral blood flow and cerebro-spinal fluid. Scand. J. Clin. Lab. Invest. **22:** Suppl. 102.
13. JØRGENSEN, P. B. 1973. Clinical deterioration prior to brain death related to progressive intracranial hypertension. Acta. Neurochir. **28:** 29–40.
14. KOREIN, J., P. BRAUNSTEIN, I. KRICHEFF, A. LIEBERMAN & N. CHASE. 1975. Radioisotopic bolus technique as a test to detect circulatory deficit associated with cerebral death. Circulation **51:** 924–939.
15. LAZORTHES, Y. & A. BES. *In* GROS.[9] : 26–27.
16. LEKSELL, L. 1955. Echoencephalography. Acta Chir. Scand. **110**(3): 301.
17. LEPETIT, J. M., J. P. PEFFERKORN & A. DANY. 1974. Echographie pulsatile et perte irreversible des fonctions cérébrales. Ann. Anesth. Franc. **15:** 101–108.
18. LOBSTEIN, A., J D. TEMPE & G. PAYEUR. 1969. La fluoroscopie rétinienne dans le diagnostic de la mort cérébrale. Doc. Ophthalmol. **26:** 349–358.
19. MACMILLAN, V. & B. K. SIESJÖ. 1971. Critical oxygen tension in the brain. Acta Physiol. Scand. **82:** 412–414.
20. MANAKA, S. & K. SANO. 1972. Study of stationary potential (SP). II. Its value in various animals and its use for the estimation of cerebral death. Brain Nerve **24:** 1573–1582.
21. MANTZ, J. M., A. LOBSTEIN & A. JAEGER. 1974. L'oeil dans le diagnostic de la mort cérébrale. Ann. Anesth. Franc. **15:** 95–100.
22. MARASASA, Y. 1973. Fundamental and clinical studies on pulsatile echoencephalography under acute intracranial hypertension. J. Wakayama Med. Soc. **24:** 59–83.
23. MINAMI, T., M. OGAWA, T. SUGIMOTO, & K. KATSURADA. 1973. Hyperoxia of internal jugular venous blood in brain death. J. Neurosurg. **39:** 442–447.
24. MISHKIN, F. 1975. Determination of cerebral death by radio-nuclide angiography. Radiology **115:** 135–137.

25. MULLER, H. R., 1966. Zur Problematik der flachen Hirnstromkurve und der Diagnose "Hirntod" nach akuter zerebraler Anoxie. Med. Klin. **61:** 1955–1959.
26. OLSSON, Y. & K. A. HOSSMANN. 1971. The effect of intravascular saline perfusion on the sequelae of transient cerebral ischemia. Acta Neuropath. **17:** 68–79.
27. OPITZ, E. & M. SCHNEIDER. 1950. Ueber die Sauerstoffversorgung des Gehirns und den Mechanismus von Mangelwirkungen. Ergeb. Physiol. **46:** 126–260.
28. PAULSON, G. W., G. WISE & R. CONKLE. 1972. Cerebrospinal fluid lactic acid in death and in brain death. Neurology **22:** 505–509.
29. PEVSNER, P. H., C. BHUSHAN, O. E. OTTESEN & A. E. WALKER. 1971. Cerebral blood flow and oxygen consumption: An on-line technique. Johns Hopkins Med. J. **128:** 134–140.
30. SHALIT, M. N., A. J. BELLER, M. FEINSOD, A. J. DRAPKIN & S. COTEV. 1970. The blood flow and oxygen consumption of the dying brain. Neurology **20:** 740–748.
31. SOKOLOFF, L. 1959. The action of drugs on the cerebral circulation. Pharm. Rev. : 1–85.
32. STARR, A. 1976. Brain-stem responses in brain death. Brain **99:** 543–545.
33. TROJABORG, W. & E. O. JØRGENSEN. 1973. Evoked cortical potentials in patients with "isoelectric" EEGs. Electroenceph. Clin. Neurophysiol. **35:** 301–309.
34. UEMATSU, S. & A. E. WALKER. 1974. Pulsatile cerebral midline echo and brain death. Johns Hopkins Med. J. **134:** 383–390.
35. VLAHOVITCH, G. & C. BOUDET. 1973. La circulation ophtalmique dans les comas dépassés. Images obtenues par l'angiographie carotidienne sous pression. Arch. Ophthalmol. **33:** 123–128.
36. YASHON, D., F. C. WAGNER, G. E. LOCKE & R. WHITE. 1970. Clinical, chemical and physiological indicators of cerebral nonviability in circulatory arrest. Trans. Amer. Neurol. Assoc. **95:** 31–35.
37. ZWETNOW, N. N. 1971. Multifokala intracerebrala injektioner av ädelgasisotop en ny klinish metod för fastställande av hjärndod. Nord. Med. **85:** 675–676.

DISCONNECTING TESTS AND OXYGEN UPTAKE IN THE DIAGNOSIS OF TOTAL BRAIN DEATH

A. Milhaud, M. Riboulot, and H. Gayet

Department d'Anesthésie-Réanimation
Centre Hospitalier Régional et Universitaire d'Amiens
F-80030 Amiens Cedex, France

Apnea is probably one of the most constant, important, and significant clinical signs for the diagnosis of brain death. The significance of apnea was recognized and described by Mollaret and Goulon in 1959 [13] and Nedey [14] in 1966 emphasized its importance. It seems useful at this point to begin to quantify apnea and to determine blood gasses at regular intervals for an entire series of patients thought to be brain-dead.

It is the further quantification of apnea that we have undertaken to study in 22 cases of brain death and our study was based on the work of Hirsch [7] in 1905 and Volhard [18] in 1908. The apnea defined in pure oxygen was called by Holmdahl [8] "apneic diffusion oxygenation," which he discussed in a remarkable 120-page study in 1956. All our patients demonstrated all of the classical signs of total brain death and had flat EEGs.

Prior to detailing the methods and results of disconnecting tests used in patients suspected of being brain-dead, we must define our terms and review some of the classical approaches. This test for apnea may be extremely significant in evaluation of other diagnostic entities as well as in evaluating the problem of brain death.

1. All medication that depresses ventilation must be eliminated. For example, circumstances that would cancel the significance of the disconnecting test include barbiturate overdose or administration of a neurosurgical "lytic cocktail." Thus, one must be certain that all types of medication that depress respiration are excluded as the primary cause.

2. The subject must have a normal temperature. Spontaneous hypothermia below 32° C, for example, may of itself produce transitory apnea (or more often a very low ventilation frequency). When craniocerebral trauma is present and the body temperature is below 32° C, it is not necessary to perform a disconnecting test since, in conjunction with the neurologic findings, such a degree of hypothermia is one of the best signs of total brain death.

3. It must be certain that the subject studied is not hyperventilated before the start of the disconnecting test.

In our series, on three occasions in two years, patients with flat EEGs had no spontaneous ventilation at the beginning of the study. During the course of the disconnecting test, a return of ventilation was noted after the persistence of apnea for more than five minutes. On one occasion, a patient had apnea for nine minutes followed by spontaneous return of ventilation. Our colleagues in neurosurgery, who have seen apnea of even greater duration than that observed in pearl divers, have asked whether we were not afraid of hypoxic aggravation [6] of pre-existing cerebral lesions in our patients. We have evaluated this problem since we have already seen two complications of accidental ventilator disconnec-

241

0077-8923/78/0315-0241 $01.75/0 © 1978, NYAS

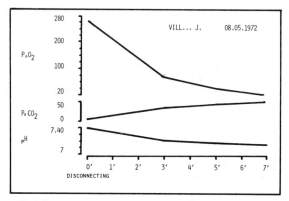

FIGURE 1. Disconnecting test without oxygen supplied to the trachea.

tion followed by circulatory arrest (less than five minutes after the onset of the apnea). Therefore we have completely stopped the simple air disconnecting test; we will give one example in which anoxia occurred as a complication.

FIGURE 1 shows the results after a disconnecting test in which the subject was ventilated with a 60 percent mixture of nitrogen and oxygen; this patient had been *without oxygen* in the trachea after disconnection. In seven minutes, the arterial pO_2 had passed from 280 mm Hg to less than 30 mm Hg.

We have forbidden this type of study since 1972 because the risk of anoxic brain damage is high when the patient is not in a state of total brain death.

For better understanding of the subject, we will review one of the basic studies in man of apnea in pure oxygen, that of Holmdahl.[8] The physiologic mechanisms are unknown.

With apnea in pure oxygen, the pO_2 in the arteries is maintained at an elevated level to avoid any desaturation. This persists for more than 30 minutes and is probably due to cardiac activity. With each cardiac systole, a certain volume of gasses comparable to the stroke volume of blood entering the lungs is equal to that ejected from the alveoli. This has been suggested by Palmiri.[4] FIGURE 2 shows a spirometric curve in which each small spike corresponds to a cardiac systole.

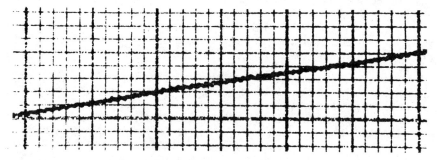

FIGURE 2. Spirometric curve in which each small spike corresponds to a cardiac systole.

In 1905 Hirsch and Volhard already noted that it was not possible for animals to live with complete apnea for several hours. Life was possible, however, if apnea was *preceded* by prolonged ventilation *in pure oxygen*. This allowed a state of sufficient nitrogen washout to be achieved. After one hour, the total body nitrogen washout is classically 50 percent.[3]

FIGURE 3 shows the simplest technique of performing the disconnecting test using pure oxygen. The technique is a relatively simple one for a physician to use, even in a small hospital without elaborate equipment. The test consists of turning the respirator off after denitrogenation has occurred by means of artificial ventilation in pure oxygen for more than one hour. Simultaneously a fine catheter is introduced at the same time into the tracheal tube. The oxygen flow through this catheter has to be at 4 or 5 liters per minute for an adult.

FIGURE 4 shows results of a disconnecting test preceded by normal ventilation in 100 percent oxygen. The arterial pO_2 falls slowly and decreases from

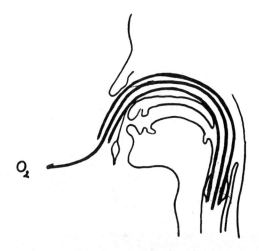

FIGURE 3. Simplest technique of performing the disconnecting test.

450 mm Hg to 95 mm Hg in nine minutes to finally stabilize at the twelfth minute. There was no true sufficient denitrogenation because the ventilation had previously been in 100 percent oxygen for only a few minutes. Because of this fact the nitrogen washout was minimal.

The technique of the disconnecting test we use today employs recordings of a spirometric curve with the spirometer full of pure oxygen (FIGURE 5). The spirometric recording is of great medicolegal interest and provides hard copy which may be placed in a patient's chart. FIGURE 6 shows a copy of an entire spirometric curve. The slope corresponds to the oxygen uptake.

FIGURE 7 shows the findings with the type of disconnecting test in pure oxygen that we currently use. Initially the p_aO_2 is at 350 mm Hg (Fio$_2$ at 100 percent for one hour of denitrogenation; the intrapulmonary shunt is not negligible). After twenty minutes of apnea the subject's arterial pO_2 does not fall below 250 mm Hg and rises to the initial level when the respirator is turned

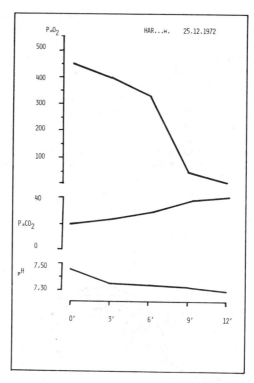

FIGURE 4. Disconnecting test with 6 liters of oxygen to the trachea without previous denitrogenation.

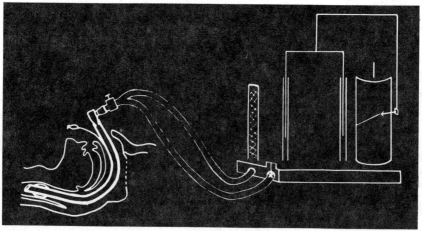

FIGURE 5. Technique using recordings of spirometric curve with spirometer full of pure oxygen.

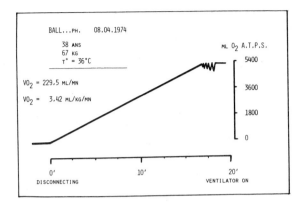

FIGURE 6. Graphic representation of oxygen uptake.

back on. If there is no return of spontaneous ventilation in spite of hypercapnic acidosis, the result of the test is positive. This is the most important datum derived from this test. In other studies no modifications of pulse, blood pressure and electrocardiographic findings were noted.

In four other patients in whom disconnecting tests were performed, similar observations were made (FIGURES 8, 9, 10 and 11). FIGURE 12 shows the mean results in 12 patients and the range of the control sample and another sample taken 14 minutes after the disconnecting test.

The arterial pO_2 never fell lower than 100 mm Hg. After 14 minutes the mean pH was 7.17 and the mean arterial pCO_2 was 61 mm Hg.

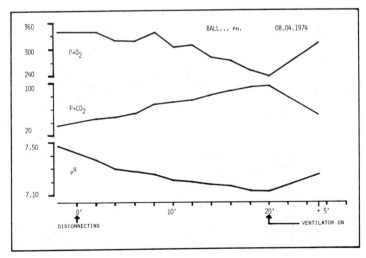

FIGURE 7. Disconnecting test preceded by denitrogenation and oxygen supply to the trachea by spirometer.

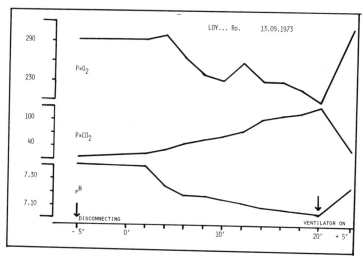

FIGURE 8. Disconnecting test preceded by denitrogenation and oxygen supply to the trachea by spirometer.

In 14 cases of total brain death we have recorded an oxygen uptake of 150 to 180 milliliters per minute. The cardiac rate and the arterial pressure did not vary during the study. The p_aO_2 was always greater than 100 mm Hg, even after 20 minutes. It was also possible to correlate hypercapnic acidosis and time (FIGURES 13 and 14).

In 22 cases the mean arterial pCO_2 increase was 2.77 mm Hg and the mean arterial pH decrease was 0.18 units per minute.

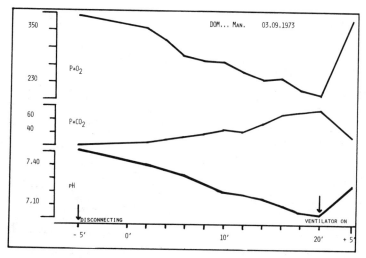

FIGURE 9. Disconnecting test preceded by denitrogenation and oxygen supply to the trachea by spirometer.

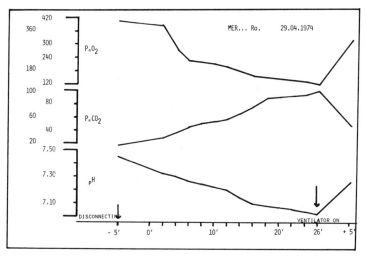

FIGURE 10. Disconnecting test preceded by denitrogenation and oxygen supply to the trachea by spirometer.

DISCUSSION

The disconnecting test to evaluate apnea may be used for a period of 15 to 20 minutes with practically no danger to the hemodynamic status. These disconnecting tests have further clinical import in addition to oxygen uptake evaluation:

1. When apnea is related to alkalosis secondary to hyperventilation and

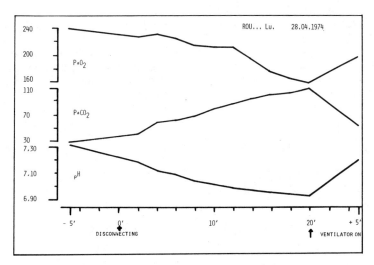

FIGURE 11. Disconnecting test preceded by denitrogenation and oxygen supply to the trachea by spirometer.

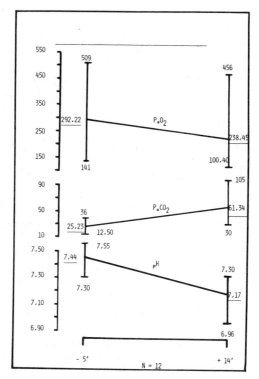

FIGURE 12. Mean results of disconnecting test in 12 patients preceded by denitrogenation and oxygen supply to the trachea by spirometer.

there is a reappearance of minimal low-amplitude respiratory activity, the diagnosis of total brain death is invalid and we continue to maintain full life-support care.

2. In the course of utilizing this test, it was possible to compare the reactions of patients in a state of total brain death with those of patients who are not brain-dead. Especially, there was no evidence of elevation of the arterial pressure linked either to apnea in pure oxygen or to the administration of a mixture of oxygen and carbon dioxide as used occasionally in carotid surgery.

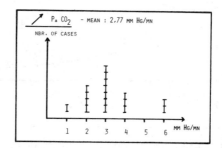

FIGURE 13. Correlation of $PaCO_2$ and time.

In patients with total brain death in our experience, the elevation of arterial pressure that normally appears after or during the first 20 minutes of apnea is totally absent.

We have never seen a false-positive response, probably because we recruit patients in whom brain death has already been diagnosed using other criteria. Moreover we do not prolong the disconnecting test for more than 15 minutes because hypercapnic acidosis can depress spontaneous ventilation. As a matter of fact, repeated blood gas determinations are essential as a control. Furthermore, prior to the disconnecting test it is necessary to hypoventilate the subject to avoid alkalosis. For example, in an adult male weighing 70 kg, we will give only 7 liters of pure oxygen at a ventilation frequency of 20 respirations per minute in order to start the disconnecting test with sufficient denitrogenation and an arterial pH close to normal. The only contraindication to the disconnecting test after one hour of ventilation in pure oxygen is when the p_aO_2 is below 100 mm Hg. Under these circumstances one cannot turn off the respirator. It does not appear that hypercapnic acidosis can cause serious brain damage.

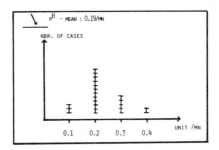

FIGURE 14. Correlation of pH and time.

CONCLUSION

The disconnecting test using pure oxygen may be utilized by general practitioners, neurologists, surgeons, anesthesiologists, and other physicians who are interested in a simple clinical complementary test for research and diagnostic purposes. Other ancillary tests are evidently useful to affirm the diagnosis of brain death, especially the EEG,[1] even if it is of relatively short duration.[11] Other confirmatory tests include measurement of arteriovenous difference in brain tissue,[2] cerebrospinal fluid examination,[9–17] electroretinography,[12] measurement of intracranial pressure,[16] echoencephalography,[10] and cerebral angiography and scintigraphy.[5]

All these subjects are treated in a special issue of the *Annales de l'Anesthésiologie Française* (1974), which was derived from a seminar held at Amiens in April 1973.*

---

* The findings reported by Milhaud and his associates have been verified in part by other investigators including Hass (unpublished data) and Fruman *et al.* (as discussed by Plum and Posner in *Diagnosis of Stupor and Coma.* 1972. F. A. Davis Co. Philadelphia), as well as by J. Schaefer and J. J. Caronna (1977. Duration of apnea needed to confirm brain death [abstract]. Neurology 27: 367).—*J. K.*

SUMMARY

The disconnecting test in pure oxygen using the apnea technique of Hirsch and Volhard (1905) and Holmdahl (1956) has been described in Amiens (1972).

This test produces transient hypercapnia without hypoxia and may be prolonged for more than 20 minutes without danger of either circulatory arrest or additional cerebral damage.

Preliminary artificial ventilation in pure oxygen has to be given for more than one hour (denitrogenation). O_2 uptake is measured using the ventilation spirograph. Arterial blood is taken every three minutes for gas measurements. The ventricular frequency and arterial pressure are monitored at the same time. In ten adults of average size, all with total brain death, we found a mean oxygen uptake of 193 ml/minute. Ventricular frequency and arterial blood pressure p_aO_2 was always higher than 100 mm Hg (even after 20 minutes). p_aCO_2 increased dramatically to more than 80 mm Hg, and the blood pH decreased to less than 7.05 units, but spontaneous ventilation was never present again. The fact that spontaneous ventilation is not present postdenitrogenation and after apnea in pure oxygen for more than 15 minutes seems to be one of the best criteria of total brain death, except in cases of acute intoxication or deep hypothermia.

REFERENCES

1. ARFEL, G. & H. FISCHGOLD. 1973. Signification du silence électrique cérébral. Electroencephalogr. Clin. Neurophysiol. **13:** 653.
2. BES, A., G. GERAUD, M. ESCANDE & J. GERAUD. 1974. La différence artério-veineuse en oxygène dans les comas dépassés. Recherche d'un critère biologique de la mort du cerveau. Ann. Anesthesiol. Fr. **XV**(III): 80–86.
3. CAMPBELL, J. A. & L. HILL. 1931. Concerning the amount of nitrogen gas in the tissues and its removal by breathing almost pure oxygen. J. Physiol. **71:** 309–322.
4. CARA, M. 1956. Influence de la circulation sur le taux alvéolaire du gaz carbonique. C. R. Soc. Biol. : 150.
5. FREREBEAU, PH. 1974. La circulation cérébrale du coma dépassé. Ann. Anesthesiol. Fr. **XV**(III): 34–40.
6. GALIBERT, P. Personal communication.
7. HIRSCH, H. Uber künsliche Atmung durch Ventilation der Trachea (dissertation). Giessen, 1905. Cited by Holmdahl.[8]
8. HOLMDAHL, M. H. 1956. Pulmonary uptake of oxygen, acid-base metabolism, and circulation during prolonged apnea. Acta Chir. Scand. (Suppl. 212).
9. LABORIT, G., A. LEGRAND & J. C. SOUFIR. 1974. Le liquide céphalo-rachidien des comas dépassés. Intérêt de l'étude enzymatique. Ann. Anesthesial Fr. **XV**(III): 48–60.
10. LEPETIT, J. P., J. P. PEFFERKORN & A. DANY. 1974. Echographie pulsatile et perte irréversible des fonctions cérébrales. Ann. Anesthesiol. Fr. **XV**(III): 101–108.
11. LEVY-ALCOVER, M. A. 1974. L'E.E.G. dans le diagnostic de coma dépassé. Annales, Anesthesiol. Fr. **XV**(III): 109–116.
12. MANTZ, J. P., A. LOBSTEIN, A. JAEGER, G. MACK & J. D. TEMPE. 1974. L'oeil dans le diagnostic de la mort cérébrale. Ann. Anesthesiol. Fr. **XV**(III): 95–100.

13. MOLLARET, P. & M. GOULON. 1959. Le coma dépassé (mémoire préliminaire). Rev. Neurol. **101**: 3.
14. NEDEY, R. 1966. Le coma dépassé (stade IV). Etude de 40 observations personnelles. Chir. **18**(1): 137–146.
15. PALMIRI, M. Cited by Cara.[4]
16. DE ROUGEMONT, J., M. BARGE & A. L. BENADID. 1974. L'égalisation des pressions intra-crânienne et artérielle systémique dans les états de mort encéphalique. Ann. Anesthesiol. Fr. **XV**(III): 117–121.
17. VOISIN, C., F. WATTEL, PH. SCHERPEREEL, B. GOSSELIN & C. CHOPIN. 1974. Apport de l'étude biochimique du liquide céphalo-rachidien au diagnostic de mort cérébral. Ann. Anesthesiol. Fr. **XV**(III): 87–94.
18. VOLHARD, F. 1908. Ueber künstliche atmung durch ventilation der trachea und eine einfache vorrichtung zur rhytmischen künstlichen atmung. Muench. Med. Wochenschr. : 55–209.

CARDIAC AND METABOLIC ALTERATIONS IN BRAIN DEATH: DISCUSSION PAPER

G. E. Ouaknine

Beilinson Medical Center
Department of Neurosurgery
Tel Aviv University Medical School
Ramat Aviv, Israel

Studies of cardiac and metabolic activities were included among 13 different tests in 52 patients who were in a state of clinical brain death (BD). These findings are presented in TABLE 1 and References 1–6. All patients were in unresponsive coma and were not breathing spontaneously. They had absent cephalic reflexes with fixed nonreactive pupils. Cardiovascular collapse, hypothermia, and polyuria usually occurred within a few days. Spinal segmental reflexes were occasionally present. The etiology in more than half the patients was head injury.

None of the patient had prior cardiac disease. Appropriate resuscitation therapy with monitoring of pulse, blood pressure and temperature was carried out on all patients. Cardiac activity in these brain-dead patients lasted for an average of 2.5 days. In 27 cases, the duration of cardiac activity was one to two days; in 23 cases, two to six days; and in two cases, seven days. Spontaneous cardiac arrest occurred in 45 patients and in seven the respirator was turned off. Progressive decline of rectal temperature to an average of 31.5° C, decrease of pulse from 86 to 55, and falling blood pressure from 110 to 60 mm Hg occurred in all cases.

Studies performed on these patients included electroencephalography, caloric testing, electronystagmography, echoencephalography, intracranial angiography, tests for cerebral blood flow and cerebral O_2 consumption, brain scan and gamma camera imaging, as well as intrathecal injection of radioiodinated serum albumin. In addition, evaluations were made on brain temperature, intracranial pressure, and pathologic studies after autopsy; see TABLE 1 and Reference 6.

This report will primarily deal with tests and findings related to cardiac activity and systemic metabolic alterations of these patients.[6-8]

ELECTROCARDIOGRAPHIC STUDIES [6-8]

In all cases a 12-lead electrocardiogram was performed. In 30 cases, continuous electrocardiographic monitoring was carried out with the aid of a Holter Avionics system until cessation of cardiac activity in 12 of them.

The electrocardiographic findings were the appearance of an additional wave (J wave) which "envelopes" the terminal part of the QRS complex and causes its broadening; prolongation of the QT interval; and depression or elevation of the ST-T segment compatible with subendocardial or subepicardial ischemia, respectively.

In the terminal phase of brain death the principal findings were progressive depression of sinus activity, atrial fibrillation, atrioventricular and intraventricu-

0077-8923/78/0315-0252 $01.75/0 © 1978, NYAS

TABLE 1

SUMMARY OF TESTS PERFORMED IN 52 PATIENTS IN BRAIN DEATH

Test	No. of Cases	Results	Remarks
Electroencephalography	38	Flat tracing even after amplification and stimulation	14 cases under oscilloscope only
Atropine test	52	No tachycardia after intravenous injection of atropine (2 mg)	42 cases under ECG
Caloric test	52	No eye movements	With ice water or ethyl chloride into the external auditory meatuses
Electronystagmography	24	Flat tracing	With ice water or ethyl chloride into the external auditory meatuses
Echoencephalography	28	No echopulsations in the oscilloscope	Demonstrated in 10 cases by photography with three different exposures
Carotid and vertebral angiography	32	Circulatory arrest at the base of the skull	Injection under pressure in five cases
Intracranial pressure	9	Very high (>100 mm Hg)	Measured by intraventricular catheter
Brain temperature	6	Brain temperature always less than rectal	Even in cases of hypothermia (e.g., $29°<32°C$)
Cerebral blood flow	9	No significant flow: <10 ml/min/100 g of brain	Xenon: 3 cases Hippuran: 6 cases
Cerebral O_2 consumption	5	<1.5 ml of O_2/min/100 ml of blood	Blood taken from carotid bifurcation and jugular bulb
Brain scanning	18	"Cold brain area" and no appearance of the superior longitudinal sinus in anterioposterior projection	Intravenous technetium
Gamma camera	12	"Cold brain area" and no appearance of the superior longitudinal sinus in anteroposterior projection	Intravenous technetium
Intrathecal injection of radioiodinated serum albumin	6	No cerebrospinal fluid flow	Even after 48 hr
Brain autopsy	28	From cerebral edema to complete lysis of brain	Corresponding to brain death duration (1–7 days)

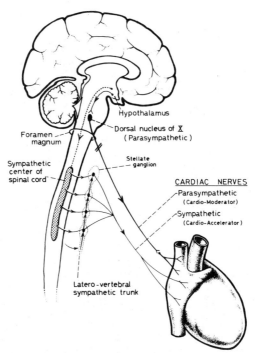

FIGURE 1. Cardiac action of the vegetative nervous system in brain death. The parasympathetic system is destroyed, while the cardiac sympathetic action continues.

lar conduction disturbances, prominent ST-T changes, and diminution of the voltage with diminution or disappearance of the J wave. In the seven cases in which the respirator was turned off (at least three days after brain death), electrocardiographic activity continued for 30 to 75 minutes.

PHARMACOLOGIC STUDIES (FIGURE 1) [6]

In the 52 cases there was no acceleration of cardiac rate after intravenous injection of 2 mg of atropine, indicating the destruction of the intracranial parasympathetic system. Normally the cardiac activity is under the antagonist influence of the intracranial parasympathetic system (vagal dorsal nucleus) and the extracranial sympathetic system. In brain death, the cardiac activity is influenced only by the sympathetic system without any regulation from the intracranial centers and by hypothermia.[7] * In 15 cases intravenous injection

---

* Although atropine has a direct effect on cardiac activity, Dr. Ouaknine appears correct in his conclusion that such small doses of intravenous atropine act centrally and are an appropriate test for brain-stem function (I. R. Innes and N. Nickerson, Chapt. 25. *In* The Pharmacological Basis of Therapeutics, 5th Ed. [1975]. L. S. Goodman and A. Gilman, Eds. : 514–523. New York, N.Y.)—*J. K.*

of 1 mg of isoproterenol always caused a marked acceleration of the heart rate and disappearance of the J waves. Intravenous injection of 2 mg of propranolol (20 cases) has always caused a slowing of the heart. Injection of propranolol after acceleration of the pulse by isoproterenol always caused a significant decrease in the pulse rate. Perfusion of aramine (50–100 mg in 500 ml) was given in 16 cases because of cardiovascular collapse; acceleration of pulse, augmentation of blood pressure and improvement on electrocardiogram were always noticed. Intravenous injection of adrenaline and noradrenaline have caused a severe arterial hypertension and tachycardia. Injection of acetylcholine and tensilon was without effect.

SYSTEMIC METABOLIC CHANGES

In four of the seven cases in which the respirator was turned off, blood was taken by cardiac puncture every 15 minutes until cessation of electrocardiographic activity. A broad range of blood chemical constituents was measured each time. The most striking modifications are exemplified by one patient. After one hour without respiratory assistance, there was a very marked increase of potassium ions, above 10 mEq/l, with increase of lactic acid from 20 mg/100 ml to 280 mg/100 ml, and pCO_2 to above 200 mm Hg; and a massive fall of the pH to 6.7 and pO_2 to 2.0 mm Hg.

Postmortem examination of the heart was carried out in 16 cases. In nine, there were no pathologic findings. Subendocardial (six cases) and subepicardial (one case) hemorrhages were found compatible with the ST-T changes on the electrocardiogram.

DISCUSSION AND CONCLUSION

The study of cardiac activity in brain death, especially in the terminal stage, has great cardiologic, neurophysiologic and pharmacologic interest.

The exceptional duration of cardiac electric activity in conditions such as we have reported (profound anoxia and acidosis) is very strange and is not described in human pathology. Exposed to the lethargic influence of hypothermia and liberated from the nociceptive influence of the parasympathetic system, the heart seems to acquire a new resistance to biological stresses. We think that these findings should be explored experimentally for a possible therapeutic application in heart disease.

In conclusion, the three bedside procedures that seem to us the more available are electroencephalography, electronystagmography, and atropine test. In recent practice, if the clinical diagnosis is evident, we may perform only the atropine test, which is the simplest test and has always proved reliable.

REFERENCES

1. GROS, C., B. VLAHOVITCH, M. BALDY-MOULINIER, G. OUAKNINE & P. FREREBEAU. 1969. Mesure du débit cérébral par clearance isotopique dans l'hypertension intracranienne. Neuro-Chir. **15:** 343.
2. OUAKNINE, G. 1973. Brain death: Clinical and laboratory criteria. Harefuah **84:** 328.

3. OUAKNINE, G., I. Z. KOSARY, J. BRAHAM, P. CZERNIAK & H. NATHAN. 1973. Laboratory criteria of brain death. J. Neurosurg. **39:** 429.
4. OUAKNINE, G., I. Z. KOSARY & M. ZIV. 1973. Valeur du test calorique et de l'electronystagmographie dans le diagnostic du coma dépassé. Neuro-Chir. **19** (4): 407.
5. OUAKNINE, G. & M. ZIV. 1974. Valeur du test calorique et de l'electronystagmographie dans le diagnostic du coma dépassé. Rev. Laryng. **95:** 445.
6. OUAKNINE, G. E. 1975. Bedside procedures in the diagnosis of brain death. Resuscitation **4:** 159.
7. DRORY, Y. & G. OUAKNINE. 1974. Cardiac activity in brain death. Harefuah **86:** 489.
8. DRORY, Y., G. OUAKNINE, I. Z. KOSARY & J. J. KELLERMANN. 1975. Electrocardiographic findings in brain death: Description and presumed mechanism. Chest **67:** 425.

EDITOR'S COMMENT

The manner in which irreversible cardiac arrest occurs in these patients is of more than passing interest and, as suggested by Dr. Ouaknine, deserves further study. In our own experience with more than 100 patients who met the criteria for brain death, we have classified three patterns which precede irreversible cardiac standstill.

The first pattern involves repeated episodes of cardiac arrhythmias which include ventricular fibrillation and periodic bizarre EKG patterns interspersed by periods of cardiac arrest. These episodes may occur repeatedly for more than 10 minutes. FIGURE 2 † illustrates the EKG of a patient meeting the cri-

† Please note that Figures 2, 3 and 4 are Dr. Korein's.

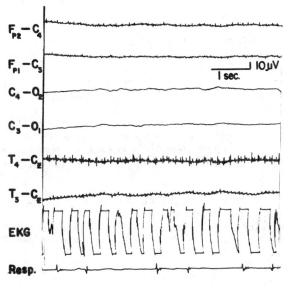

FIGURE 2

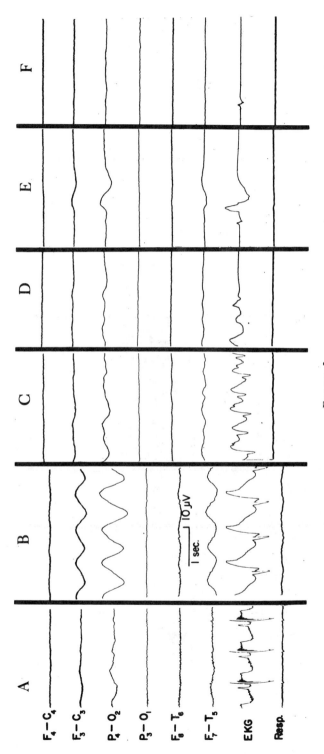

FIGURE 3

257

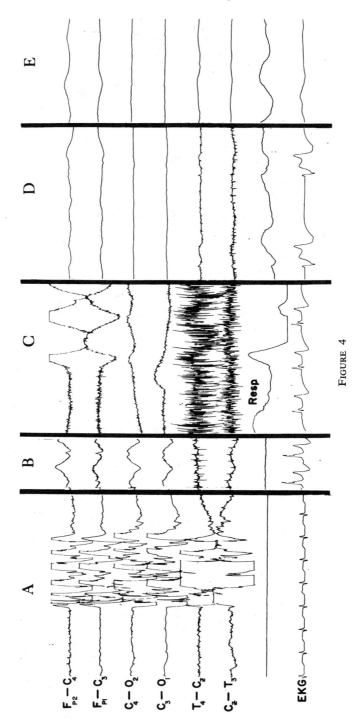

FIGURE 4

teria of brain death, showing a bizarre, tachyarrhythmia that occurred repeatedly prior to irreversible cessation of cardiac activity. This patient was being maintained on a respirator.

A second pattern is illustrated in FIGURES 3A to F. In this situation, the patient met all criteria of brain death and was taken off the respirator. The illustrations are representative samples of the gradual slowing and distortion of the EKG wave form which finally slowed down, becoming intermittent until it ceased completely. Each sample is approximately 1.5 minutes apart. (Note the EKG artefact in the EEG tracings in FIGURE 3B-E.)

The third pattern is illustrated by FIGURES 4A to E. In this situation, the patient initially did not meet the criteria for brain death and bursts were seen in the EEG (FIGURE 4A). The subsequent illustrations (FIGURES 4B to E) represent samples through a 25-minute period during which the patient met the clinical criteria of brain death and the EKG progressively slowed with concomitant distortion of the wave form; however, there were no episodic phenomena observed prior to the termination of EKG activity. Artefacts in EEG channels in FIGURE 4B were related to the EKG changes and the respirators. At one point (FIGURE 4C) there was a transient increase of EMG artefact. The respirator was not disconnected. The monitoring channel for respirations (FIGURES 4D and E) was erratic. This was due to movement of the tracheotomy tube, which was used as the source to record the activity of the respirator.

—*Julius Korein*

DISCUSSION

GOODMAN: One thing that hasn't been brought out in the discussion of ancillary tests and the diagnosis of brain death is that such a test should be one that a nonneurologic physician can utilize. I do not believe that brain death occurs that frequently on a busy intensive care ward. The diagnosis should not necessarily require evaluation by a neurophysiologist. We need a test that the average physician in the ICU can use. It should be readily available, inexpensive, easily performed, and completed quickly. Further, it should result in a hard copy that enables one to obtain a permanent record that can be placed in the patient's chart for future evaluation. The evidence for brain death should be perfectly clear.

We have had eight years of experience using the isotope angiogram. In patients with brain death the intracranial circulation stops. If you can demonstrate this, you can avoid all the previously mentioned pitfalls, especially those relating to the performance of EEGs and even parts of the clinical examination.

It is preferable to use a portable gamma camera to obtain the isotope angiogram, but most hospitals have similar nonportable equipment that may be utilized. Some illustrations of applications of this technique are presented: DISCUSSION FIGURE 1 reveals a normal portable isotope angiogram in a comatose patient. DISCUSSION FIGURES 2A and B show a portable isotope angiogram in a child before and after brain death. The third example is of a woman who had intracerebral hemorrhage documented by computerized tomography scan and who subsequently went into respiratory arrest. The patient was then given Pavulon and became decerebrate. She was also on gentamicin, which poten-

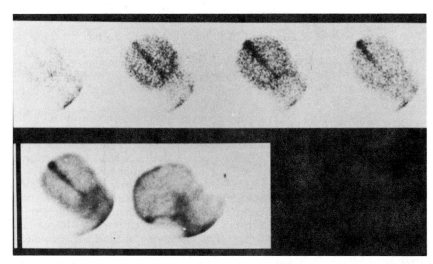

DISCUSSION FIGURE 1. Normal portable isotope angiogram taken in a 47-year-old woman who was resuscitated after cardiac arrest. An inexperienced house officer made a diagnosis of brain death, even though all clinical criteria were not present. EEG was flat. Portable isotope angiogram showed arterial flow in the distribution of the anterior and middle cerebral arteries and early filling of sagittal sinus. Static scan (*lower panel, right*) performed after several minutes showed venous sinuses.

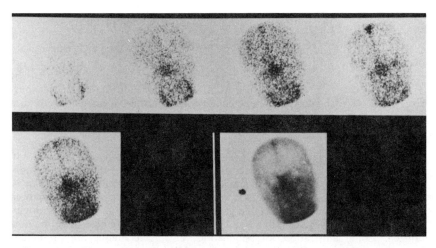

DISCUSSION FIGURE 2A. The patient was a 3-year-old girl with smoke inhalation who underwent cardiopulmonary resuscitation. A portable isotope angiogram (*above*) was normal.

tiated the neuromuscular blockade caused by Pavulon. She had high doses of barbiturates for seizures and she was hypothermic. These factors would have made clinical examination and the EEG very difficult to interpret. By use of the gamma camera, one can visualize absence of intracranial blood flow within 10 minutes (DISCUSSION FIGURE 3). The intracranial sinuses do not fill. The visual "picture" of the results of this test can be pasted on the patient's chart, and can be shown to the family, the nurses, etc. It is the simplest ancillary test that I know of to confirm brain death.

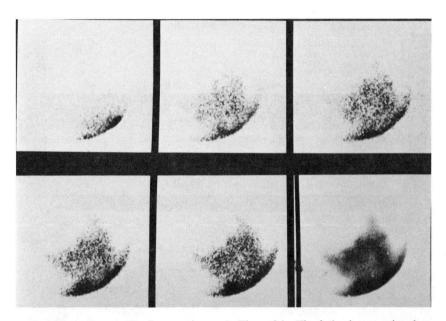

DISCUSSION FIGURE 2B. Same patient as in Figure 2A. The following morning there was clinical brain death and a repeat isotope study showed no flow above the base of the skull. An electroencephalogram at this time showed artefacts.

PLUM: It seems to me that this is a rather straightforward problem. When any organ dies, including the brain, there is blood-vessel necrosis that occurs along with tissue death. The organ loses its capability for autoregulation. As a result of brain death, intracranial pressure necessarily must equal the blood pressure, which is now striking a passive vascular bed. As the capillary circulation of that passive bed fails, one will no longer be able to pass isotopes or any other tracer through that circulation. This is not to say that this is the cause of brain death. Several experimental studies have demonstrated that the no reflow phenomenon occurs after the tissue dies, and so this is not the cause of tissue death. Nevertheless, it does become an accurate indication that the particular organ under study has not been viable for at least 30 to 60 minutes from the time of cessation of circulation. Under the circumstances that we encounter it may be very difficult to tell whether or not someone in an ICU is brain-dead. Therefore a test of intracranial circulation, such as one using isotopes, is about as simple and quick as one could hope for. It is difficult to find fault with such a test. I would appreciate other opinions.

SUTER: We have struggled with the problem of obtaining such studies on intracranial blood flow and have met with opposition, lack of interest and lack of availability of equipment. This appears to be a practical problem at this point. I believe that further controlled studies would be required. In principle, I have no opposition to such tests for intracranial circulation.

PLUM: As a clinical investigator, I am apalled at the lack of experimental

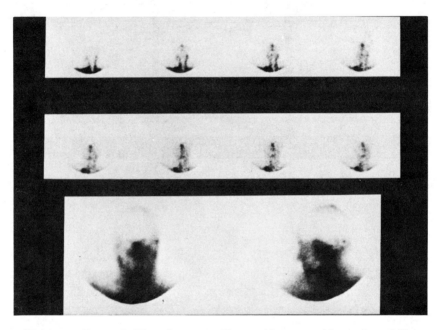

DISCUSSION FIGURE 3. The paient was a 50-year-old woman with a prolonged illness and metabolic encephalopathy who developed a spontaneous intracerebral hemorrhage demonstrated by CT scan. Hypothermia was also present. The isotope angiogram and subsequent static scans (*bottom row*) are typical of brain death.

work to support any of the particular viewpoints that have been advanced.

SUTER: I think that the experimental design in evaluating these tests of intracranial circulation would have to be specified. The EEG, which we are more familiar with, despite the pitfalls described, which can often be overcome, should be used in any controlled study. We do have an extremely large quantity of data on the EEG in brain death which affords a reliable comparison to other ancillary techniques used to aid in diagnosis. The test described by Dr. Goodman may be worthwhile, especially in patients who are in coma but are not brain-dead. We would not eliminate the performance of EEGs on patients who are brain-dead if the results are validated.

BRAUNSTEIN: All I can say about a controlled study is that many thousands of brain scans are performed every day, including an isotope flow study and delayed scans. Our own experience and inquiries to other departments of nuclear medicine have resulted in complete confirmation that there is no condition other than brain death where one sees no blood entering the head and absent sinuses.

PLUM: It seems to me that you are attempting to resurrect the brain scan, which is being replaced by the CT scanner, from its approaching obsolescence. In our institution, it is difficult for me to understand the role of the brain scan except in situations such as this. We have computerized axial tomography available 16 hours a day.

WALKER: The question was raised as to what ancillary technique might be used in the ordinary hospital where sophisticated neurologic and physiologic equipment may not be available. The answer to this is relatively simple. One can confirm brain death by either further examinations, such as we have mentioned, or by further observation of the patient. In following patients who had all clinical manifestations of brain death for a period of three days, we have found no patient who has recovered after that time. Therefore, in the ordinary hospital without the use of electroencephalography or any of these examinations that I have mentioned, one could determine brain death simply by the additional clinical observation of the patient. Insofar as the use of scans is concerned, in the future computerized tomography may replace scans for the determination of brain death. As I have indicated, it is possible by means of computerized tomography using enhancement to demonstrate the intracranial vessels. This is possible if blood is passing through them and they are opacified. It is now rather common for patients coming into the emergency room to go directly to the CT scanner and have a picture made. This is probably going to replace many of the other examinations that we are currently performing for the determination of brain death.

GOLDMAN: Dr. Milhaud, do you recommend using the disconnecting test in patients with post-traumatic pulmonary insufficiency or metabolic acidosis, which we frequently see in the military?

MILHAUD: Are you asking whether we use the test in patients with cranial and pulmonary trauma?

GOLDMAN: Correct, or in patients who have multiple trauma where they have post-traumatic pulmonary insufficiency—the adult respiratory distress syndrome.

MILHAUD: In these situations, it is important to have a good result of blood gas measurement before starting the tests. If the initial pO_2 is below 70 mm Hg, for example, I don't recommend the test, of course.

WALKER: Dr. Milhaud, what do you do if you have a rare case with a combination of chronic obstructive pulmonary disease in an advanced stage and brain death? Do you worry then about the lack of hypoxic drive for the apnea test?

MILHAUD: If the initial pO_2 is too low, below 100 mm Hg it is necessary to be very prudent because hypoxia will be present anyway. Of course, the disconnecting test does not cause hypoxia except if the initial arterial pO_2 is markedly decreased. I was asked whether or not high pCO_2 causes brain damage. Can one be sure that one is not aggravating a pre-existing neurologic lesion with high pCO_2? We cannot be positive. However, in previous experience with other patients, we have not caused lesions of the nervous system when the pH is low and the pCO_2 is high.

WALKER: This question has been debated extensively in this country. Our concern has not been so much for the brain because these tests are done at a time when we consider the brain to be dead. The question has been raised as to whether an increased arterial pCO_2 might not be toxic to other organs. In our series of patients with brain death, 25 percent had irreversible cardiac arrest due to cardiac lesions such as infarction. If the patient had an increased pCO_2 and a decreased arterial pH, for example, would we not then damage these other organs?

MILHAUD: It is possible, but the majority of the patients in whom we performed the disconnecting test were young and had no cardiac disease. They were candidates for organ transplantation. We never saw arrythmia or aggravation of cardiac activity during the test.

CARONNA: Dr. Severinghaus and Dr. Comroe, using patients who were paralyzed, raised the pCO_2 levels to 100 mm Hg without any permanent deleterious effects. I have two further comments to make. First, we have frequently used this type of oxygenation test for apnea. Drs. Plum and Posner have alluded to it in their book, and the only caveat is that we have used it in patients after cardiac arrest. However, if a patient is on dopamine you must continue to increase the dopamine since the acidosis causes hypotension. Second, my only point of disagreement is that I do not believe that you have to keep increasing the arterial pCO_2 indiscriminately. Drs. Comroe, Severinghaus, Truman and others have shown that pCO_2s above 70 depress brain function, although this is reversible. In addition, a pH below 7.0 depresses respiration. Since there is debate about the subject and a pCO_2 of about 60 gives maximal stimulation to respiratory effort, I do not see any reason to allow the pCO_2 to rise into the hundreds, possibly causing CO_2 narcosis.

MORPHOLOGY OF DEFECTIVELY PERFUSED BRAINS IN PATIENTS WITH PERSISTENT EXTRACRANIAL CIRCULATION

John Pearson, J. Korein, and P. Braunstein

Departments of Pathology, Neurology, and Radiology
New York University Medical Center
New York, New York 10016

The advent of efficient machines for the artificial support of respiration coupled with clinical reliance on cessation of heart beat as an indicator of death has made it commonplace for pathologists to find evidence that the brain of a comatose patient has died long before the rest of the body. The dead brain has softened and may even have disintegrated while heart function has continued (FIGURE 1). The heart is a resilient muscular pump, a component of the mechanical and chemical support systems of the body. Within the cerebrum of the brain neuronal function gives rise to such human attributes as complex emotion, abstract thought, foresight, and precise communication. Cognitive function can occur when the heart and lungs are replaced by machines; the brain cannot be replaced by a machine. Without a brain a carcass can have no interest in its own continuance. Such a carcass functions at an incomplete low level and cannot support itself. It cannot actively contribute to the welfare of other human beings, but its presence can certainly contribute to their misery and exhaustion.

Physicians using life-support machinery during the perimortem period may unintentionally find themselves caring for a biological preparation with no other human attributes than physical form. Since they initiate use of such machinery physicians should be willing to retain the sole responsibility for switching it off. It is unfair to transfer emotional stress and possible feelings of guilt to those who love or know the patient by asking them to participate actively in the decision to terminate care. In order that family and friends can be spared this burden physicians must have well-defined and legally accepted evidence that human life has ceased.

A strong plea has been made for the inclusion of irreversible loss of cognitive function in statutory definitions of death.[1] Since surcease of all essentially human attributes must occur with the death of the brain, it would seem reasonable to base a definition of the time of human death on the death of the brain rather than that of other organs. Such a definition could be further narrowed to concentrate on death of the cerebrum alone since it is in the cerebrum that cognitive and communicative functions are centered, with the remainder of the brain serving mainly in conductive and regulatory roles. Some states accept the concept of brain death when it can be shown that the entire brain within the skull including the brain stem is dead. Experience indicates that in the majority of such cases the spinal cord within the spinal column will not have died. If death can be certified while the spinal reflexive and conductive component of the central nervous system is still alive, then it would seem reasonable to certify death when the reflexive and conductive elements of the infratentorial brain are alive, but the supratentorial sentient brain is dead. There is nothing

265

0077–8923/78/0315–0265 $01.75/0 © 1978, NYAS

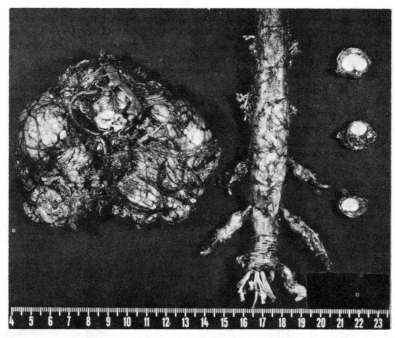

FIGURE 1A. The cerebellum is necrotic and partially macerated, particularly adjacent to the medulla, which itself is soft, discolored and abnormally low in position. The dural sac surrounding the lumbar spinal cord is distended.

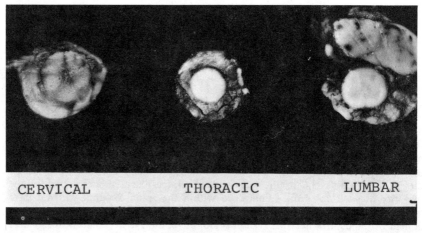

CERVICAL   THORACIC   LUMBAR

FIGURE 1B. Closeups of the spinal cord in cross section show that the distension is due to avulsed necrotic brain fragments displaced into the cerebrospinal fluid space.

intrinsically significant in the intracranial location of the infratentorial brain. Infratentorial structures cannot by themselves generate consciousness.

There is widespread support for the certification of death when the entire brain is dead (brain death) while other organs continue to function. More controversial is the concept that such certification is justified when the cerebrum alone is dead (cerebral death) while other parts of the brain and general soma continue to function.

When the cerebrum is dead, there can be no return of a cognitive state. Cerebral functioning can, however, be clinically undetectable for prolonged periods when in fact the cerebrum is alive and potentially capable of regaining good function.[2] Electroencephalographic activity may be below recordable levels during temporary intoxication.[3] Thus, lack of primary and reflexive cerebral function or of detectable electrical activity may not be reliable indicators of cerebral death.

Persistent absence of cerebral circulation should be a good indicator of cerebral death since intrinsic energy reserves of the brain are sufficient for only a few minutes of life.[4] A simple bedside technique has been developed for the detection of critical deficits in cerebral blood flow.[5] The passage of a bolus of radioactive technetium through the systemic and cerebral circulations is monitored. If cerebral blood flow is less than 20 percent of normal, no bolus trace is recorded from the head. Angiographic studies indicate that the bolus technique reliably detects absence of significant blood flow through the cerebrum.[6] Neuropathologic changes in comatose, apneic patients on whom repeated bolus studies were performed at least 20 hours prior to cardiac death confirm that the absence or presence of a head bolus distinguishes two distinct subsets of patients.[7]

PATHOLOGIC OBSERVATIONS IN PATIENTS STUDIED WITH THE BOLUS TECHNIQUE

In the absence of a bolus a critical deficit in cerebral blood flow was predicted. The brains from six patients with absence of bolus were diffusely swollen, congested and cyanotic. They were extremely soft, and the demarcation of gray from white matter was diminished. The pressure exerted by the swollen brain had caused some of the necrotic tissue to be squeezed into abnormal positions in a process known as herniation. Parts of the cerebrum were displaced into space normally occupied by lower parts of the brain. Parts of the cerebellum were forced into the spinal canal. In some instances fragments of dead brain had broken off and were floating free in the cerebrospinal fluid around the spinal cord in the lower part of the back. Microscopically no evidence could be found for persistent blood flow. The necrotic brain was autolysed as evidenced by breakdown of intrinsic cells without any contribution from factors dependent on blood supply. Red cells, lining cells of blood vessels, supportive cells of brain and neurons were all involved in the autolytic process. The autolytic changes involved the cerebellum and brain stem as well as the cerebrum. Thus, it was found that the entire brain was dead when a persistent critical deficit in cerebral blood flow had been shown by absence of a head bolus 20 hours prior to cessation of cardiac activity. Autolysis of the degree found indicated that the brains had been kept warm after their deaths. Such autolysis can be mimicked by keeping dead animal brain at 37° C for 20 hours prior to fixation (FIGURE 2). The pathologic changes demonstrated that the brains of

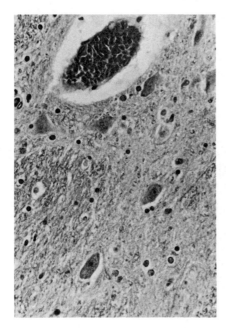

FIGURE 2A. Human brain cooled prior to fixation: Normal neurons, astrocytes and oligodendroglia are present. (This figure and FIGURES 2B, C, D, and E are all stained with hematoxylin and eosin; magnification ×252.)

FIGURE 2B. Rat brain fixed immediately after death: Normal neurons, astroglia, oligodendroglia and vessels are present.

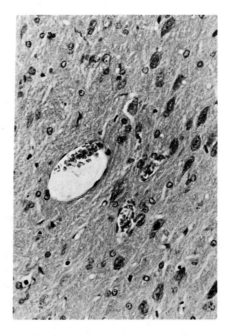

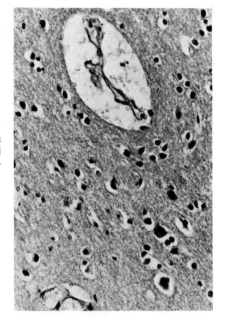

FIGURE 2C. Autolysed human brain from a "no bolus" patient: Neuronal detail is obscured. Glial nuclei are condensed. Vessels are degenerated.

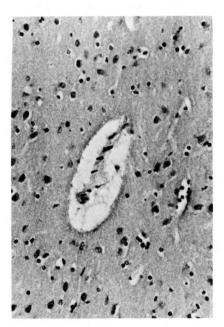

FIGURE 2D. Rat brain kept in the dead head and permitted to autolyse at 37° C for 20 hours prior to fixation: Neuronal detail is obscured. Glial nuclei are condensed. Vessels are degenerated.

the six patients without bolus traces were without blood supply and were dead while mechanical and chemical functions required to maintain body temperature were intact or replaced by artificial systems.

In six patients with a head bolus present 20 hours before cardiac standstill pathologic changes were less severe and were focal rather than diffuse. Widespread softening and herniation were not present. Necrotic tissue was never displaced into the spinal canal. In all six patients there was microscopic evidence of persistent blood flow in focally necrotic regions. Red cells within blood vessels were intact; vascular endothelium was swollen and reactive. Scavenger cells had migrated into the necrotic zones to begin the active process of removal of debris. Astrocytes were generally reactive rather than necrotic. A few places were found in which minor degrees of autolysis indicated local absence of blood flow. The cerebellum and brain stem were generally undamaged.

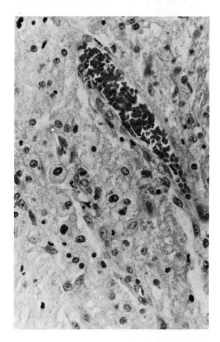

FIGURE 2E. Reactive changes in human brain from a "bolus present" patient: Blood vessel endothelium is prominent. Astroglial nuclei are enlarged. Macrophages are present.

COMMENT

The bolus technique has been shown to be capable of detecting critical deficit in blood flow in adults.[6] Pathologic studies support the clinical prediction that in the persistent absence of adequate blood flow there is diffuse cerebral necrosis. If a bolus is absent during studies repeated at a one-hour interval, it can be confidently predicted that the cerebrum is dead and that cognitive function will never return. Results to date indicate that the hindbrain is also dead, but more experience is needed before it is known that this will always be the case. A more extensive study demonstrated that no patient lacking a bolus ever survived.[6] In the absence of a bolus it would appear that efforts to support a comatose patient are futile.

In the presence of a bolus it is likely that parts of the brain are morphologically intact and at least potentially capable of recovery of function. The eventual outcome will depend on the nature and extent of the focal brain damage and the integrity of other organ systems. While many comatose, apneic patients with a bolus present do die,[6] intensive therapeutic efforts on their behalf are justified.

We have not had the opportunity to test the bolus technique in a comatose patient with reversible suppression of brain electrical and metabolic activity caused by toxins such as barbiturates. There is no theoretical reason, however, to suspect that cerebral blood flow would be absent in such a patient even though oxygen uptake may be minimal. It is anticipated that a bolus would be present and that potential for recovery would thus be correctly predicted.

There are several categories of patients in whom the bolus technique has not been sufficiently evaluated. These include infants and young children, patients with apallic syndromes or persistent vegetative state, and patients within six hours of inception of cerebral insult. The bolus technique does not test brainstem viability; such testing requires other clinical and laboratory methods.

The bolus technique is a valuable predictor of the presence or absence of diffuse cerebral death in comatose respirator-supported patients. Cerebral death associated with local failure of blood flow can be detected while the mechanics of extracerebral circulation remain intact. The bolus technique can be used to confirm whether or not there has been death of that part of the brain which is essential for the continuance of the cognitive and communicative functions that are most characteristic of human life.

REFERENCES

1. BERESFORD, H. R. 1977. The Quinlan decision. Problems and legislative alternatives. Ann. Neurol. **2:** 74–81.
2. ROSENBERG, G. A., S. F. JOHNSON & R. P. BRENNER. 1977. Recovery of cognition after prolonged vegetative state. Ann. Neurol. **2:** 167–168.
3. POWNER, D. 1976. Drug associated isoelectric EEG's—a hazard in brain death certification. JAMA **236:** 1123.
4. MYERS, R. E. & M. YAMAGUCHI. 1976. Effects of serum glucose concentration on brain response to circulatory arrest. J. Neuropath. Exper. Neurol. **35:** 301.
5. BRAUNSTEIN, P., I. KRICHEFF, J. KOREIN & K. COREY. 1973. Cerebral death: A rapid and reliable diagnostic adjunct using radioisotopes. J. Nucl. Med. **14:** 122–124.
6. KOREIN, J., P. BRAUNSTEIN, A. GEORGE, M. WICHTER, I. KRICHEFF, A. LIEBERMAN & J. PEARSON. 1977. Brain death: I. Angiographic correlation with the radioisotopic bolus technique for evaluation of critical deficit of cerebral blood flow. Ann. Neurol. **2:** 195–205.
7. PEARSON, J., J. KOREIN, J. H. HARRIS, M. WICHTER & P. BRAUNSTEIN. 1977. Brain death: II. Neuropathological correlation with the radioisotopic bolus technique for evaluation of critical deficit of cerebral blood flow. Ann. Neurol. **2:** 206–210.

PATHOLOGY OF BRAIN DEATH

A. Earl Walker

Department of Surgery
Division of Neurosurgery
University of New Mexico School of Medicine
Albuquerque, New Mexico 87123

INTRODUCTION

A number of reports on the pathologic changes found in the brains of persons maintained on a respirator have appeared in the last few years.[2, 3, 5, 7, 8, 10, 13, 17, 19, 21, 23] These studies have emphasized the varied alterations that develop under such circumstances. To illustrate this point a brief summary of the findings in 226 brains from the Collaborative Study of Cerebral Death * will be presented.[22]

Gross Findings

The mean weight of the brains examined was 1450 ± 196 grams, a figure within the range of a series of brains from persons matched for age and sex. However, if the series is broken down into those cases meeting the basic criteria of a dead brain and those with some evidence of cerebral viability, the former group has, on the average, heavier brains.

Appearance of the Brain

In many cases, the gross appearance of the brain was more the result of the secondary reactions than the primary pathologic lesion. In this series, approximately 10 percent of the brains looked normal. The remainder were swollen, soft, and discolored to a greater or lesser degree. Herniations at the tentorial notch were present in 67 percent of the patients, especially in those who had been on the respirator for 24 hours or more.

Spinal Cord

The spinal cord was the best-preserved part of the nervous system, appearing grossly normal in 60 percent of the cases. Sections of the spinal cord stained for cells and myelin were usually normal. In about 10 percent of the cords examined, fragments of cerebellar tissue were found in the spinal subarachnoid space. Little or no inflammatory reaction was noted at the site of these folial deposits. The most prominent myelopathy was seen at the junction of the

---

* The terms "cerebral death" and "brain death" are usually used interchangeably in this article.—*J. K.*

0077–8923/78/0315–0272 $01.75/0 © 1978, NYAS

cervical cord and the medulla oblongata where tonsillar herniations occur. Moreover, at this site there is blood supply from both the cerebral and spinal circulations, so that even if the cerebral supply is blocked, "demarcating reactions" consisting of localized edema and petechial hemorrhages may be produced by the spinal vascular system. In this series, 54 of 127 cases examined had localized edema, necrosis, infarction, or hemorrhage at the cervicomedullary junction. In 51 spinal cords, at other levels, there was edema, neuronal loss, neurolysis of anterior horn cells, hemorrhage, and (rarely) infarction.

Brain Stem

The brain stem had a variety of lesions. The medulla oblongata, bearing the brunt of the pressure and distortion due to displacement and compression by the cerebellar tonsils, was flattened, edematous, and had neuronal fallout. In some cases, the pons was the site of edema, necrosis, neurolysis, and/or petechial hemorrhages, usually on the periphery. Mesencephalic displacement, distortion, and compression by transtentorial herniations were common and were accompanied by edema and hemorrhages. The sites of these midline or periaqueductal bleedings were often flame-shaped and confluent.

Cerebellum

The cerebellar pathology, although prominent, was variable in degree. In 36 cases (16 percent) there was no apparent abnormality in the cerebellum. The caudal displacement of the cerebellar tonsils was often associated with necrosis and laceration. In some cases, a rostral shift produced compression and secondary necrosis of the culmen. Histologically, the changes were mainly in the cerebellar folia. Necrosis of the granular layer was associated with varying degrees of neurolysis of the Purkinje cells and pericellular edema. In all, about 80 percent of the cases had some such, and in the majority of cases quite pronounced, alterations in the little brain.

Diencephalon

The structure of the diencephalon was preserved, but neuronal edema or lysis were common. Small hypothalamic or thalamic infarcts or softenings, probably due to displacement and compression by a transtentorial herniation, were frequently encountered.

Cortex

The cerebral cortex was most consistently (94 percent of the cases) involved by pericellular edema, necrosis, neuronal loss, hemorrhage, and infarction. The extent of the lesions varied, in some cases being diffuse and in other cases patchy.

The neuropathologic findings in the patients dying within the first six hours were more related to the acute lesions precipitating the morbidity than to anoxic phenomena. Cardiac disorders and trauma accounted for 22 of the 35 persons dying in the first 24 hours on the respirator. Gross and petechial hemorrhages, subarachnoid bleeding, and edema of the hemispheres and brain stem were commonly seen in these brains. Lytic or necrotic changes in this early period were difficult to identify.

The constellation of pathologic findings termed "respirator brain" (RB) has been considered the substrate of cerebral death.[11] The pathologic picture described as respirator brain was present in approximately 40 percent of the cases in the series. Such brains are characterized by swollen cerebral hemispheres, brain stem and cerebellum, with herniations into the foramen magnum caudally and the incisura rostrally. Rarely (1 percent of cases) the brain is mushy, but often it is so soft that it is difficult to remove from the calvarium without tearing the brain stem. The cerebellum, particularly the tonsils, may be necrotic and fragmented, with pieces of tonsillar tissue displaced and lodged along the spinal cord anywhere from the cauda equina to the cervical segments. Even though the brain is placed in a fixative soon after death, the tissues may not harden well. Microscopically, there is necrosis of many parts of the brain, particularly the cerebellar folia and the cerebral cortex. The basal ganglia and the diencephalon are less affected than most other areas of the brain. In spite of the severe necrosis, there is little or no inflammatory or cellular reaction, although occasionally gliosis may be present. The cerebellar folia (particularly the granular layer and, in varying degrees, the Purkinje cells) are edematous and necrotic. Pyknotic nuclei and eosinophilic neuronal cytoplasm are usually evident in histologic preparations from all parts of the cerebrum. Endothelial changes occlude many cortical capillaries, but frank thromboses are rarely encountered. As a result, ischemic changes of the cortical neurons—"red neurons"—are present.[4, 6] A marked decrease in nerve cells is present in places, amounting to a laminar necrosis. Generally, the cerebral cortex is more severely involved than the white matter.

The brains of patients on the respirator for several weeks, especially if some cranial nerve function or biological activity in the EEG remained, show patchy multiple lesions of the gray and white matter that usually do not fulfill the requirements of a respirator brain.

DISCUSSION

It is obvious that the state of the brain of persons suspected of cerebral death varies greatly from minimal to severe necrotic changes. None of the brains are normal, but only 1–2 percent are completely necrotic and mushy. But there is a gradation in the alterations found in brains from patients suffering from similar conditions and for essentially the same length of time. This does not mean that these factors play no role in the pathologic findings. Certainly the time the patient is on the respirator before death has an influence upon the pathologic changes in the brain.

However, the period of artificial ventilation is only a rough estimation of the time the brain was anoxic, for the pathologic alterations are secondary to anoxia as the result of cessation of cerebral blood flow (CBF). If the latter could be more accurately determined, the correlation between no CBF and RB might be greater.

Time on Respirator

Of the brains from persons on artificial respiration for up to 12 hours, only two of 15 were classified as respirator brains; of the 19 brains from those on the respirator 12 to 23.9 hours, five met the criteria for respirator brains; and of 65 brains in patients artificially ventilated for 24 to 47.9 hours, 32 were considered respirator brains. Thereafter, in patients on the respirator for a further 96 hours, approximately half (36) of the 74 brains were classified as respirator brains. After that time, the number dropped to approximately 33 percent. One interpretation of this sequence might be that a respirator brain requires approximately 24 hours to develop.†

TABLE 1

CORRELATION OF CLINICAL, EEG, AND PATHOLOGIC FINDINGS IN SUBJECTS
ON THE RESPIRATOR AT LEAST 24 HOURS

State of Cephalic Reflexes and EEG on Final Examination	Respirator Brain	Nonrespirator Brain	
Absent cephalic reflexes and ECS	69	38 *	
Absent CR and not ECS	3 †	20	
Present CR and ECS	1 ‡	3	
Present CR and not ECS	5 §	33	
	78	94	172

* These cases had the following mitigating factors: (1) absent CR and ECS developed less than 24 hours before death in 24 cases and at an unknown time in two cases; (2) brain-stem damage was the primary lesion in seven cases; (3) cortical lesions were present in four cases; (4) the histopathology was unknown in one case.

† Two of these patients had so much electrocardiographic and muscle artefact in their records that neither BA or ECS could be diagnosed; the record on the other patient was made five hours before death.

‡ The last clinical examination on this patient was made 30 hours before death.

§ EEGs and clinical examinations were made 1, 9, 60 and 208 hours before death in four cases; the fifth had brain-stem damage.

The Clinical State

Assuming that the encephalic changes considered typical of a respirator brain require approximately 24 hours to develop, a respirator brain would not be expected unless a person had been artificially ventilated for at least a day. Accordingly, to ascertain the real correlation between the absence of clinical and electroencephalographic (EEG) evidences of death and the respirator brain, one should analyze only those cases that had been aerated for at least 24 hours. One may assume that the state of the cephalic reflexes (CR) is an index of the clinical condition. In TABLE 1, the CR and EEG are related to the neuro-

† It would appear, as Dr. Walker previously mentioned, that the critical factor in development of the "respirator brain" is not the time on the respirator, but other factors such as cessation of cerebral blood flow.—*J. K.*

pathology as defined by the RB. It is apparent that absence of CR and biological activity in the EEG is associated with a RB in 65.5 percent of cases. However, if the 38 nonrespirator brain cases are analyzed, certain mitigating factors become apparent. Of these patients with absent cephalic reflexes and ECS whose brains did not meet the criteria of a respirator brain, 24, and possibly 26, had had these clinical findings for less than 24 hours, so that they might not have had sufficient time to develop RB. An additional seven patients with severe brain-stem damage might have had spurious signs as the result of low blood pressure. Thus, a more accurate figure for cases with nonrespirator brains would be obtained by eliminating these 33 cases; there remain five anomalous cases, which gives a correlation of 93.2 percent between absence of cephalic reflexes, ECS and RB.

In the other categories corrections might also be made for the mitigating factors which would improve the correlation.

It should be recognized that a brain may have irreparable and lethal changes without necessarily meeting all criteria for cerebral death. This would be particularly true if the major site of insult were along the brain stem, where vital functions have their anatomic loci. These considerations may explain the few cases that do not seem to follow the general rule that absent function is associated with morphological brain changes.

The principal point of controversy regarding the changes in the brain in cerebral death, in particular the respirator brain, relates to its pathogenesis.[1] Because the changes described above as characteristic of the respirator brain may be found in nonventilated patients as the result of delayed fixation or inadequate refrigeration of the cadaver, some neuropathologists do not accept the concept, but regard the condition as postmortem autolysis. Although some changes—a swollen, discolored brain, and "red" neurons—are particularly prominent in the respirator brain, and other alterations—softening and necrosis —in the autolysed brain, perhaps the only distinctive feature is the presence in the respirator brain of fragments of cerebellar tissue in the subarachnoid or subdural space. These fragments break off from the macerated cerebellar, usually tonsillar, herniations that result from swelling of the intracranial contents.[18] Presumably, because the respirator causes repetitive pressure changes (pulsations) in the spinal subarachnoid space, the necrotic herniation becomes fragmented and pieces of cerebellar tissue traverse the subarachnoid or subdural space to be deposited among the nerve roots.

To understand the different concepts regarding the neuropathologic substrate of cerebral death, it is necessary to consider the biochemical changes that occur in postmortem autolysis.

Usually this process results from the biochemical release of intracellular enzymes which are normally within mitochondria, lysosomes or microsomes. As the result of unbalanced action of phosphatase and anaerobic glycolysis, lactic and other acids accumulate, producing an acidosis which destroys lysosomes releasing a protein-splitting enzyme—cathepsin. Thus, in autolysis the long-chain molecules of protein are broken down into smaller elements which increase the osmotic activity, and water is drawn into cells and interstitial tissue. If these enzymes are destroyed by preheating the fresh tissue to 55° C or by cellular poisons, these changes do not occur and the brain tissue retains its normal appearance and staining reactions.

With this concept of autolysis, we may consider the alterations that occur in cerebral deaths. If one assumes, as often occurs, that cerebral death is the total infarction of the brain, the changes evolving, as Lindenberg has stated, would depend upon the premortal state of the central nervous system. If the brain was hypoxic prior to arrest of circulation and had exhausted its supply of oxygen and the enzymes associated with Krebs cycle, the encephalic structures would undergo little necrosis in the postmortem period. Under such conditions the phosphocreatinine, ATP and ADP would be depleted and what glucogenic substance was present could not be utilized, even anaerobically, so that little lactic acid would be produced. On the other hand, if the brain had a large supply of enzymes and glucose, in the absence of oxygen, anaerobic glycolysis would produce lactic acid. Lindenberg calculated that acidosis might develop at the rate of 0.15 of 1 pH/minute, thus creating an optimal environment for the release of hydrolytic enzymes normally contained within lysosomes. Thus, a disturbance of the osmotic balance would induce a marked uptake of water by cells and interstitial tissue. Further evidence for this hypothesis has come from the work of Myers and Yamaguchi,[12] who showed that food-deprived monkeys may recover from a 10-minute arrest of cerebral circulation, whereas glucose-infused animals develop myoclonic seizures and die within two days. The food-deprived animals have a moderate decrease in ATP to 0.08 μmol/g (control 2.08), moderately increases in lactate to 12.08 μmol/g (control 3.01), and an increased Na, K-activated ATPase activity. In glucose-infused animals, 10 minutes of circulatory arrest decrease ATP only to 0.1 μmol/g, but markedly increase cerebral lactate to 32.5 μmol/g. The brains of the food-deprived animals have no significant changes, whereas the brains of the fed monkeys are edematous and swollen and have an impaired blood-brain barrier resembling the RB.

It is thus apparent that autolysis and the changes produced by cerebral anoxia, although differing in degree, may be somewhat similar. Moreover, since both are dependent upon enzymatic activity, they may be modified by conditions that alter or deplete cellular enzymes or metabolites.

In the early stages of anoxia, as long as some circulation is present, lactic acid produced by the anaerobic cellular metabolism may be picked up and carried away by the blood stream, thus lessening the tendency to acidosis. However, if the trend is not balanced within six hours, osmotic acidosis causes swelling of the vascular endothelium that reduces the size of the lumen. In another 12 to 48 hours, the capillaries are plugged by swollen endothelium, blebs or erythrocytic debris. This state further aggravates the oxygen supply to the brain. The vicious circle is thus completed.

These changes require time for their evolution. Since the alterations decrease the density of the brain tissue, they might be followed by serial computerized tomography. Only a few reports have appeared on this subject. They have indicated that the varying pathologic changes that occur in cerebral death give inconstant findings in computerized tomograms. Theoretically, if the brain became a homogenous gelatinous mass as the result of autolysis, with obliteration of the cerebral ventricles by the swollen cerebral tissue, tomograms should demonstrate a generalized reductions of the attenuation of the brain. However, Rådberg and Söderlundh [16] found no such generalized reduction nor obliteration of the cerebral ventricles, even when an examination was made four to five days after the establishment of the diagnosis of cerebral death. Localized attenuation in cases of cerebral infarction is detectable at times after eight hours, although several days may pass before such changes become evident.

In life, the difference in attenuation between grey and white matter is probably due to the greater vascularity of the grey matter. With the congestion of the cortex found in cerebral death, the attenuation may increase early, as it does in the grey matter of cadavers, although prolonged obliteration of the capillaries by endothelial swelling and subsequent autolysis might decrease the attenuation level. Obviously, more studies of the changes seen by computerized tomography over a period of time are necessary to establish the characteristic findings and the variations that occur in time.

REFERENCES

1. ADAMS, H. 1976. Letter to editor—"the respirator brain." Arch. Neurol. **33:** 589–590.
2. ADAMS, R. D. & M. JÉQUIER. 1969. The brain death syndrome—hypoxemic panencephopathy. Schweiz. Med. Wochenschr. **99:** 65–73.
3. BERTRAND, I., F. LHERMITTE, B. ANTOINE & H. DUCROT. 1959. Nécroses massives de système nerveux central dans une survie artificielle. Rev. Neurol. **101:** 101–115.
4. BRIERLEY, J. B., B. S. MELDRUM & A. W. BROWN. 1973. The threshold and neuropathology of cerebral "anoxic-ischemic" cell damage. Arch. Neurol. **29:** 367–373.
5. FUGIMOTO, T. 1973. "Brain death" and vital phenomena: Autopsy findings in cases maintained on a respirator for a prolonged period. Jap. J. Clin. Med. **31:** 700–706.
6. GREENFIELD, J. G. & A. MEYER. 1963. General pathology of the nerve cell and neuroglia. In Greenfield's Neuropathology, 2nd ed : 29–34. Williams and Wilkins. Baltimore, Md.
7. KJELDSBERG, C. R. 1972. Respirator brain. In Pathology of the Nervous System. J. Minckler, Ed. **3:** 2952–2961. McGraw-Hill. New York, N.Y.
8. KRAMER, W. 1970. Acute lethal intracranial hypertension Clinical and experimental observations. Psychiat. Neurol. Neurochir. **73:** 243–255.
9. LINDENBERG, R. 1972. Systemic oxygen deficiencies: The respirator brain In Pathology of the Nervous System. J. Minckler, Ed. **2:** 1583–1617. McGraw-Hill. New York, N.Y.
10. MOLLARET, P., I. BERTRAND & H. MOLLARET. 1959. Coma dépassé et necroses nerveuses centrales massives. Rev. Neurol. **101:** 116–139.
11. MOSELEY, J. I., G. F. MOLINARI & A. E. WALKER. 1976. Respirator brain: Report of a survey and review of current concepts. Arch. Pathol. Lab. Med. **100:** 61–64.
12. MYERS, R. E. & M. YAMAGUCHI. 1976. Effects of serum glucose concentration on brain response to circulatory arrest. J. Neuropath. Exp. Neurol. **35:** 301.
13. NICHOLSON, A. N., S. A. FREELAND & J. B. BRIERLEY. 1970. A behavioural and neuropathological study of the sequelae of profound hypoxia. Brain Res. **22:** 327–345.
14. NORDLANDER, S., P. E. WIKLUND & E. ASARD. 1973. Cerebral angioscintigraphy in brain death and in coma due to drug intoxication. J. Nucl. Med. **14:** 856–857.
15. PEARSON, J., J. KOREIN, J. H. HARRIS, M. WICHTER & P. BRAUNSTEIN. 1977. Brain death: II Neuropathological correlation with the radioisotopic bolus technique for evaluation of critical deficit of cerebral blood flow. Ann. Neurol. **2:** 206–210.
16. RÅDBERG, C. & S. SÖDERLUNDH. 1975. Computer tomography in cerebral death. Acta Radiol. (Suppl.) **346:** 119–129.
17. SCHNEIDER, H., W. MASSHOFF & G. A. NEUHAUS. 1969. Klinische und morphologische Aspekte des Hirntodes. Klin. Wochenschr. **47:** 844–859.

18. SCHNEIDER, H. & F. MATAKAS. 1971. Pathological changes of the spinal cord after brain death. Acta. Neuropath. **18:** 234–247.

19. STEEGMANN, A. T. 1968. The neuropathology of cardiac arrest. *In* Pathology of the Nervous System. J. Minckler, Ed. **1:** 1005–1029. McGraw-Hill. New York, N.Y.

20. TORACK, R. M., H. ALCALA, M. GADO & R. BURTON. 1976. Correlative assay of computerized cranial tomography (CCT), water content and specific gravity in normal and pathological postmortem brain. J. Neuropathol. Exper. Neurol. **35:** 385–392.

21. TOWBIN, A. 1973. The respirator brain death syndrome. Hum. Pathol. **4:** 583–594.

22. WALKER, A. E., E. L. DIAMOND & J. MOSELEY. 1975. The neuropathological findings in irreversible coma. J. Neuropathol. Exp. Neurol. **34:** 295–323.

23. ZANDER, E., D. T. RABINOWICZ & N. TRIBOLET. 1971. Etude anatomo-clinique de la mort cérébrale. Schweiz. Med. Wochenschr. **101:** 1225–1234.

DISCUSSION

HUGHES: In association with the NIH Collaborative Study, Dr. Litz and I have been working on pathologic, clinical and EEG correlations in brain death patients. We expected, of course, that when Dr. Litz looked through his microscope we would obtain some outstanding correlations between the clinical and the pathologic pictures. In fact, it did not turn out that way. I can summarize the findings thus far, which are as yet unpublished. The gross pathologic findings appear to correlate better with the clinical findings than do the observations obtained by microscopy. Dr. Pearson, do you have any comments on that?

PEARSON: Let me ask you these questions: Were you correlating your results with the presence or absence of blood flow clinically? Did you have any measurement of intracranial blood flow? If there was absent blood flow and you allowed a 20-hour period so that the pathologic changes could occur, did you still find confusion?

HUGHES: Cerebral radioisotope angiograms were taken in only a certain portion of our patients, so I can't give you statistics on a large number in whom blood flow studies have been done. However, we were reviewing patients who met the criteria of brain death from other points of view compared to those who did not meet these criteria.

PEARSON: In that case confusion is likely to arise. When we first reviewed our own data in a manner essentially similar to the way in which you reviewed yours, we had the same problem. Only when you select a subgroup of patients in whom you have a specific indication of when the CBF has ceased (or decreased below a critical level), and in whom you have allowed specific time for pathologic changes to pass, can you derive a distinct set of neuropathologic findings that correlate with the clinical and EEG criteria for brain death. Our own study is limited in number of patients, and I would welcome further studies by others that would either confirm or refute our observations.

MOLINARI: Was there any difference in the gross brain weight between those patients who had a bolus and those who did not?

PEARSON: I do not advocate weighing the brain at all. Normal brain weight varies greatly. There was no variation of significance that we detected. In another neuropathologic study relating to drug addiction, in which I knew brain edema to be present in the addict, brain weight was not a useful indicator of the presence or absence of edema. One must remember that the ventricles contain fluid. If the brain is compressed and the fluid squeezed out, the brain weight will be significantly altered. Therefore, weight is not a useful measure.

MOLINARI: That is my point. Did you have a greater degree of herniation in patients without a bolus?

PEARSON: We did tend to have greater degree of variation.

MOLINARI: Where did the increased volume, which causes increased intracranial pressure, come from if there was no circulation?

PEARSON: This is a game everybody plays; where is the increased volume? How quickly can it happen?

PLUM: Absent circulation only tells you the end point. It does not tell you the stages in between. There is an abundant opportunity for water to move into those necrotic tissues before the circulation stops. The arrested circulation does not precede the ultimate death of the brain; it follows it.

MOLINARI: Your statement is not consistent with experimental models in which death of the cells occurred rather quickly after the brain was deprived of circulation. I still have a problem in explaining edema in such a rapidly collapsing system.

PAMPIGLIONE: This question is addressed to those who have experience with the bolus technique: Will there be a period when intracerebral and intracranial circulation will reappear with return of the bolus or does this imply permanent loss of the cerebral circulation?

PLUM: The question of whether the bolus will reappear once it is absent is significant.

BRAUNSTEIN: In our series, the head bolus has never reappeared once it was found absent. A study in Minnesota of 15 infants and children in whom a modification of the bolus technique was used showed reappearance of the bolus in one case (Ashwal, S., A. J. K. Smith, F. Torres, M. Loken and S. N. Chou. Radionucleide angiography: A technique for verification of brain death in infants and children. J. Pediat. In press). Consequently we feel very strongly that the bolus test must be repeated after an appropriate time interval. The case described was that of a four-day-old infant who met the clinical criteria of brain death, had increased intracranial pressure, and a phenobarbital level of 8 mg/ml. The EEG showed "no electrical activity except during photic stimulation" and the head bolus was absent. After the infant was treated with mannitol, dexamethasone, and acetazolamide for one day, spontaneous respiration returned, intracranial pressure decreased, and the head bolus returned. The infant subsequently recovered, but was severely brain-damaged.

PLUM: Earlier Dr. Goodman spoke about utilization of isotopic imaging and the performance of a single test for intracranial circulation, and Dr. Fein described return of circulation using cerebral angiography. I am not familiar with such data relating to return of flow in the literature on angiography or isotope studies.

GOODMAN: Although we have not been repeating the isotope scans, we perform the procedure after the patient has received appropriate medication, such as mannitol. In addition, we wait a long enough time prior to and during the procedure, and therefore feel justified in performing a single study.

TRANSITORY ISCHEMIA/ANOXIA IN YOUNG CHILDREN AND THE PREDICTION OF QUALITY OF SURVIVAL

G. Pampiglione, Jane Chaloner, Ann Harden, and Judith O'Brien

Department of Clinical Neurophysiology
The Hospital for Sick Children
London WC1N 3JH, England

INTRODUCTION

When rigor mortis has set in, the person is dead according to all criteria. If exceptions occur, these are probably due to errors of observation and judgment, as, sad to say, miracles are no longer fashionable.

The central nervous system is particularly sensitive to alterations in general body metabolism, including the oxygen and carbon dioxide content of the perfusing blood. The electrical activity of the brain, as recorded from scalp electrodes, may be considered a running commentary of the functional state of the underlying brain, which largely depends on the metabolic state of cerebral tissues. The range of cerebral tolerance for alterations in acid/base balance, calcium, potassium, or blood sugar levels is relatively wide in comparison with alterations in hydration and plasma sodium level, which affect brain function over a much narrower range, of the order of 10 percent.

The electroencephalogram (EEG), like any other physical sign in medicine, should not be interpreted in isolation but together with other clinical data such as the biochemical, respiratory and circulatory condition of the patient. Correlations between EEG changes and more general metabolic events may be misleading if the electrophysiologic and biochemical data are not sampled concurrently. This is particularly important in the intensive care situation and following resuscitation procedures, when the assessment of cerebral function determines subsequent management.

The concept of "death of the brain" and its relevance to death of other organs was carefully studied by Marie François Xavier Bichat, who in 1800 published in Paris a concise book entitled *Recherches Physiologiques sur la Vie et la Mort*.[1] He explained the importance of brain function in the process of death, listing the sequence of events in the rest of the body following death of the brain. He made an important distinction between the functions of "animal life" (consciousness, sensation, voluntary movement) and "organic life" (cardio-respiratory, digestive, liver and kidney function).

In comparison with present-day knowledge, however, two aspects were missing from Bichat's outstanding observations: (1) the possibility that with the improvement of medical and nursing techniques resuscitation of the heart could become a fairly common event; and (2) that the development of investigational procedures, such as electroencephalography, would enable us to assess important aspects of brain function that cannot be otherwise measured. Bichat would have been fascinated by the reports presented at this meeting of The New York Academy of Sciences!

When blood perfusion to the brain becomes suddenly inadequate, as when cardiac arrest occurs, there is only a *narrow margin of time* between reversible and irreversible changes in brain function.

0077-8923/78/0315-0281 $01.75/0 © 1978, NYAS

The innumerable papers that have appeared during the last 20 years on "brain death" and those being discussed at this symposium show how many different ways may be used to prove that permanent loss of cerebral function has occurred when the patient is technically maintained as a heart-lung "preparation"—a state that may provide a fortune to some doctors and lawyers, but that represents a serious strain on hospital resources and the patient's relatives.

The present paper is based on observations made over the last 20 years on 636 children who were resuscitated following a transitory episode of ischemia/ anoxia. Its emphasis is on the possibility of predicting the quality of survival in those patients whose EEG showed a variety of phasic activities in the early postresuscitation period.

MATERIALS AND METHODS

The 636 patients were selected according to criteria parallel to those already published by Pampiglione and Harden [2] and include 406 cases of complete cardiocirculatory arrest which required a period of cardiac massage (327 of

TABLE 1

RESUSCITATION AFTER TRANSITORY ISCHEMIC/ANOXIC EPISODES IN 636 BABIES AND CHILDREN (APRIL 1957–APRIL 1977)

	No.	First EEG within 24 Hours	First EEG Later
Cardiocirculatory arrest	406	326	80
Severe cardiorespiratory difficulties	230	134	96
Total	636	460	176

these patients had the first EEG taken in the first few hours after resuscitation) and a further 230 patients with cardiorespiratory difficulties in whom EEG investigations were also carried out (TABLE 1).

All the patients were admitted to the Hospital for Sick Children, London, under the care of various physicians and surgeons. We did not include all those patients in whom cardiac arrest was a deliberate part of surgical procedures, nor patients with severe head injuries or acute poisoning.

A total of 2,180 EEGs were taken at the patient's bedside with mobile apparatus using Offner 8-channel type T, Beckman Accutrace 8-channel, and more recently a Grass 8–10 model using techniques previously described.[3] In each patient a minimum of 7 channels was used for the EEG and one for the electrocardiogram. The stick-on electrodes, carefully selected, were applied with collodion and left in place for subsequent EEGs in the next few hours or days. The amplification system allowed a margin of increased sensitivity to reach 1 microvolt/millimeter pen-deflection and noise level not exceeding 2 microvolts.

The general condition of each patient at the time of the EEG was noted together with the results of various biochemical investigations with emphasis on the following: state of consciousness; heart-rate (whether spontaneous or paced); spontaneous versus assisted respiration; blood pressure changes; body temperature; presence or absence of voluntary, involuntary, or elicited movements; flaccidity or stiffness of the muscles of the face, jaw, limbs and tongue at rest or in response to various stimuli; size of pupils and response to light; fundoscopic examination; occurrence of any seizures; drugs administered. The interval between the first and later EEGs was determined by a variety of individual circumstances and each record lasted from 10 minutes to 2 hours, usually repeated over the first 24 hours.

Some reconstruction of the timing of events during the dramatic phase of resuscitation was always attempted, but the total duration of the estimated period of inadequate cerebral perfusion could not be precisely ascertained in the majority of patients. The sequence, duration, and efficacy of the resuscitation maneuvers in the first few minutes and the therapeutic management in the first few hours or days after the re-establishment of circulation and respiration were difficult to evaluate either at the time or retrospectively. Only in exceptional circumstances, as other workers have found, could accurate timing of the events be achieved. Moreover, there was considerable individual variability in the pre-existing metabolic, respiratory, renal and cardiocirculatory conditions. Factors related to the range of age covered in this study added further complexity to the comparative evaluation of apparently similar cases. The presence of congenital cardiocirculatory or respiratory disease occurred in less than half of the cases and in some patients this was discovered only at postmortem examination. The long-term follow-up study of each child depended largely on individual circumstances.

RESULTS

From experience gained recording EEGs in the operating theater during cardiothoracic surgery it was found that the EEG changes after circulatory arrest with precisely timed re-establishment of cardiocirculatory functions were closely related to the duration of the period of inadequate cerebral perfusion.[4-8] The re-establishment of heart action during resuscitation and the re-establishment of respiration (whether or not assisted) *are easy to achieve,* but the re-establishment of cerebral function represents a substantially different problem.

Cardiocirculatory arrest of 10–30 seconds caused, with a latency of 6–10 seconds, increasingly slow activity in the EEG and this change tended similarly to affect various areas of the brain, although this finding was slightly more obvious in the initial phase over the anterior half of the two hemispheres. This may be followed by decreased amplitude of the traces, sometimes reaching equipotentiality; but with prompt resuscitation the sequence of events is rapidly reversed.

Cardiocirculatory arrest lasting as long as 3–4 minutes caused initially the same EEG changes as above, but total loss of phasic activity (electrocerebral silence) always follows. However, if cerebral circulation and oxygenation were promptly restored, phasic activity would reappear, beginning with irregular, slow waves, usually within minutes, while later, over a period of several hours, the original EEG features would return.

Cardiocirculatory arrest lasting between 5–8 minutes again caused electrocerebral silence, but phasic EEG activity returned in less than 2 hours after the re-establishment of circulation, with initially intermittent, very slow waves, generalized, reaching 200 or more microvolts. This activity, although fluctuating in amplitude at first, gradually became continuous. The evolution of this very slow activity in the following days varied from case to case.

Cardiocirculatory arrest of about 8–10 minutes again led to a period of electrocerebral silence of less than 2 hours followed by the appearance of phasic activity in the form of bursts of large-amplitude sharp waves, spikes and irregular slow components reaching over 0.5 millivolt. Each burst lasting 1–4 seconds was separated from the next burst by a period of 4–20 or more seconds of equipotentiality. This periodicity could continue for many hours, during which time stereotyped seizures would occur,[9] but total equipotentiality returned over a period of less than 2 days. This electrocerebral silence was then permanent.

Cardiocirculatory arrest lasting more than 10 minutes was never followed by the return of any phasic EEG activity.

From such experience in the operating theater under exceptional circumstances of continuous EEG monitoring before, during and after cardiothoracic surgery with periods of arrested cerebral perfusion in children of various ages, it became possible to extrapolate such EEG findings in relation to the occurrence of unexpected and largely untimed spontaneous cardiocirculatory and respiratory troubles.

In general the main clinical and EEG aspects were similar, whether altered cerebral function was due to ischemia (as in cardiocirculatory arrest) or to anoxia (as in respiratory arrest without necessarily gross circulatory impairment). The EEG features after resuscitation mainly fell into one of four groups (FIGURE 1). In some patients other features than those seen in FIGURE 1 were seen, such as gross asymmetries between the activities of the two hemispheres, multifocal spikes or sharp waves occurring independently in various areas of each hemisphere, or an area of persisting equipotentiality while the activity elsewhere was well preserved. In these cases the occurrence of emboli, particularly in patients wih congenital heart disease, was suspected although sometimes difficult to prove.[10, 11]

However, the presence of isolated spikes, without much alteration over a period of several days, was in keeping with the possibility that the EEG alterations might have been present already before the cardiocirculatory arrest and resuscitation procedures, representing an already pre-existent cerebral pathology. This could be confirmed in the occasional patient who had had an EEG prior to cardiocirculatory arrest and resuscitation. It was also found that when resuscitation was carried out in patients who were known to have a cerebral disease such as an encephalitis and who had EEGs prior to the cardiac arrest, the outcome in both clinical and EEG features represented the combined effect of the original cerebral disease plus the acute insult due to the transitory inadequate cerebral perfusion. In addition, patients who had multiple periods of anoxia/ischemia, whether relative or total, such as in repeated cardiac arrests, may sustain further cerebral insults which modify substantially the final outcome.

We soon learned that no rule applied to every situation because each patient and the circumstances that led to the ischemic/anoxic episode, followed by reestablishment of heart action and a period of intensive care, are very difficult to assess at an early stage, while the subsequent course of the illness may vary from one patient to another in relation to factors that we are often unable to either recognize or quantify. It became apparent that when EEG studies began between 2 and 24 hours after resuscitation, comparison with subsequent EEGs, especially during the first week, became much more valuable for both management and prognosis (data for the patients who had EEG investigations beginning

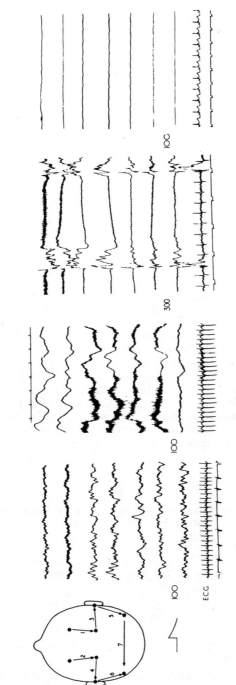

FIGURE 1. Patterns of prognostic value of main EEG features seen 2–24 hours after resuscitation from cardiac arrest in children. (A) EEG taken one hour after resuscitation in 3-month-old infant. There was recovery of consciousness within 12 hours, excellent survival, and no cerebral damage. (B) EEG taken 6 hours after resuscitation in 7-year-old child. Consciousness did not return, but spontaneous respiration did. (C) EEG taken 4½ hours after resuscitation in 9½-year-old child. Repetitive seizures began 4 hours after resuscitation. Consciousness did not return and death occurred within 2 days. (D) EEG taken 7 hours after resuscitation in 8-year-old child. There was no return of consciousness, and the child, who was maintained on a respirator, died on the fourth day after cardiac arrest. Necropsy showed extensive cerebral necrosis. From Pampiglione and Harden.[2] Reproduced by permission of the publisher.)

TABLE 2A

TABLE 2A

CARDIOCIRCULATORY ARREST (FIRST EEG WITHIN 24 HOURS)

Age	No.	Dead in Less than 2 Weeks
0–1 month	65	55
1–6 months	80	50
6 months–2 years	78	42
Over 2 years	103	61
Total	326	208

more than 24 hours after resuscitation were too varied in timing to be comparable).

Some data are shown on the 326 patients resuscitated after cardiocirculatory arrest (TABLES 2A and B) and 134 resuscitated after severe cardiorespiratory difficulty (TABLES 3A and B), all with EEG investigations in the first 24 hours. The outcome was first evaluated at the end of two weeks; the figures demonstrate some trends, but tabulation of individual cases is impossible.

For example, among the group of children who were dead two weeks after resuscitation, there were some who had well-preserved EEGs and were clinically recovering, but death followed a further ischemic/anoxic episode, from which they could not be resuscitated. Among the patients who survived more than two weeks, severe neurologic sequelae were present in half of the children with persisting irregular, very slow activity in the EEGs. In contrast, of a total of 121 survivors with rapidly improving EEGs over the first few days, only six had residual severe neurologic sequelae (TABLES 2B and 3B).

In 29 children with EEGs taken soon after resuscitation there were features such as a persistent asymmetry between homologous areas of the brain or focal discharges without an excess of slow activity, unlike those known to occur after general ischemic/anoxic episodes. It was presumed in these cases, even in the

TABLE 2B

CARDIOCIRCULATORY ARREST (FIRST EEG WITHIN 24 HOURS) IN PATIENTS
ALIVE MORE THAN 2 WEEKS

Age	No.	EEG Improving in 1 Week	Slow Activity Persisting	Miscellaneous EEG Abnormalities
0–1 month	10	5 (1)*	0	5 (1)
1–6 months	30	21 (1)	2 (2)	7 (2)
6 months–2 years	36	20 (0)	11 (4)	5 (3)
Over 2 years	42	34 (1)	5 (3)	3 (0)
Total	118	80 (3)	18 (9)	20 (6)

* Number of patients surviving with severe neurologic deficit are shown in parentheses.

TABLE 3A

SEVERE CARDIORESPIRATORY DIFFICULTIES (FIRST EEG WITHIN 24 HOURS)

Age	No.	Dead in Less than 2 Weeks
0–1 month	39	24
1–6 months	33	20
6 months–2 years	15	9
Over 2 years	47	29
Total	134	82

absence of a previous EEG, that other cerebral disorders had been present prior to the cardiocirculatory arrest.

The formulation of an early prognosis as to the probable quality of survival after resuscitation was primarily based on the evolution of early EEG findings, and the postresuscitation period was divided into three stages:

Stage 1 covered the period of the first week after resuscitation; during this period the four main groups of EEG features as shown in FIGURE 1 were found to be valid. The prognosis was good in terms of both survival and satisfactory cerebral condition in Group A (rapid EEG improvement), but was totally unfavorable in Groups C and D. Those of Group B (persisting, irregular slow activity) were more complex, particularly when gross alterations in water and electrolyte balance or problems of inadequate ventilation complicated the picture. Improving EEG features during the first week were in keeping with a much more favorable prognosis than was persisting, irregular slow activity.

Stage 2 covered the period from the end of the first week to the end of the first month. The evolution of EEG features during this period gave a clearer idea of the probable subsequent clinical evolution, Group A having recovered from the cardiocirculatory arrest, and Groups C and D being either dead or remaining in a state of total loss of "animal life." Evolution in Group B, how-

TABLE 3B

SEVERE CARDIORESPIRATORY DIFFICULTIES (FIRST EEG WITHIN 24 HOURS) IN PATIENTS ALIVE MORE THAN 2 WEEKS

Age	No.	EEG Improving in 1 Week	Slow Activity Persisting	Miscellaneous EEG Abnormalities
0–1 month	15	12 (2)*	0	3 (0)
1–6 months	13	10 (1)	1 (1)	2 (1)
6 months–2 years	6	4 (0)	0	2 (1)
Over 2 years	18	15 (0)	1 (0)	2 (2)
Total	52	41 (3)	2 (1)	9 (4)

* Number of patients surviving with severe neurologic deficit are shown in parentheses.

ever, tended to vary, either improving and predicting a fairly satisfactory re-covery or continuing to show grossly irregular slow activity (although often diminishing in amplitude), implying the possibility of permanent severe cerebral damage.

Stage 3 covers the period after the end of the first month. The general clinical features are usually much clearer than in the earlier phases of the inten-sive care period and the contribution of EEG investigations is now much more limited (i.e., for evaluation of specific problems, such as what areas of the brain might remain more affected than others).

In all these stages, and particularly during Stage 1 (first week after resuscita-tion), the type of evolution of the EEG features was the most relevant indica-tion of prognostic value. Any deterioration would suggest additional compli-cating factors to the initial insult such as respiratory, metabolic or cardiocircu-latory troubles, whether spontaneous or due to excessive therapeutic enthusiasm.

DISCUSSION

In the last 20 years intensive care units have rapidly multiplied all over the world and many lives have been saved, although many resuscitated patients are left with gross disabilities. Others may be kept as heart-lung preparations and the definition of their state is part of present-day legal debate. It is, however, during the intensive care period and particularly during the first week after resuscitation that EEG studies give information that is unobtainable with other methods of clinical examination.[2, 5, 12-17]

Many neurosurgeons, neurologists or psychiatrists in Europe, and particu-larly in England, do not have adequate training in clinical neurophysiology, are not accustomed to neurophysiologic investigations in the intensive care situation, and may be unaware of the pitfalls in interpretation of EEG data. Permanent electrocerebral silence is now accepted as evidence of unrecoverable brain func-tion (loss of "animal life") and, provided the recording techniques are adequate, there is no reason to doubt its reality. The increasing skills of anesthetists, nurses, cardiothoracic surgeons, and others in the resuscitation team with par-ticular experience in liver or kidney function are able to preserve for a long time a heart-lung preparation with completely unrecoverable cerebral function. The complex legal situation in the United States of America is somewhat different from that in the European Economic Community; and in England the National Health Scheme has made it possible to carry out repeated investigations without financial problems for the family. From the medical point of view, however, our duties remain the same on either side of the Atlantic. In our specialty we try to assess cerebral function as an integral part of the information that guides the correct management of the patient.

A great deal of discussion has been going on over the last few years on permanent electrocerebral silence. This is a practical situation which from the medical point of view corresponds to what Bichat had called the total loss of animal life, synonymous with death of the individual at a stage when some function of other organs, such as growth of hair and nails, is still possible even in spite of rigor mortis.

In the intensive care situation, after resuscitation, we have adequate means, not only to establish that "brain death" has occurred, but equally, if not more important, to assess the chances of survival and to some extent also the quality of survival. This concept had been proposed many years ago and has stood the test of time.[5]   The present paper shows that from serial EEG studies during Stage 1 and to some extent Stage 2, a persisting excess of irregular slow activity in the EEG without appearance of rhythmic components indicates severe and persisting neuropsychiatric sequelae. There is, however, little doubt that the prognostic considerations have to be assessed in the knowledge of individual factors and not at statistical level because many possible complicating factors may remain unspecifiable.

It is important to remember that a period of EEG equipotentiality, followed by an increase in slow activity, is a common feature after a relatively brief episode of cerebral ischemia/anoxia, a severe head injury, or after administration of some drugs. However, in the context of resuscitation following cardio-circulatory and respiratory arrest (i.e., excluding head injuries and poisoning) when some phasic activity returned in the EEG of some of our patients, EEG investigations had to be repeated at intervals of a few hours at first and later every few days to achieve a meaningful prognostic evaluation. The medically qualified neurophysiologist responsible for EEG studies after resuscitation should always be present at the time of each investigation. Adequate experience of this type of clinical problem cannot be improvised and full awareness of technical pitfalls as well as of differential diagnostic problems is essential.

The large proportion of babies under one month of age who did not survive in our series is difficult to interpret; it would be easy, but probably wrong, to argue that the brain of a young baby is more easily damaged by ischemia/anoxia than that of an older child. It seems more likely, instead, that such high mortality was only due to the circumstances in which the cardiorespiratory arrest and resuscitation had occurred and to the very high percentage of organ malformations found at autopsy in this very young age group.

During Stage 1 (the first week after resuscitation) other factors than anoxia may modify the EEG features with an increase in slow activity. The interpretation of some of these features is often difficult, but the period of inadequate ADH function with hyponatremia is usually accompanied by an increase in slow activity more obvious over the posterior half of the two hemispheres and is particularly marked after cardiac surgery.[3, 18] In general, during hypoglycemia, hyperventilation and to some extent hypoxia, the increase in slow activity is slightly more marked over the anterior half of the head in contrast with the case of hyponatremia. Again, at this stage it is essential to establish the type and severity of the metabolic upset before deciding that the increase in slow activity in the EEG might be due to primary intracerebral complications. Equally relevant is to know the oxygen saturation of the blood and base excess at the time of the EEG investigations and to make sure that there are no severe complications in the lung, liver or kidney. Many other organs in addition to the brain may be affected by episodes of ischemia/anoxia, creating a vicious circle where the metabolic upset secondary to ischemia of the kidney, for example, affects brain function.

In our experience the persistence of grossly irregular slow activity (Group B) during Stage 1 and particularly during Stage 2 after resuscitation is much less common than the features of Groups A, C and D. This may be due to the very narrow, critical time factor between fully reversible and totally irreversible cellular damage. This time factor is one of the most important missing links in the great majority of spontaneous ischemic/anoxic episodes that require resuscitation. It is, therefore, the evolution of the EEG features of Group B during the first and second week that allows a reasonable forecast of the subsequent evolution of cerebral complications of each patient.

The electrical activity of the brain utilized as a sensitive monitoring system after resuscitation is of great help, not only for a long-term prognosis, but also for an immediate correct evaluation of therapeutic procedures in the intensive care situation, including appropriate artificial ventilation, assisted cardiac action and the use of some drugs.

As emphasized in the literature,[2, 16, 19] any investigation of cerebral activity limited to one or two areas of the brain is inadequate in most instances and may lead to misinterpretation of data. The utilization of a single-channel monitoring (as recommended by some anesthetists and others unaccustomed to the differential diagnostic problems of the intensive care situation) should be firmly discouraged.

There is no doubt that the information offered by properly performed neurophysiologic investigations does not duplicate any of the other clinical signs in medicine and offers direct information about some aspects of cerebral function that cannot be achieved by other methods of physical examination; this is relevant when we try to forecast survival and to some extent the quality of survival. The complex interplay between the clinical conditions, the results of laboratory investigations and the EEG findings in relation to the final outcome defies any statistical approach. However, *there is little doubt that no EEG or biochemical service at all is much better than an unreliable and misleading service.*

When it was possible to start the EEG investigations between 2–12 hours after the cardiorespiratory arrest, the prognostic evaluation was more accurate than when such an evaluation was based on first EEGs taken a few days after the episode. In our experience repeated EEG investigations over the two weeks following resuscitation from an episode of ischemia/anoxia offer a reliable guide to favorable prognosis as to recovery of brain function when EEG improvement occurs. However, more care and longer-term studies are required when the EEG features do not improve or suggest the occurrence of complicating factors.

ACKNOWLEDGMENTS

We are grateful to our colleagues at the Hospital For Sick Children for their interest in our studies and in particular to past and present members of the cardiothoracic unit. We are indebted to Miss Elizabeth Moore for her secretarial assistance.

REFERENCES

1. BICHAT, M. F. X. 1800. Recherches Physiologiques sur la Vie et la Mort (1st ed.)., Paris.
2. PAMPIGLIONE, G. & A. HARDEN. 1968. Resuscitation after cardiocirculatory arrest; prognostic evaluation of early EEG findings. Lancet i: 1261–1265.
3. PAMPIGLIONE, G. 1965. Electroencephalographic and metabolic changes after surgical operations. Lancet ii: 263–265.
4. PAMPIGLIONE, G. 1960. Neurophysiological aspects of cerebral ischaemia. Proc. Roy. Soc. Med. 53: 329–332.
5. PAMPIGLIONE, G. 1962. EEG studies after cardiorespiratory resuscitation. Proc. Roy. Soc. Med. 55: 653–657.

6. PAMPIGLIONE, G. & D. J. WATERSTON. 1958. Preliminary EEG observations during partial and complete occlusion of cerebral blood flow. Electroenceph. Clin. Neurophysiol. **10**: 354.
7. PAMPIGLIONE, G. & D. J. WATERSTON. 1961. EEG observations during changes in venous and arterial pressure. *In* Cerebral Anoxia and the EEG. H. Gastaut & J. S. Meyer, Eds. : Charles C Thomas, Springfield, Ill.
8. HARDEN, A., G. PAMPIGLIONE & D. J. WATERSTON. 1966. Circulatory arrest during hypothermia in cardiac surgery: An EEG study in children. Brit. Med. J. **2**: 1105–1108.
9. PAMPIGLIONE, G. 1963. Crises après réanimation. Rev. Neurolog. **109**: 323–324.
10. PAMPIGLIONE, G., & A. HARDEN. 1965. Local cerebral complications during cardiac surgery possibly related to emboli. Riv. Patol. Nerv. Ment. **86**: 268–275.
11. ARFEL, G., J. PASSELECQ & C. CASANOVA. 1968. Embolies gazeuses en chirurgie cardiaque. Anesth. Analg. Réanim. **25**: 175–177.
12. WERTHEIMER, P., M. JOUVET & J. A. DESCOTES. 1959. À propos du diagnostic de la mort du systèm nerveux central. Presse Méd. **67**: 87–88.
13. FISCHGOLD, H. & P. MATHIS. 1959. Obnubilations, comas et stupeurs. Electroencéph. Clin. Neurophysiol. (Suppl. 11) : 126.
14. PAMPIGLIONE, G. 1973. Neurophysiological studies in some aspects of the intensive care situation. Proc. Assoc. Europ. Paediat. Cardiol. **9**: 47–53.
15. PAMPIGLIONE, G. 1975. Early neurophysiological assessment after insult to the central nervous system. *In* Ciba Foundation Symposium No. 34. Elsevier-Excerpta Medica-North-Holland. Amsterdam.
16. ARFEL, G. 1970. Problèmes EEG de la Mort. Masson. Paris.
17. PRIOR, P. F. 1973. The EEG in Acute Cerebral Anoxia. Excerpta Medica. Amsterdam.
18. HARDEN, A., G. H. GLASER & G. PAMPIGLIONE. 1968. Electroencephalographic and plasma electrolyte changes after cardiac surgery in children. Brit. Med. J. **4**: 210–213.
19. BENNETT, D. R., J. R. HUGHES, J. KOREIN, J. K. MERLIS & C. SUTER, Eds. 1976. Atlas of EEG in Coma and Cerebral Death. : 244. Raven Press. New York, N.Y.
20. PAMPIGLIONE, G. 1970. The electrical activity of the brain in sick children resuscitated after cardiac arrest (in Russian). *In* Recovery Period after Resuscitation. : 212. Symposium, November 1968, Moscow.

DISCUSSION

SUTER: Is it true that, excluding children with trauma and poisoning, you have not had a child with an isoelectric EEG who recovered?

PAMPIGLIONE: That is correct.

PLUM: I believe that this is a universal experience. Many observers, including myself, think that the diagnosis of brain death is really not a very big problem. As Dr. Pampiglione indicated, this has been editorialized in a leading British journal. He and other investigators have indicated that if one needs information to supplement the clinical findings, the electroencephalogram may be sufficient. If the prerequisite of appropriate recording and interpretation is made by individuals of experience, and if drug poisoning can be excluded, the value of the isoelectric EEG as an ancillary test to confirm brain death is virtually fail-safe. Controversies have occurred in situations where drug intoxication and other reversible etiologies have not been ruled out.

Rather than the problem of brain death, the issue of cognitive death, with its attendant ethical and medical difficulties, is far more serious. These problems have been considered in greater depth by European investigators and will require further research in the future. Aspects of these problems have been discussed at this meeting. Exactly what we can anticipate as the medical contribution to this gloomy condition is uncertain.

THE VEGETATIVE STATE AND ITS PROGNOSIS
FOLLOWING NONTRAUMATIC COMA *

D. E. Levy, R. P. Knill-Jones,†‡ and F. Plum

Coma Unit and Department of Neurology
New York Hospital-Cornell Medical Center
New York, New York 10021; and the
† Hospital Health Services Research Unit
University Department of Medicine (Western Infirmary)
Glasgow, Scotland

INTRODUCTION

Modern medical techniques can assure the survival of many acutely ill, comatose patients who never regain apparent psychological awareness. Many of these patients, however, retain sufficient function of their respiratory, cardiovascular, gastrointestinal, and urinary systems to sustain a vegetative existence. They may open their eyes and move their limbs, face, and eyes in a reflex manner in response to environmental stimuli, but they fail to communicate in any symbolic manner with others, nor do they initiate complex behavior. These patients thus pass from the sleep-like state of coma into a state in which they can be said to be awake but not aware. Jennett and Plum [1] described such patients as being in a "persistent vegetative state," and this clinical designation has achieved increasing acceptance over the subsequent five years.

Wakefulness is easy to recognize, but deciding whether another person is aware can be difficult. Nonetheless, it may be even more difficult to deduce whether specific pathologic lesions are present, and Jennett and Plum explicitly noted that the vegetative state described behavior and "presumed neither a particular physio-anatomical abnormality nor a specific pathological lesion." [1] Not all patients who are in a vegetative state have identical clinical features, and one recent publication [2] has divided patients in the vegetative state into different groups on the basis of their clinical signs.

The clinical variability of patients with altered states of consciousness forms the basis of an international cooperative effort to provide guidelines for predicting neurologic outcome from coma. Patients with coma secondary to trauma have been studied by Drs. Bryan Jennett, Graham Teasdale and others in Glasgow, by Drs. Braakman and Minderhoud in the Netherlands, and by Dr. T. Kurze and associates in Los Angeles. [3] Patients in nontraumatic coma have been investigated by Dr. Plum's Department at Cornell and by Drs. David Shaw, Niall Cartlidge, and David Bates in Newcastle-upon-Tyne; Dr. John Caronna helped to organize the study and has extended it to San Francisco since 1975. Dr. Robin Knill-Jones has conducted the data analysis. Of the 310 subjects so far fully analyzed in the nontraumatic group, 12 percent sub-

* This study was supported by National Institutes of Health Contract No. NO1-NS-42328 and by the Josiah Macy, Jr. Foundation.

‡ Supported in the Hospital Health Services Research Unit by grants from the Nuffield Provincial Hospitals Trust and the Scottish Home and Health Department.

sequently recovered wakefulness, yet remained in the vegetative state. Analysis of these patients permits us to consider two important questions: (1) Can one predict which comatose patients will pass into the vegetative state? and (2) Can one predict the ultimate outcome of patients in the vegetative state?

METHODS

The present report is based on a detailed examination of adult patients in coma not caused by trauma or drugs.[4] Patients whose coma was believed secondary to drugs or alcohol were excluded since almost all such individuals should recover fully with supportive treatment. To eliminate from consideration the transient unresponsiveness of syncope or the preterminal state, only patients in coma lasting at least six hours were included.

Coma was defined operationally as sleep-like unresponsiveness; patients in coma were unarousable and gave no evidence of psychological awareness of the self or the environment. Such patients (1) did not open their eyes, either spontaneously or in response to any verbal stimulus, (2) expressed no comprehensible words, and (3) neither obeyed commands nor moved their extremities appropriately to localize or resist noxious stimuli. This definition emphasizes the sleep-like quality of coma. Verbally unresponsive patients whose eyes were open were not admitted to the study.

The operational definition of the vegetative state was similar to that for coma, with the exception that the eyes would open, usually spontaneously but occasionally only in response to verbal stimuli. (A few patients appeared to be in the vegetative state immediately after cardiac or respiratory arrest, but they never entered sleep-like coma, and were excluded from the formal study. One such patient remained vegetative for 36 hours and then died of a second cardiac arrest, and another regained consciousness so that within 12 hours he followed commands, but he too died of a second cardiac arrest one day later.) The expression of any comprehensible words was by definition incompatible with the vegetative state. Slightly more elaborate motor responses were permitted than for coma, so that as long as patients did not obey commands or imitate the examiner either with their limbs, with their eyes, or with other parts of their face, they were considered to meet the motor criteria for the vegetative state.

All patients were evaluated in accordance with a Neurologic Profile that included appraisal of forebrain and brain-stem function using criteria developed by Plum and Posner[5] and Teasdale and Jennett.[6] The components were graded approximately from best to worst (TABLE 1) and recently have been described in detail.[4] The clinical evaluation was performed at onset of coma and daily thereafter. A temporal profile of the patient's course was developed by indicating on special forms the best and worst responses during successive time intervals of 24 hours, 2 to 3 days, 4 to 7 days, 8 to 14 days, and 15 to 28 days.

We recorded the level of recovery attained one, three, six, and 12 months after the onset of coma. Many patients in coma from medical diseases are desperately ill and often have terminal medical complications. Because we were primarily interested in the potential for neurologic recovery with optimal treatment, we recorded the best level of recovery attained within each interval as well as the actual level of recovery at the end of each interval. Five outcome grades were defined by Plum and Caronna[7] and Jennett and Bond[8]: *Good recovery* meant the patient could resume normal life, and even at times return to work; *moderate disability* was applied to patients disabled for employment but independent in daily activities; *severe disability* implied that the patient depended on others for daily support (paralyzed patients who communicated only with the eyes as in the "locked-in" syndrome [5] were included in this group); patients in the *vegetative state* and those who *died without recovery* from coma comprised the final two outcome categories.

TABLE 1

NEUROLOGIC PROFILE USED TO ASSESS COMATOSE PATIENTS

1. *Verbal responses*
   Oriented speech
   Confused conversation
   Inappropriate speech
   Incomprehensible speech
   No speech

2. *Eye-opening*
   Spontaneous
   Response to verbal stimuli
   Response to noxious stimuli
   None

3. *Pupillary reactions*
   Present
   Absent

4. *Spontaneous eye movements*
   Orientating
   Roving conjugate
   Roving dysconjugate
   Miscellaneous movement
   Lateral deviation at rest
   Dysconjugate at rest
   None

5. *Oculocephalic responses*
   Normal
   Full
   Minimal
   None

6. *Oculovestibular response*
   Normal
   Tonic conjugate
   Minimal
   None

7. *Corneal responses*
   Present
   Absent

8. *Respiratory pattern*
   Regular
   Periodic
   Ataxic

9. *Motor responses*
   Obeying commands
   Localizing
   Withdrawal
   Abnormal flexion
   Abnormal extension
   None

10. *Deep tendon reflexes*
    Normal
    Increased
    Absent

11. *Skeletal muscle tone*
    Normal
    Paratonic
    Flexor
    Extensor
    Flaccid

RESULTS

Preliminary analysis of 450 patients in nontraumatic coma identified 55 (12 percent) who opened their eyes but never displayed any convincing evidence of awareness at any time during the first month after the onset of coma. Only the first 310 patients in coma, however, have been analyzed in detail (TABLE 2); 36 of these recovered only to the vegetative state within the first

TABLE 2

TABLE 2

BEST ONE-MONTH OUTCOME FROM NONTRAUMATIC COMA IN 310 PATIENTS

Outcome	Patients	
	Number	Percent
No recovery	183	59
Vegetative state	36	12
Severe disability	41	13
Moderate disability	15	5
Good recovery	35	11

month, and these 36 patients form the nucleus for the following description, although there were others who appeared to be in the vegetative state earlier in their course and who subsequently improved. There were 15 men and 21 women in the group, and the mean age was 57 years. Three patients who were "locked-in" are excluded from the present report.

Nontraumatic Causes of the Vegetative State

Most of these 36 patients sustained some form of diffuse hypoxic-ischemic brain injury, usually from cardiac arrest (TABLE 3). Seven patients had focal brain infarcts, usually progressing to coma after 24 to 36 hours; the coma appeared to result from brain-swelling with consequent widespread cerebral and upper brain-stem dysfunction. The cause of coma could not be determined in two patients.

TABLE 3

NONTRAUMATIC CAUSES OF THE VEGETATIVE STATE

Cause	Number of Patients
Diffuse hypoxia-ischemia	22
Cardiac arrest	15
Profound hypotension	4
Respiratory failure	3
Cerebrovascular disease	10
Brain infarct	7
Brain hemorrhage	2
Subarachnoid hemorrhage	1
Other	4
Herniation from tumor	1
CNS infection	1
Unknown	2

*Clinical Features of 36 Patients with Best One-Month Outcome of the
Vegetative State*

The 36 patients destined to become vegetative generally had intact brain-stem function almost as early as when first examined. Many awakened from coma within a few days, by which time several had orienting eye movements, moved their limbs in response to a noxious stimulus, or groaned. Early differentiation of these patients from those who later regained awareness was difficult.

Verbal Responses

Speech could not be evaluated in 11 patients because they were intubated at admission. Most of the remaining patients never made any sounds, but four patients were groaning within one day after the onset of coma. Even after a month, however, none of these four uttered any comprehensible words.

TABLE 4

EYE-OPENING RESPONSE

Days after Onset	Eye-opening Response	
	Spontaneous	to Noise
1	5	0
3	10	5
7	20	3
14	20	2
28	19	0

Eye-opening

Spontaneous eye-opening developed quickly in many of the vegetative patients: five of the 36 had spontaneous eye-opening within one day and more than half opened their eyes by the end of a week (TABLE 4). A smaller number of patients opened their eyes only in response to verbal stimuli.

Pupillary Reactions

As a sign of relatively well-preserved brain-stem function, most of these patients had pupils that reacted to light. Nonreactive pupils at admission were present in only two patients. Pupillary responses returned in one of these after five days, a woman who opened her eyes the following day but never moved in response to commands or even in response to pain. She died after another four weeks. The other patient never regained pupillary responses; she had undergone cataract surgery a few days prior to cardiac arrest but was said to have had intact pupillary reactions postoperatively.

Spontaneous Eye Movements

Roving conjugate eye movements developed quickly in many of these patients (TABLE 5), nearly half of the 36 patients achieving roving eye movements
at one week. Three patients appeared to have orienting eye movements within
three days, usually following moving objects or looking toward sound, but none
of these ever followed commands either with their eyes or with their extremities,
and they never spoke, even over a one-month period.

Oculocephalic and Oculovestibular Responses

Three-quarters of the 36 patients developing the vegetative state had conjugate tonic responses of their eyes to ice-water oculovestibular stimulation at
the onset of coma. Rare patients even exhibited a few erratic beats of nystagmus superimposed on conjugate tonic eye deviation. This response was seen in
two patients at one day, in four at three days, and in nine at one week, and
differs from that seen in awake patients who instead have rapid sustained
nystagmus but no conjugate tonic deviation. We term this abnormality an
"atypical conjugate tonic" response.

TABLE 5

SPONTANEOUS EYE MOVEMENTS

	Eye Movements	
Days after Onset	Orienting	Roving Conjugate
1	1	12
3	3	13
7	3	16

Corneal Responses

Corneal responses were absent in five patients at admission; three of these
five had sustained cardiac arrests but were also under the influence of sedatives
(alcohol, anticonvulsants, or anesthesia), and the corneal response returned
within two days.

Respiratory Pattern

Periodic respirations were relatively uncommon, being noted in only five
of the 36 patients at any time in their course.

Motor Responses

Motor responses varied greatly (TABLE 6). The most common response in
all time periods was withdrawal of the limbs from a noxious stimulus; extensor

TABLE 6

MOTOR RESPONSES

Days after Onset	Motor Responses				
	Localizing	Withdrawal	Flexor	Extensor	None
0	—	11	8	10	7
1	1	13	9	8	5
3	2	12	6	9	6
7	2	13	7	10	3

responses were the next most frequent response in most time periods. Two patients displayed localizing motor responses to noxious stimuli, but they never improved any further and remained in the vegetative state throughout the first month.

Deep Tendon Reflexes and Skeletal Muscle Tone

Absent deep tendon reflexes or flaccid tone were more common in patients who never awakened than in those who became vegetative. Only 3 of the 36 vegetative patients had absent reflexes at admission, whereas reflexes could not be elicited in 41 of the 176 who died without awakening. Eleven patients who became vegetative had reduced muscle tone at admission, while 78 of those who died without recovery had toneless muscles.

Early Prediction of the Vegetative State

Many of the responses in the Neurologic Profile measure the state of brain-stem function, which was often relatively preserved in patients who entered the vegetative state. As the preceding description implies, few early responses reliably predicted which comatose patients would awaken but remain vegetative (TABLE 7). There were 89 patients who failed to move their extremities in response to noxious stimulation at the onset of coma, and most of these (78)

TABLE 7

EARLY SIGNS CORRELATING WITH POOR ONE-MONTH OUTCOME

Day	Sign	No Recovery	Vegetative State	Severe Disability	Moderate Disability/ Good Re- covery
0	Absent motor responses	71	7	6	5
1	Absent corneal responses	81	4	0	0
7	Roving eye movements (hypoxia-ischemia)	3	12	1	5
7	Persistent coma	5	17	16	4

never regained awareness. Nonetheless, absent motor responses cannot be considered a reliable predictor since this pattern was also present in 11 of the 41 patients who regained awareness. Absent corneal responses at one day invariably heralded a poor outcome, but realization that sedative drugs might blunt the corneal response should discourage early reliance on this sign. Although many of the vegetative patients awakened within a few days, coma persisted for at least one week in 42 of the 310 patients in the study. Fifteen of the 32 patients in hypoxic-ischemic coma who still had roving conjugate eye movements after one week never improved beyond the vegetative state. Seventeen of these later awakened but remained vegetative, a proportion (42 percent) more than three times that in all the patients at the onset of coma (12 percent).

Short-Term Outcome of Early Vegetative Patients

We have determined the best one-month outcome in patients who awakened within a few days but appeared to be in a vegetative state (TABLE 8). Thus far, 450 patients in nontraumatic coma have undergone preliminary analysis; of these, there were 34 who at 24 hours opened their eyes either spontaneously or in response to verbal stimuli but did not obey commands or speak comprehensible words and were thus, at least briefly, in a vegetative state within one day. Only 11 of these 34 patients ever recovered any degree of independence, and 12 more required assistance for all daily activities. Eleven of these 34 "early vegetative" patients (32 percent) failed to improve beyond the vegetative state, an incidence more than twice that among the 450 patients at the onset of coma (12 percent). Poor motor responses in these patients increased the likelihood of their remaining in the vegetative state. Seven of these 34 awake patients had absent, extensor, or flexor motor responses at one day; five remained vegetative, and two became severely disabled. Once awake, failure to regain motor function within a few days also increased the likelihood of remaining in the vegetative state: 15 of the 34 patients who were awake at one day had poorer than localizing motor responses after three days, and none of these 15 achieved a moderate disability or good recovery, whereas nine of the 15 (60 percent) remained in the vegetative state.

There were 39 patients who appeared to be vegetative at the end of one week, and only one did even moderately well. Nearly two-thirds (25) failed to regain awareness by the end of the first month, and 12 were severely disabled. No patient achieved a good recovery, and of the two who survived a month with a moderate disability, one was dead within three months.

TABLE 8

BEST ONE-MONTH OUTCOME OF PATIENTS IN EARLY VEGETATIVE STATE

	Vegetative State	Severe Disability	Moderate Disability	Good Recovery
Vegetative at one day	11	12	3	8
Vegetative at seven days	25	12	2	0

TABLE 9

LONG-TERM OUTCOME OF PATIENTS IN THE VEGETATIVE STATE

Months after Onset	Dead	Vegetative	Aware	Incomplete Follow-up
1	30	25	—	—
3	44	7	2	0
6	47	4	2	2
12	48	3	0	4

Long-Term Outcome of Patients in the Vegetative State

We have evaluated the long-term outcome in comatose patients who did not improve beyond the vegetative state within one month of the onset of coma (TABLE 9). Preliminary analysis of data obtained from 450 patients in non-traumatic coma identified 55 such patients. Thirty of the patients died within the first month, leaving 25 survivors. Of these, 14 died by the end of three months, seven remained vegetative, and two uttered occasional comprehensible words but never followed commands. An additional three patients died by the end of six months, and one of those who had spoken died by the end of the first year. The other patient had not yet survived one year from the onset of coma. None of 25 patients surviving in the vegetative state one month after the onset of coma ever regained any form of independence in daily activities.

DISCUSSION

Patients in the vegetative state can display a wide range of clinical signs—from absent motor responses to noxious stimuli to localizing movements toward such stimuli and from absent spontaneous eye movements to apparent orienting eye movement. The common denominator is the appearance of wakefulness without any external evidence of communication or complex behavior. The development of the vegetative state as early as one week seems a bad prognostic sign, although some patients might have died before the full potential for neurologic recovery was realized.

One point to discuss is the inclusion of those patients whose eyes appear to follow moving objects. Such eye movements were included among the clinical features of vegetative patients studied by Jennett and Plum,[1] and Higashi *et al.*[2] reported eye following movements in more than 40 percent of 130 patients in the vegetative state. Bricolo[9] states that "the presence of (ocular) fixation and pursuit movements indicates integrity of the occipito-mesencephalic pathways." Nyström,[10] however, described a 10-year-old girl who survived 14 months after the onset of traumatic coma; after three weeks, she opened her eyes, and after six months, she seemed to move her eyes and reach out her hand "when greeted loudly." She died after an epileptic seizure, and the cerebral hemispheres were "pathological in all preparations," the left hemisphere being the more damaged. Denst *et al.*[11] reported a patient who appeared to have been in the vegetative state but whose eyes "on occasion seemed to follow the examiner." At autopsy 10 months later, the brain was found to have extensive cortical thinning and neuronal loss throughout the cerebral hemispheres, including the occipital lobes. Thus, although orienting eye movements may be a relatively better sign than absent eye movements or roving conjugate eye movements, they can occur in patients without evident psychological awareness and with extensive brain damage.

Desirable as it would be to predict at onset which patients in coma will enter and remain in the vegetative state, present data fail to indicate that this is possible for all patients. Several unfavorable signs or combinations of signs have been noted: (1) absent motor responses at admission; (2) absent corneal responses at one day; (3) poor motor responses at three days, despite awakening at one day; (4) persistent roving conjugate eye movements at one week in patients with coma caused by diffuse hypoxia-ischemia; (5) persistent coma for one week; and (6) the vegetative state at one week. Some of these signs have received attention by other investigators: Bell and Hodgson [12] reported that only 5 of 46 patients in coma for more than three days after cardiac arrest were ever discharged from the hospital, and three of these were severely disabled, whereas one of the others was an 11-month-old child, and the presence of uremia contributed to coma in the fifth patient. Willoughby and Leach [13] reported that "reflex" motor responses even as early as one hour after cardiac arrest heralded a poor outcome; of 18 such patients, nine died without improvement, one died after some unspecified neurologic improvement, one survived in a vegetative state, six appeared to have been severely disabled, and one was able to work under supervision. These two reports highlight the importance of many of the clinical signs that seem predictive in the present study, but persistence of coma or poor motor signs cannot be considered to be fully reliable predictors of a poor outcome from coma.

Patients with nontraumatic coma who have not regained awareness by the end of one month have little likelihood of subsequently demonstrating sentience and no apparent chance of an independent existence. This is consistent with the report of Higashi et al.,[2] who followed 110 patients in the vegetative state. Only three of these patients recovered and survived for three years, but none of them were able "to resume activity as a social human being." Most other reports are on small numbers of patients. Jacobsen [14] reported on five patients with protracted unconsciousness after injury to the head. Although reconstruction of the details is incomplete, three of these patients seem to have been in the vegetative state after a month (Nos. 1, 3, and 5), and two later recovered speech; one had a vocabulary of 10 words, and the other was able to verbalize requests, but he was wheelchair-bound, aggressive, and dependent on others for daily support. Two of the four patients with the "complete apallic syndrome" described by Ingvar and Brun [15] died, and the other two were unchanged after one year.[16] Snyder et al.[17] identified 13 patients who were in coma for at least two days after cardiac arrest, the end of coma being defined as the time the patient began "responding to voice." None of these patients ever regained the ability to sustain an independent existence, but the precise number who were in a vegetative state is not given. Anecdotal rumors of dramatic recovery are common, but such cases are seldom reported in detail, a recent exception being that by Rosenberg et al.[18] They described a 43-year-old man who remained in a postanoxic vegetative state for approximately one and a half years before improving. Although he reportedly did not open his eyes or have any motor response to noxious stimuli for six months, he was then noted to awaken and remain vegetative until about one year later, when he began to speak and follow commands. After two years, he scored 100 on the verbal section of the Wechsler Adult Intelligence Scale, but even then he was paralyzed in three extremities and remained severely disabled.

The term "vegetative state" describes the behavior of a group of patients sharing the feature of wakefulness without giving evidence of awareness of self and environment. Their clinical features vary, but it may become possible to identify some of those in coma who will .become vegetative. Present data indicate that the condition at seven days is rarely associated with return of independence, and at 30 days, essentially never.

SUMMARY

The vegetative state is a condition of wakefulness without awareness. Clinical features of 36 patients in coma who did not improve beyond the vegetative state in one month were evaluated as part of an international collaborative prospective study of 310 patients with nontraumatic coma. The vegetative group included 22 subjects with diffuse hypoxia-ischemia, seven with focal brain infarction, two with brain hemorrhages, one each with subarachnoid hemorrhage, infection, and cerebral herniation caused by tumor, and two in whom the precise cause of coma was unknown. The vegetative group had signs of good brain-stem function but little function of cerebral cortex. Many patients awakened quickly after the onset of coma: five opened their eyes within one day, 13 within three days, and 16 within one week. Roving conjugate eye movements were prominent. Nineteen of the 36 vegetative patients died within one month; 32 died by the end of one year. Only two patients ever regained any evidence of psychological self-awareness (both improving within three months), but both remained completely dependent for daily care. Patients in coma may develop the vegetative state within a few days, but if they are still vegetative after a month, the chance of regaining independence is negligibly small.

REFERENCES

1. JENNETT, B. & F. PLUM. 1972. Persistent vegetative state after brain damage. A syndrome in search of a name. Lancet 1: 734–737.
2. HIGASHI, K., Y. SAKATA, M. HATANO, S. ABIKO, K. IHARA, S. KATAYAMA, Y. WAKUTA, T OKAMURA, H. UEDA, M. ZENKE & H. OAKI. 1977. Epidemiological studies on patients with a persistent vegetative state. J. Neurol. Neurosurg. Psychiat. 40: 876–885.
3. JENNETT, B., G. TEASDALE, S. GALBRAITH, J. PICKARD, H. GRANT, R. BRAAKMAN, C. AVEZAAT, A. MAAS, J. MINDERHOUD, C. J. VECHT, J. HEIDEN, R. SMALL, W. CATON & T. KURZE. 1977. Severe head injuries in three countries. J. Neurol. Neurosurg. Psychiat. 40: 291–298.
4. BATES, D., J. J. CARONNA, N. E. F. CARTLIDGE, R. P. KNILL-JONES, D. E. LEVY, D. A. SHAW & F. PLUM. 1977. A prospective study of nontraumatic coma: Methods and results in 310 patients. Ann Neurol. 2: 211–220.
5. PLUM, F. & J. B. POSNER. 1966. Diagnosis of Stupor and Coma. Davis. Philadelphia, Pa.
6. TEASDALE, G. & B. JENNETT. 1974. Assessment of coma and impaired consciousness. A practical scale. Lancet 2: 81–84.

7. PLUM, F. & J. J. CARONNA. 1975. Can one predict outcome of medical coma? In Outcome of Severe Damage of the Central Nervous System (Ciba Foundation Symposium, 34, new series): 121–139. Excerpta Medica. Amsterdam.
8. JENNETT, B. & M. BOND. 1975. Assessment of outcome after severe brain damage. A practical scale. Lancet 1: 480–484.
9. BRICOLO, A. 1976. Prolonged post-traumatic coma. In Handbook of Clinical Neurology. P. J. Vinken & G. W. Bruyn, Eds. Vol. 24: 699–755. American Elsevier. New York, N.Y.
10. NYSTRÖM, S. 1960. A case of decortication following a severe head injury. Acta Psych. Neurol. Scand. 35: 101–112.
11. DENST, J., T. W. RICHEY & K. T. NEUBUERGER. 1958. Diffuse traumatic degeneration of the cercbral gray matter. J. Neuropath. Exp. Neurol. 17: 450–460.
12. BELL, J. A. & H. J. F. HODGSON. 1974. Coma after cardiac arrest. Brain 97: 361–372.
13. WILLOUGHBY, J. O. & B. G. LEACH. 1974. Relation of neurological findings after cardiac arrest to outcome. Brit. Med. J. 3: 437–439.
14. JACOBSON, S. A. 1956. Protracted unconsciousness due to closed head injury. Neurology 6: 281–287.
15. INGVAR, D. H. & A. BRUN. 1972. Das komplette apallische Syndrom. Arch. Psychiat. Nervenkr. 215: 219–239.
16. INGVAR, D. H. 1973. Cerebral blood flow and metabolism in complete apallic syndromes, in states of severe dementia, and in akinetic mutism. Acta Neurol. Scand. 4: 233–244.
17. SNYDER, B. D., M. RAMIREZ-LASSEPAS & D. M. LIPPERT. 1977. Neurologic status and prognosis after cardiopulmonary arrest: 1. A retrospective study. Neurology 27: 807–811.
18. ROSENBERG, G. A., S. F. JOHNSON & R. P. BRENNER. 1977. Recovery of cognition after prolonged vegetative state. Ann. Neurol. 2: 167–168.

DISCUSSION

INGVAR: I have a question concerning eye movement. In some of the patients with apallic syndrome, which I previously described, in whom there was proven destruction of the neocortex, we also observed eye movement and eye-opening. There was a noticeable absence of roving, looking, orienting eye movements. Would you say, Dr. Levy, that the neocortex is a prerequisite for such roving, orienting movements? Also, what were the EEG findings in these patients?

LEVY: In response to your second question, the premise of this study generally was to try to provide a framework that would be available to virtually any center anywhere, namely, the simple observation of the patient. For this reason the EEG was not evaluated in as much detail as described by others in this volume. EEGs were, of course, obtained on these patients, but the detailed analysis and correlation of the results with outcome has not yet been completed.

In response to the first question, there were three patients who appeared to have some sort of orienting eye movement. One of these patients did come to postmortem examination. The findings were extremely complex. This patient had a myocardial infarction, cardiac arrest with anoxia and multiple emboli. He had occipital lobe involvement, multiple contusions, and a small subarachnoid hemorrhage. Any precise correlation of his ocular activity with this pathology would be somewhat difficult.

MOLINARI: Dr. Ingvar's question was also about roving eye movements and the neocortex.

LEVY: If that was the sense of your question, I misunderstood it. As far as we can tell, one does not require the neocortex for roving eye movement. Dr. Plum had previously indicated this in 1972. Dr. Nyström has described a patient who, in fact, actually appeared to move her eyes toward the examiners. At autopsy there appeared to be pathologic damage to the entire cortex. Denst *et al.* also reported a similar situation with extensive damage throughout the cerebral hemispheres. Therefore, I believe these types of eye movements may not require the neocortex.

MOLINARI: What was your evidence for sleep-wake cycles if you did not use the EEG? Was it just eye-opening and -closing?

LEVY: It was usually clinical observation. In most patients, these observations were casual.

PLUM: The behavioral observations on sleeping and waking are fairly reliable, unless patients have bilateral third nerve weakness.

LEVY: I think it is more difficult to determine whether a patient is aware and cognitive. Determination of wakefulness did not seem quite as difficult.

WALKER: I noted that the corneal reflexes were particularly sensitive. Did they come back after a longer period of time, and was their return correlated at all with subsequent recovery?

LEVY: Generally, in the entire group of 310 patients, any patient whose corneal response did not return within 24 hours was destined to do badly. Although I cannot answer that question precisely, I remember one patient who had come in under the influence of alcohol, whose corneal reflexes returned after two days; nonetheless the patient remained vegetative. I do not have the exact information on hand on the prognosis of those patients in whom the corneal reflexes did return.

PAMPIGLIONE: The fact that so many patients in this group die is a very important point. I suppose that this justifies the term "vegetative," analagous to vegetables, which perish, in contrast to plants, which continue to grow. Obviously, there is a tremendous interplay between the results of such qualitative investigation—in your case, observation of the patients—and the degree of management that will enable a patient in this condition to survive. It is difficult for me to evaluate the significant factors in the survival of the patients of your study.

LEVY: Most of these patients are desperately ill, and even some of those who achieved "good" recovery were dead by the end of the month. We felt it was more important to evaluate the best level of outcome of these patients in order to obtain some index that would guide us in the selection of those patients in whom maximal efforts would be rewarded by recovery to the level of an aware, social human being. Although I do not remember precisely, I believe that more patients in the vegetative state died earlier than did other patients in this group.

PLUM: I think that Dr. Pampiglione wants to know whether one is dealing with self-fulfilling prophecies. It should be noted that the observations were not made by the personnel who took care of the patients. The patients were cared for in independent intensive care or neurosurgical units. The observation and the relationship of the observations to potential outcome were not shared with those people who were taking care of the patients. It was assumed that

under the circumstances of this study, all patients would receive maximal care
to whatever degree required.

There was evidence, in fact, that this was so. However, if one looks at the
outcome between Rotterdam, Glasgow and Los Angeles, where very different
energies were expended in terms of the care of patients with head injuries, the
results were essentially the same for all three groups of patients. You can draw
a number of conclusions from this fact, but the important one would be that
no one voluntarily decreased care and influenced the outcome.

THE DEFINITION OF DEATH: ETHICAL, PHILOSOPHICAL, AND POLICY CONFUSION

Robert M. Veatch

Research Group on Death and Dying
Institute of Society, Ethics and The Life Sciences
The Hastings Center
Hastings-on-Hudson, New York 10706

In the early days of the Karen Ann Quinlan case it was suggested by some not closely involved in the case that she was dead according to a new definition of death.[1-3] Those who made the claim seem to have been confused. They apparently did not realize that although Ms. Quinlan's brain was severely damaged, it was not dead. Nor did they realize that even if her brain were dead, the State of New Jersey had not changed its definition of death to make it legal to pronounce a person dead solely because the brain is destroyed. Because of this confusion, the use of brain criteria for the pronouncement of death might have led to prosecution. Furthermore, these claimants did not realize that it would still be possible to decide to let a patient die even if she were not dead according to new concepts of death.*

Significant confusion remains over the technical, ethical, philosophical, and policy questions raised by the definition-of-death debate. The confusion began well before the appearance of the report of the Ad Hoc Committee of Harvard Medical School on the Definition of Brain Death a decade ago.[4] That report stated in its first sentence that "Our primary purpose is to define irreversible coma as a new criterion for death [4] (p. 337). It said this in spite of the fact that nowhere following that sentence was there ever a hint of an argument—much less a convincing demonstration—that irreversible coma was synonymous with the death of the person as a whole. Clearly the content of that report was quite different from such an argument. It reported in detail what the Committee thought were empirically accurate predictors of irreversible coma. It did not deal at all with the more difficult question: "If a person is in irreversible coma, should he be treated as if he were dead?"

"Brain death" itself is a confusing term. It can have a noncontroversial meaning: the irreversible destruction of the brain tissue. It can also have a radically different meaning, one that is more philosophically and politically controversial. It can also mean "the death of the person as a whole as measured by the functioning of the brain." This ambiguity is the reason why I and many others would strongly recommend that the term "brain death" be abandoned.

The term reflects the ambiguity revealed in the Harvard report. Brain death can focus on technical, empirical criteria for the irreversible destruction of the brain. That was approximately the meaning of the term as used by the Harvard Committee. On the other hand it can be used at a more conceptual level, as

---

* See the Editor's Comment at the end of the discussion of this paper.

0077-8923/78/0315-307 $01.75/0 © 1978, NYAS

in arguments about whether the person as a whole should be considered dead when the brain has died.

The same linguistic point can be made about the term "cerebral death." It can mean the death of the cerebrum (leaving open the question of whether the person is dead when the cerebrum is dead) or it can mean the death of the person based on the destruction of the cerebrum. To make matters even more confusing "cerebral death" can be confused with "brain death." Sometimes, in spite of the obvious significant difference between the two, the terms are used interchangeably. This can lead to statements that the brain is dead when only cerebral activity has ceased. (No current law would permit pronouncement of death when only cerebral activity has ceased.) It can also lead to insistence on more rigorous criteria than necessary for measuring the prognosis of a person in irreversible coma or with irreversible loss of cerebral function.

The source of much of our confusion is the ambiguity of the term. We must keep separate three distinct questions. The empirical question is, "What are the best technical measures of the destruction of the brain?" The philosophical, conceptual question is, "What is it that is so essential to our concept of human life such that when it is lost we should treat the individual as dead?" The policy question is, "When should our laws and our courts regard a person as dead and when should a medical professional be authorized to pronounce a person dead?" Previous papers in this Conference have dealt primarily with the first question. Clearly no amount of biological, neurologic evidence will ever be decisive in deciding what it is an individual has lost when he has lost what is essential to our concept of humanness. The contribution to the discussion of the neurologists acting as neurologists should be empirical evidence of empirical predictors of the functioning of the brain and the likelihood of recovery of function once lost.

We should take pause when we realize that the Harvard Report, which *de facto* was limited to this empirical, biological task, may have been wrong even at this level. It appears that the Committee did not distinguish between criteria for irreversible coma, which it claimed to be identifying, and criteria for irreversible destruction of the brain, which would be relevant for any ethical or legal judgments based on the death of the whole brain. Whether the so-called Harvard criteria measure the destruction of the brain, or whether they measure irreversible coma, is a question that is primarily in the hands of those with appropriate neurologic skills. It appears, however, basing our judgment on the earlier papers at this Conference, that the Harvard criteria may be precise measures of neither of these.

The important questions for those of us who are not specialists in those empirical disciplines are much more at the levels of concept and policy. At the conceptual level we ask, "What does it mean to be dead?" At the policy level we ask, "Under what circumstances should we call a person dead?"

FOUR CONCEPTS OF DEATH

Even if we know precisely the predictors of the destruction of the brain, it is still an open question whether we ought to call a person dead when his brain is destroyed. In general terms an entity is considered dead when there is a complete change in the status of that entity characterized by the irreversible loss of those characteristics that are essentially significant to it.[5, 6] †

Throughout history, in various times and cultures, many answers have been given to the question of what is essentially significant to the human. Four answers remain as plausible to large numbers of people. Each involves the irreversible loss of some essential characteristic.‡ The four essential characteristics are the presence of the soul, the flowing of "vital" body fluids, the capacity for bodily integration, and the capacity for consciousness and social interaction.

The Irreversible Loss of the Soul

Probably more people in world history, and even more of those alive today, have believed that death means the irreversible loss of the soul than have held all of the other concepts we shall consider. The link between the departure of the soul and death can be either analytical or synthetic. If the soul is simply *defined* as the element that departs at death, then we learn nothing about what holders of this concept of death thought death to be. It seems clear, however, that large numbers of people, including classical thinkers in Greek, some Christian, and most secular Western thought, until recently had a more synthetic notion of the relationship between the soul and death. The soul was the animating principle of thought and action in man and was identified with mental, emotional, and sometimes (but not always) with spiritual functions. It was nonmaterial, but nevertheless a metaphysical reality. It was important to nurture the soul and know its locus. Descartes, for instance, held that although the soul is united to all the portions of the body "there is yet . . . a certain part in which it exercises its functions more particularly than in all the others." [7] He was convinced that this was in the brain, "not the whole of the brain, but merely the most inward of all its parts, to wit, a certain very small gland which is situated in the middle of its substance," that is, the pineal body.

Although this view continues to be held by many people throughout the world, it is largely abandoned by most thinkers trained in the world view of Western science. It is beyond the pale of empirical scientific study and does not lend itself to the precision necessary for secular clinical and legal judgment. We shall abandon this concept, although some of its characteristics may be more plausible than other, more modern conceptions of what it means to be dead. The classical notion that both an organic component (called the body) and a nonorganic component must be present for a human to be alive is still accepted by many twentieth-century persons. This is a condition that some other concepts of death cannot satisfy. The insight of Descartes, that it is not the whole brain that is the locus of the most critical functions, but only a small part of it, is also challenging to contemporary thought. To these two dimensions of the

---

† For a fuller development of the argument see my book *Death, Dying, and The Biological Revolution.*[5]

‡ Because the loss is irreversible, all of the current talk about out-of-body and life-after-death experiences are really a confusion. It would be better to talk about apparent afterlife experiences while living, but with certain vital functions temporarily suspended. Certainly if death is the irreversible loss of function, then individuals who are still alive are not, and never have been, dead.

classical concept of death as the departure of the soul from the body we shall have to return.

The Irreversible Stopping of the Flow of "Vital" Body Fluids

When modern man secularized his philosophical understanding of his nature, he had to find another, more biological formulation of what it meant to be dead. In answer to the question, "What is it about human life that its loss is so essential that the individual who loses it ought to be called dead?," modern man began to give answers focusing on the heart and lungs. We may try to deduce his concept of death from the empirical measures he made to determine whether an individual is dead. We could identify visual and tactile observations of respiration, pulse, and heart beat. More recently these have been made more sophisticated by the use of an electrocardiogram, but the tests are basically the same. They only tell us, however, that functions related to the heart and lung seem to be important.

If we ask what it is about the heart and lungs that is so important, it becomes clear that it is not their functioning per se that was thought essential. Consider the case of a patient whose lungs are permanently destroyed and who is maintained on a respirator or a blood oxygenator. Clearly he was and still is thought to be alive. Even the hypothetical person whose heart and lungs are permanently destroyed but who is maintained on a heart-lung machine would still be alive beyond any doubt. The critical function is not the heart and lung activity, but the flowing of the vital fluids—the blood and breath—that these organs normally produce.

The decisive problem with this concept of the essence of life is that it is not only simplistic, but biologically reductionistic. It makes no distinction between the human and the human's body. It is a vitalistic, animalistic notion of the human as essentially a biological species in which the biological functions of respiration and circulation are critical.

It is important to realize that there is no scientific or medical argument against that position. It is fundamentally not a scientific or medical question. If some individuals and some religious and philosophical schools of thought choose to answer the question "What is essential to the human's nature?" by pointing to respiration and circulation, no laboratory evidence will ever refute the stance. This position is, however, in conflict with the view of virtually every religious and philosophical group in human history.[8, 9] It can at least be said for the defenders of the idea that death occurs when the soul departs from the body, that they recognized that a human is more than his body and some of its lesser functions.

Irreversible Loss of Bodily Integration

The new possibility of maintaining circulation and respiration in the absence of any brain activity has led many, but not all, to re-examine their concept of what it means to be dead. Henry Beecher, the chairman of the Harvard Committee, revealed his philosophical disdain for these functions when he considered the problem of hopelessly comatose patients. He asked, "Are these hopelessly comatose patients really still alive?" In answering his own question he contrasted the definition in *Black's Law Dictionary* to an alternative focusing on functions that are believed to relate to the activity of the brain. The functions he mentioned were "the individual's personality, his conscious life, his unique-ness, his capacity for remembering, judging, reasoning, acting, enjoying, worry-ing, and so on." [10] He went on to argue that "We have proof that these and other functions reside in the brain, proof through studies of damage to the brain by surgery, or accident, or disease. . . . It seems clear that when the brain no longer functions, when it is destroyed, so also is the individual destroyed; he no longer exists as a person: he is dead." [10]

Note that he says we have proof that these functions reside in the brain, but when he attempts to establish that these functions are the critical ones for deciding that a person should be treated as dead, he must shift to language such as "one believes" or "it seems clear." He is no longer in the realm of the scientific.

That he has shifted to the realm of metaphysics or ethics, however, does not necessarily mean that he is any less sure of himself. It is appropriate for him to say with confidence—with philosophical certainty—that the functions he has identified are more significant than the circulatory and respiratory functions.

The technical criteria that the Harvard Committee have identified imply that the integrative functions of the nervous system are implicitly the activities that defenders of a concept of death related to brain function see as man's essence. Spontaneous respiration, bodily reflexes, and response to stimuli are all integrative activities. Thus, according to this view, it makes sense to speak of the death of the person as a whole at the point when the person loses the ability to integrate his body as a whole.

It seems that this concept of death as the irreversible loss of bodily integrat-ing capacity is philosophically preferable to the two previous concepts of death. It appeared that the battle was about over. Some who were raised prior to the asking of the more precise philosophical questions would continue romantically to hold onto the heart as the seat of the soul, the *sine qua non* of life. But it appeared that eventually all reasonable people would come to accept a concept of death that sees loss of integrating capacity as decisive. To be sure this could not be proved in any scientific empirical sense, but it was nevertheless taking on the character of a reasonably well-established philosophical certainty.

Then the neurologists began to differentiate cases more clearly and the philosophers began to ask their questions more carefully. Brierley and his col-leagues reported two cases in which patients were apparently in irreversible coma—there was neurologic and histologic evidence that the cerebrum was destroyed—yet the patients breathed spontaneously and had intact lower brain centers.[11] These were a challenge to the Harvard criteria as perfect predictors of irreversible coma. The criteria may not ever classify someone in irreversible coma when he is not. That was the original fear. It appears, however, that they may be classifying some people as not in irreversible coma when they are. The criteria may predict something other than irreversible coma. They may predict destruction of the brain, or some third state in which more of the brain is destroyed than if the patient were only in irreversible coma. If so, the criteria may not be perfect predictors of either whole-brain or cerebral death.

This possibility is a real challenge. It is a challenge to what was thought to be a carefully derived empirical consensus. (Beecher said at one point, "It is clear that we have a definition of irreversible coma.") It is also a challenge at the philosophical or conceptual level. Is it really integrating capacity of the human body that is essential to his being treated as alive or is it something more specific, something residing in a more limited portion of the brain?

Irreversible Loss of Consciousness or Capacity for Special Interaction

If one examines more closely the list of functions that Beecher takes as essential to being alive, it is clear that they are related to activities of the brain, but it is also clear that they do not relate to the brain as a whole. They are all what have sometimes been called the "higher brain functions": consciousness, remembering, judging, reasoning, enjoying, and the like. Neurologically we are left with the question, "Is it possible that all the essential functions could be irreversibly lost even though some of the brain cells remain alive?" Conceptually we must ask, "Is it really the integrating functions of the brain that are so essential or is it perhaps some other brain functions?"

We have found fault with the concept of death that focuses on the functions of respiration and circulation, in part because it is biologically reductionistic: it sees man as essentially animalistic. It abandons the earlier view that saw man as having both organic and nonorganic components—both body and soul. Yet everything that can be said in this regard against the concepts of death that focus on respiration and circulation can be said also against a concept that focuses on integrating capacity. Perhaps bodily integration is in some sense a more noble function than respiration and circulation, but it is still biologically reductionistic. If an individual who has irreversibly lost higher functions can still retain major integrating capacities because his lower brain centers are intact, such an individual would not meet the Harvard criteria; he would not have experienced death of the entire brain. It is still possible, however, that one could decide to call such an individual dead.

If the essential characteristic is not the vitalistic integrating capacity, then what is it? It could be capacity for consciousness—a capacity that seems to underlie most if not all of the higher functions that Beecher listed. That formulation takes cognizance of the mental capacities we have found lacking in the two previous concepts of what it means to die.

The Judeo-Christian tradition, however, has not seen man primarily as an isolated mentally functioning unit. Both Aristotle and the Judeo-Christian tradition have seen the human as essentially a political or social animal—one who has the capacity for social interaction with his fellow humans. Capacity for social interaction may then be the essential element whose loss constitutes death of the person as a whole. There is a danger that we may tend to evaluate social capacities qualitatively. The same risk exists, however, for the criteria of consciousness, integrating capacities, and even respiratory and circulatory function. Any capacities for social interaction must be a sign of life, no matter how rudimentary. In anatomic and physiologic perspective this may be identical to the capacity for consciousness. To have consciousness without capacity for some kind of social interaction seems impossible; to have social interaction without consciousness is equally implausible. So for questions of technical measurement of brain function, the distinction may not be important. It remains, however, crucial in considerations of the human being's essential nature.

We have criticized concepts of death that identify loss of fluid-flow and integrating capacities as the essential characteristics. These concepts share the quality of being excessively biological; they are organically reductionistic. Yet reliance on capacities for consciousness or social interaction by themselves, may err on the side of not giving enough of a place for the human body. The Judeo-Christian tradition that emphasizes man as a social animal still sees him as an animal. The body is an essential element. While avoiding the biological reductionism of other concepts of death, we should not slip into a Manichaeism that could accept the possibility of a living person free of his body. I doubt that the notion of disembodied consciousness will ever be more than a figment of the science fiction writer's imagination. Nevertheless, it is clear that a disembodied consciousness, conceivable, say, as a transferral of a memory to a magnetic tape equipped with sensory input and some kind of outputs, would not have all the necessary characteristics of humanhood. The body, the physical features, are necessary, if not sufficient, conditions.

Many have assumed that the struggle over the definition of death was about over. Advocates of concepts of death centering on heart and lung function will give way to advocates of concepts centering on central nervous system function. The real question today is not the choice between heart and brain, but rather which part or parts of the nervous system are so essential to human function that their irreversible loss would constitute death of the person as a whole. Once one realizes that there are several brain functions that are potentially chosen as central, it is clear the philosophical debate is far from over. Reasonable people will disagree over whether a person should be pronounced dead when it is confirmed that only some portion of his brain is destroyed. The question becomes even more complex when one realizes that individual brain cells may live on after the most rudimentary brain functions have been lost. Thus, it makes little sense to hold out for the death of the entire brain in the sense of every cell's being dead. If one is going to hold to a concept of death based on brain function, it seems that at least some function above the cellular level ought to be present for a person to be considered alive. Yet if some functions—at least intracellular functions—are to be excluded when deciding which functions are significant, how does one go about deciding just which functions are necessary conditions for being considered alive? The ethical, philosophical, and theological issues remain crucial. Only when there is some degree of consensus, at least temporarily, on those issues can the more technical questions of measures of brain function and the more policy-oriented questions of when society should permit or require death to be pronounced be taken up in the context of the definition-of-death debate.

NEW CONFUSIONS IN THE DEBATE

Logically both the technical and policy questions in the definition of death are derived from the conceptual or philosophical questions. The links of the conceptual to technical and policy questions, however, are quite complex. One cannot determine whether technical measures or criteria such as the Harvard criteria are criteria *for death* until one has some answer to the conceptual question—at least to the point of being convinced that functioning of the brain has something very relevant to do with deciding whether a person is dead. Likewise, one cannot answer the policy question of when society should permit or require that death be pronounced until one has some idea what it means to be dead. The links among these levels in the debate need not be direct, however. Several problems remain.

The Link Between Conceptual and Technical Questions

Deciding the condition of certain body organs is important for many questions other than that of the pronouncement of death. But only after one has decided what it means to die can one begin to link technical measures of organ condition to the pronouncement of death. For some concepts of death, the technical measures follow quite easily. If the fluid flow through the body is crucial, the pulse, the heartbeat, the flowing of the breath through the nostrils become relatively straightforward tests.

If the loss of capacities for bodily integration is crucial, and one decides that the brain as a whole is the organ with decisive responsibilities for bodily integration, then tests to measure the irreversible destruction of the brain, or at least the irreversible loss of all brain function, become important.

Under these assumptions, if the Harvard criteria measure irreversible coma rather than complete destruction of the brain, the four technical measures would not be definitive in deciding to pronounce death. If, however, what they measure is closer to destruction of the whole brain, they are relevant in spite of the original decision to call them criteria for irreversible coma.

More recently attempts have been made to determine the appropriate tests or criteria for measuring irreversible loss of consciousness, capacity for social interaction, or some other combination of higher brain functions. The EEG alone, for instance, may be a better test of loss of the critical functions. The bolus techniques described at this meeting may be, as well. There is no *prima facie* reason why brain-stem activities such as spontaneous respiration or reflexes would have to be absent in order to measure loss of higher brain function. If mental functions are necessary conditions for being alive, then we may have a problem quite analogous to the one that existed when the departure of the soul was the indicator of death: the processes may not be directly observable. Charron [12] and others have argued that whatever our concept of death, the technical measures used must be of a publicly verifiable state. There is a major debate about whether mental processes can be reduced to physical states.[13-15] Even if one makes the assumption that reduction of a complex mental process like consciousness to physical structures is possible, the physical structures may be so complex that no tests of their functioning are plausible.[16, 17] Certainly the electroencephalogram, which has been proposed as a measure of cerebral function, is at best a crude measure. The possibility that there could be electroencephalographic activity from some portions of perfused cortex, without the possibility of the person's ever regaining consciousness, suggests that much more precise technical measures would be required to avoid the possibility of classifying some individuals as alive when they are really dead according to concepts of death based on consciousness.[11]

We must come to grips with the possibility, indeed the probability, that we shall never be able to make precise physiologic measures of the irreversible loss of mental processes. In this case we shall have to follow safer-course policies of using measures to declare death only in cases in which we are convinced that some necessary physical basis for life is missing, even if this means that some dead patients will be treated as alive. But the fear of treating an occasional dead patient as alive was the reason we abandoned heart and lung measures. This suggests that the arguments for moving beyond heart and lung measures may be suspect, even if we are convinced at the level of concept that a person should be considered dead if he has lost integrating capacities or capacity for consciousness and social interaction. Only when we are convinced that our measures will not falsely consider someone dead, should the measures be used. It appears that the Harvard criteria or similar tests of entire brain function may have reached that level of certainty if death is to be pronounced when the entire brain is destroyed. (There appears to be very little evidence, however, to demonstrate that there really is destruction of the entire brain rather than certainty that the patient will not recover any of the functions being tested when the Harvard criteria are met.) We shall have to ask the technically competent people whether tests such as the electroencephalogram alone provide certainty that there will never be a recovery of consciousness if we choose to use a concept of death based on loss of that function.

The Link Between Conceptual and Policy Questions

Just as the key technical questions for purposes of pronouncing death are derived from the philosophical decisions at the conceptual level, so the policy questions will also be derived from our philosophical conclusions about what it means to be dead. Normally our public policy dealing with when death should be pronounced should reflect our philosophical stand. There may be grounds for deviation, however. In a simpler era, our policy that death "occurs precisely when life ceases and does not occur until the heart stops beating and respiration ends" implied a policy that may not have been based precisely on our understanding of what it means to be dead. (Whether it does or not depends on the degree to which the use of old heart-lung measures were based on a concept of death related to fluid-flow and the extent to which they were mere short-cut tests for determining when integrating capacities or capacities for consciousness had been lost.)

Now we may be in a similar position regarding the choice between whole-brain-oriented policies and policies that focus on loss of consciousness and social interaction. Even if we believe that a person should be considered dead when he has lost the capacity for consciousness, we might favor legislation requiring pronouncement of death when and only when the entire brain is destroyed. We might do this because we are philosophically uncertain about the more progressive concept of death or we may do so for technical reasons. We may be convinced that there are no precise and accurate measures of the irreversible loss of consciousness. Then a policy embodying the concept should not be written into law lest some neurologists might pronounce death too quickly, attempting to use measures of loss of consciousness even if the lower portions of the brain remained intact. We might oppose writing such a policy into law because we believe in principle that no such measures can be devised. If, however, we are convinced of the philosophical principles leading to the conclusion that a person is dead when he loses capacity for consciousness, we should, in principle, be willing to use tests of that capacity for pronouncement of death even if parts of the brain remain viable. Thus, some tests might be devised that measure the absence of a necessary condition for consciousness even if they do not measure the sufficient conditions.

There is another reason why our policy for pronouncement of death may not correspond precisely with our philosophical understanding of what it means to be dead. If the conceptual issues are philosophical and theological in nature and not verifiable in a scientific sense, some difference of opinion will likely remain in the society. Some laws would permit (but not require) physicians to pronounce death when all brain functions (or the relevant parts) are irreversibly destroyed. This is based, presumably, on a respect for the conscience of the individual physician. I see no basis for respecting that conscience in this way, however. To grant to the physician the option of not pronouncing death when socially accepted criteria are met is to violate the rights and the autonomy of others involved and the dignity of our memory of the patient who may have supported the social consensus. Certainly a physician should have the right to withdraw from his obligation to pronounce death in a case where he is personally convinced, based on his own religious or philosophical positions, that the patient is still alive. He cannot, however, use those personal values to continue treating a corpse as alive or a living person as a corpse.

The problem of personal conscience vis-à-vis the patient and his family is quite another matter. A substantial portion of our population now accepts each of the concepts of death I have discussed. One recent survey of residents of the state of Missouri can be interpreted as implying that only 7 percent of the respondents held that a person should be considered dead if his brain is destroyed, while other, larger groups held more conservative and more liberal positions (Ref. 12, p. 1006). If any one concept is institutionalized in law, in cases in which these concepts are critical, the majority of the population will probably have death pronounced on them using some concept of death other than the one they personally hold. Our traditional pluralistic solution to the problem of individual variation on questions of philosophy and theology is to grant a limited right of conscientious objection. The case should be no different here. Thus a state could choose to write a law specifying that a person should be considered dead if there is complete absence of brain function; and it might also recognize the plight of the Orthodox Jew or bible-belt Baptist who had felt very strongly that he should be considered alive if his brain was destroyed, but his heart continued to beat. This is not to say that such persons would really be alive or dead based on personal choice. Rather they would be *treated* as dead or alive on this basis. The only policy solution is to select the most plausible concept of death and adopt it as policy for purposes of pronouncement of death, but then allow limited conscientious objection for individuals who have strong objections to that concept of death. The individual might be permitted to write a document specifying that the consensus definition of death should not be used in his case, but some other definition selected from a number of options. The law might require pronouncement of death when there is irreversible loss of the function of the entire brain or the cerebrum, the capacity for consciousness, or some other specified function. It could permit an individual to execute a document specifying in his case that the older heart and lung criteria be used. In cases in which the individual has not executed such a document, we might follow the precedent of the Uniform Anatomical Gift Act and permit family members to exercise their judgment about what the patient would have wanted unless there is evidence of the patient's wishes to the contrary. The safer course might be to retain the older heart-lung oriented concept of death in cases in which the patient or his family do not express wishes to the contrary. That may, however, be sufficiently implausible as a social consensus that we should take the somewhat riskier course and adopt one of the other concepts of death, again permitting individual selection of some other concept of death. In any case, if individual discretion is permitted, it would have to be limited by the bounds of reasonableness to avoid having family members deciding that a patient with heart, lung, and brain function was dead or that a patient with none of these functions was alive.

Once we realize that the basic issues are philosophical and theological in nature—that the critical question is what is it that is so essential to the human's nature that its loss constitutes death—it makes sense to recognize the individual and cultural variations in the answers to that question. No technical information alone can ever answer the conceptual and policy questions (although it may well tell us the state of particular portions of the body). The confusions that exist among the technical, philosophical, and policy questions will require our devoting careful attention not only to the basic question of what is essential to the human's nature, but also to its implications for technical and policy matters.

REFERENCES

1. 1976. In the matter of Karen Quinlan, an alleged incompetent. Superior Court of New Jersey. Opinion. November 10, 1975. *Cited in* In the Matter of Karen Quinlan. : 541. University Publications of America. Arlington, Va.
2. ODEN, THOMAS C. 1975. *The National Observer,* November 8 : 24.
3. SULLIVAN, JOSEPH F. 1975. *The New York Times* October 3 : 39.
4. 1968. A definition of irreversible coma. Report of the Ad Hoc Committee of the Harvard Medical School to Examine the Definition of Brain Death. JAMA **205:** 337–40.
5. VEATCH, ROBERT M. 1977. Death, Dying, and the Biological Revolution. : 21–76. Yale University Press. New Haven, Conn.
6. VEATCH, ROBERT M. 1975. The whole-brain-oriented concept of death: An outmoded philosophical formulation. J. Thanatol. **3**(1): 13–30.
7. DESCARTES, RENÉ. The passions of the soul. *In* The Philosophical Works of Descartes, Vol. 1. : 345. Cambridge University Press (1911). Cambridge, England.
8. VEITH, FRANK J. *et al.* 1977. Brain death. I. A status of medical and ethical considerations. JAMA **238:** 1651–55.
9. VEITH, FRANK J. *et al.* 1977. Brain death. II. A status report of legal considerations. JAMA **238:** 1744–48.
10. BEECHER, HENRY K. 1970. The new definition of death: Some opposing views. Unpublished paper presented at the meeting of the American Association for the Advancement of Science, December 1970.
11. BRIERLEY, J. B. *et al.* 1976. Neocortical death after cardiac arrest. Lancet September 11 : 560–65.
12. CHARRON, WILLIAM C. 1975. Death: A philosophical perspective on the legal definitions. Washington University Law Quart. (4): 979–1008.
13. SMART, J. J. C. 1963. Philosophy and Scientific Realism. Routledge and Kegan. London.
14. FEIGL, HERBERT. 1967. The "Mental" and the "Physical." University of Minnesota Press. Minneapolis, Minn.
15. O'CONNOR, JOHN. 1969. Modern Materialism: Readings on Mind-Body Identity. Harcourt, Brace and World. New York, N.Y.
16. SNYDER, S. H. 1972. Catecholamines in the brain as mediators of amphetamine psychosis. Arch. Gen. Psychiat. **27:** 169–79.
17. HILGARD, E. R. & G. H. BOWER. 1966. Theories of Learning Appleton-Century-Crofts. New York, N.Y.

DISCUSSION

A. S. MORACZEWSKI (*Pope John XXIII Medical-Moral Research and Educational Center, St. Louis, Mo.*): I want to make two brief comments, one of which regards the conceptual problem. We have a basic difficulty, because underlying the conceptual problem of death is a more basic one that has to do with the nature of man. Obviously, many different concepts of man's nature exist and because of the variation in concepts, we're going to have a variation of what we mean by a dead human being. And so further research on this level is needed.

Secondly, we must note that these problems are being discussed in a pluralistic society. The papers presented earlier at this Conference presented empirical data. It might be fruitful to approach the problem asymptotically, that is, to take one of two extremes where there is no question that the person is dead. If a person is decapitated by a guillotine, for example, I expect that the vast majority would agree that that person is dead. On the other hand, if a person is asleep, or in a reversible coma, most individuals would say that that person is alive. The idea would be to evaluate that area of certitude and expand it to regions of increasing uncertainty, which is where the problem lies. Then more attention could be focused on the limited area, having eliminated extremes to see whether it is possible in our culture to achieve general agreement. An empirical approach to the problem may be derived in this manner from the extreme situation.

I appreciate the fact that an attempt was made in the previous papers to clarify the notion of brain death and to recognize that some confusion still exists. The attempt to define the problem both conceptually and operationally in terms of the words used takes cognizance of the confusion that is evident in the literature so far.

VEATCH: I agree that this is the defined task. We certainly must set the boundaries. The alternatives include treating the putrefying body if it were alive and treating patients who are mentally retarded as if they were dead.

I am not optimistic, however, about the possibility of reaching a consensus, given the amount of variation that exists. I am convinced that there is virtual unanimity in this group that if a person's brain is destroyed, we should treat him as dead. However, I do not think there is a consensus when we move out beyond those present. This is clearly apparent if we contrast the "classical" definition of death with that of cerebral death. I'm not at all optimistic that a consensus will emerge around any one concept no matter what it might be.

T. LEAFFER: My question concerns ethical issues in human experimentation on persons with irreversible brain syndromes, in particular, those in long-term-care institutions who may not have next-of-kin. Would it be considered ethically justifiable to perform research that may be of high risk but that does not relate directly to their condition? Would it be more ethically acceptable if the research were restricted to their condition, particularly since there is the problem of informed consent?

VEATCH: The question deals with research on patients who are either alive or dead, depending on how we settle the conceptual question. I have no difficulty with the ethics of research on either living patients in irreversible coma, or the recently diagnosed cadaver in which respirations are present.§ I do believe that there are serious questions pertaining to consent that can be raised. It may well be that much of the research that we would contemplate on scientific grounds would not be possible because consent could not be obtained.

Many among us have signed cards saying that our bodies may be used for research after we are dead, and I certainly have no objections to consent of that type.

R. NESBAKKEN (*Rikshospitalet, Oslo, Norway*): In my country we have legislation and definition of death based on the total destruction of the brain. The traditional criteria, that is, the arrest of systemic circulation and respiration, are still valid. I think the total concept of brain death may be misleading to the public. There is only one definition of death, although it may be diagnosed in various ways.

Let me take the traditional diagnosis of death, which includes circulatory arrest and arrest of spontaneous respiration. These criteria are no longer universally applicable; for example, during open heart surgery the respiration and the heartbeat may be stopped for prolonged periods of time, and the patient is not dead. Therefore, additional criteria to diagnose death are necessary. The present Norwegian regulations state that "The diagnosis of death is based on the following definition: death has occurred when there is a total destruction of the brain, with complete and lasting cessation of all functions in the cerebrum, the cerebellum, and the brain stem. This definition is generally valid and covers all causes of death." Death can be diagnosed in two different ways. The first may be called the traditional way, which will include the criteria that are used in the majority of cases—irreversible cessation of cardiac and respiratory activity. If these functions are artificially maintained, the following six criteria must be fulfilled: (1) the presence of known intracranial disease, which will compromise the intracranial circulation; (2) total unconsciousness; (3) arrest of spontaneous respiration; (4) absence of cephalic reflexes; (5) cessation of all electrical activity in the brain; and (6) supply to the brain as demonstrated by four-vessel craniocerebral angiography.

Therefore, we have one definition of death diagnosed in two different ways, either in the traditional or in the classical way, or, by a new way, which includes definite proof that the intracranial circulation has come to a halt.

VEATCH: I would emphasize that there is a concept behind both the Norwegian and the American effort. There is a rough consensus that a person should be pronounced dead when and only when there is some kind of evidence of the death of the brain, either cardiorespiratory findings or evidence directly measuring brain function, indicating that the brain is irreversibly destroyed. If one does not accept the premise that death should be pronounced when and only when the brain is irreversibly destroyed, then some radically different legislative and ethical stance would be required, for instance, if the view were held that even if the brain was destroyed but the heart continued to beat that the person still existed in all his essence. There is no amount of laboratory research that can refute that stance. You might enter into a theological argument about the fundamental nature of man, and it is that type of argument that must be resolved.

Likewise if one believes the individual is dead even though some brain activity (e.g., brain-stem activity) remains, there is no biological argument that can refute this, although there may well be persuasive philosophical arguments.

NESBAKKEN: I believe we should evaluate the problem of patients in persistent vegetative states and consider the ethical problems involved. In contrast, the problem of brain death is well-defined and demands appropriate legislation.

VEATCH: There is indeed a legitimate dispute here, if not between neurologic and heart function, at least on the question of which neurologic functions are essential. We can eliminate that problem by hypothesizing one or more stances, but that will not be any more satisfactory than a hypothesis of death when a person's foot is amputated.

I would like to make a few additional remarks in the form of questions that will highlight the lack of precision in our terminology. What is meant by conciousness? The definitions are not clear-cut, which is also true for every other concept of death we have discussed. What do you mean by circulation? Does 5 percent blood flow to the brain count as circulation or not? What do you mean by respiration, systemic respiration or cellular respiration? What do you mean by loss of integrating capacity? If the cord is intact but everything above the cord is destroyed, is there still some residual integrating capacity?

Similarly, the problem of conciousness is not a problem that is unique to my formulation. It is required that all of these be spelled out operationally.

When we say the complete destruction of the brain, do we really mean that? Do we mean every neuron has to die? Or do we mean something else? And if we mean something else, what is it? There are questions of precision in formulation that need to be addressed no matter what stand one takes on each of these positions.||

EDITOR'S COMMENT

"In the matter of Karen Ann Quinlan, an alleged incompetent," one must guard against the inherent confusion due to imprecision, distortion and frequent lack of complete information that is communicated to the public by means of many news media. In order to clarify some pertinent issues, the results of neurologic evaluation of Ms. Quinlan, which was performed at the request of the Quinlan family and their attorneys (P. Armstrong and J. Crowley), will be presented. My examination was performed on October 10, 1975, approximately six months after her initial episode of anoxia due to transient respiratory arrest as indicated by review of her entire medical record up to that date. Ms. Quinlan was not brain-dead at that time nor was she ever pronounced brain-dead. She met none of the criteria of brain death but was in a persistent vegetative state. There had been no evidence of cognitive function from the onset according to previous examiners and there was none during this examination. The patient did have a complex repetoire of cephalic reflexes, decerebrate posturing and, when not stimulated, she was apneic. With repetitive noxious stimuli, reflex patterns and eye-opening occurred in a stereotyped fashion; random, slightly disconjugate extraocular movements were noted as well as spontaneous breathing with overriding of the respirator. Multiple examinations always re-

---

|| It should be noted that papers elsewhere in this volume attempt to answer more precisely many of the questions Dr. Veatch asks in the discussion.—*J. K.*

vealed electroencephalographic activity, and normal intracranial circulation was confirmed by angiography. These facts are a matter of public record as testimony in the form of the transcript of the legal proceedings of the trial. Two major problems were dealt with in these proceedings and may be paraphrased as follows: First, who was the legal guardian? Second, could the withdrawal of "extraordinary care" procedures, including removal of the respirator, be permitted at the request of the guardian of this patient who was in an irreversible noncognitive state? The difficulties related to the judicial decisions as a result of these legal proceedings are discussed by Dr. Beresford elsewhere in this volume.

—*Julius Korein*

THE SOCIAL EFFECTS OF CHANGING
ATTITUDES TOWARDS DEATH

James P. Carse

Department of History and Literature of Religion
New York University
New York, New York 10003

It is the thesis of this paper that we are seriously mistaken when we suppose that it is the recent sophistication of our health-care technology that has led us into the moral dilemmas of knowing when it is appropriate to terminate a life. The moral issue did not arise as the result of the technology. On the contrary, as I shall argue, the technology was developed in response to a deeper and a prior moral concern. To see how this is the case it will be necessary to step back for a moment to look into the sources of the moral attitude toward death in the Western world.

If one were forced to make a quick comparison between attitudes toward death in the East and those in the West, one might reasonably respond that in the East death is generally understood as a metaphysical phenomenon, while in the Western world it has been more frequently regarded as a moral phenomenon. In both Hinduism and Buddhism, for example, the path from birth to death follows the normal course of natural events. Death does not come as the result of a transgression against the divine, nor is it an unnecessary condition imposed on living things by a malevolent deity. It is not even a particularly evil fate. In fact, in Hindu mythology there occurs a story of the gods' decision to lift the burden of mortality from all living persons. They soon regretted this decision, however, and promptly rescinded it, for they discovered that universal immortality would have the effect of overpopulating the earth, and that, what is still worse, it would lead to insufferable boredom and immorality. If one could look forward to an endless existence, almost any act could be put off indefinitely, causing a great torpor to descend upon the whole race and leading them to the permanent neglect of their duties.

In the Western imagination death is not as much a general condition of human existence as it is the result of a deep violation against the proper order of things. There is a double edge to this view. On the one hand, death is a flaw in human existence, a profound fault. Something has gone terribly wrong and existence is not what it should be. Its original nature has been seriously damaged. The overcoming of death is therefore a matter of returning to what once was the case, of restoring the integrity, or healing the wounds of existence. On the other hand, this unnatural flaw in human existence comes from human existence itself. It is not imposed on us from without. We did it to ourselves. We have freely violated our own original nature.

Agamemnon's death at the hands of his wife Clytemnestra and her lover Aegisthos was in no sense an accident of history. Agamemnon got precisely what he deserved from his earlier immorality—he had insulted a goddess—and even that was the consequence of a long succession of immoral acts by persons in his own family. Clytemnestra and Aegisthos were in turn savagely done in by Orestes out of revenge for the murder of his father. None of these deaths has behind it a natural necessity of the sort described by Hindus and Buddhists,

0077-8923/78/0315-0322 $01.75/0 © 1978, NYAS

and all of them originate in a free choice. We can make the same point about
the view of death among the ancient Hebrews, for Adam and Eve would certainly have been deathless had they not violated the injunction of the Lord God
and eaten of the Tree of the Knowledge of Good and Evil. Christians, in their
belief that the wages of sin is death, adopted the Jewish view whole.

If the way into death is moral, so is the way out. By acts of love, or faith,
or by perfect righteousness, the original state of existence might be restored.
The Greeks seemed to have rather modest expectations of this sort, however,
for they remain silent on the fate of those souls who strove for perfection.
Socrates speculated that he might have the "amusing" privilege, if he survived
his death, of speaking with the departed sages of the past and searching their
minds, "to find out who is really wise among them, and who only thinks that
he is." He certainly offered no resplendent vision of a repaired human nature.
In one of the great Egyptian myths, by way of contrast, the passionate love of
Isis for the murdered Osiris was undiminished even when she learned that the
body of her beloved had been dismembered and hidden throughout the Nile
valley. The ultimate joyous resurrection of Osiris is not a phenomenon of
unaided nature, but the triumph of Isis' loving intention to restore him to life.
The Christian myth of the resurrection also has a deeply moral element. The
raising of Jesus from the dead is a manifestation of the love of God, and of
God's gracious desire to restore the whole human race to its original purity in
spite of its continuing disobedience. The Resurrection of the faithful will not
follow automatically, however, but only when they have bound themselves in
loving union with the risen Christ.

The subject of this paper is the social effects of changing attitudes toward
death. I have begun with these reflections on the distinction between moral
and natural attitudes toward death for several reasons. To begin with, the
assumption that death is a flaw in human existence that ought to be removed
has a strong influence on the medical practitioner; it tends to make his role less
functional than spiritual. Physicians are no longer expected to do nothing more
than correct physical disorders; they are also expected to achieve the redemption
of existence itself.

It is well to remember that this exalted role of the physician is not the
consequence of the aggrandizing of profit-hungry individuals giving the public
the hard-sell on costly therapies for maladies they probably do not even know
they have, and may not even have; and much less is it the creation of isolated
geniuses working in their dimly lit garages and basements with exotic chemicals
and primitive laboratory equipment paid for out of their own pockets—all in
the selfless commitment to pure knowledge. The present shape of the medical
profession is largely the result of swelling social demand. High individual fees,
steadily increasing insurance premiums, generous bequests from the estates of
the wealthy, and politically popular governmental largesse all constitute a kingly
patronage that continues to underwrite the astounding growth of the profession
and its institutions. There are, to be sure, frequently heard complaints about
the costs of medical care or the antihuman environment and policies of caring
institutions. But these are insignificant when compared to the social push, at
the other end, demanding increased medical service, and medical service in
certain favorite areas, such as dying and death. However much the public has
complained, they nevertheless have the kind of medical profession they demanded and paid for.

The point of these latter remarks is to suggest that society wants something more than simply the treatment of disease. If it is true that in the Western imagination death is primarily a moral rather than a metaphysical phenomenon, then this vast patronage has somewhere behind it the desire to recover our lost immortality. Death is not a limit within which we are to develop our humanity, according to this view, but the very enemy that robs us of our humanity, and therefore an enemy that must be destroyed in the interest of rescuing that humanity. It is no accident that we speak of "fighting" an epidemic or "hunting out and conquering" the cause of a crippling disease. The medical profession is not a public service subvened to make our lives more pleasant; it is an army engaged in combat with a rapacious and malevolent force. Moreover, it is an army we are determined to train and equip well enough that it will be sure to win. Responsible medical scientists are already speaking freely of the time in which all disease will have been vanquished, and a large part of the public's fascination with DNA research surely rises from that tiny possibility that someone will pull the winning ticket in the genetic lottery and offer all of us eternal youth.

Having said this, we must complicate this brief account of the traditional morality concerning death by admitting that it is certainly likely that most persons engaged in some one of the many fields concerned in some way with dying and death—and there are many such fields—will not recognize themselves in this caricature. They may well protest that what impels them is not the glamour of moral combat, but the palpable excitement of intellectual adventure. This protest has its own tradition in the Western world. Not all great systems of thought that we have inherited from the past are committed to a moral view of death. The ancient Epicureans, for example, argued that death was a perfectly natural phenomenon that came when the organization of atoms in the body suddenly simplified itself. We would not distort the Epicurean philosophy on this point if we translated their teaching into modern scientific argot and said that death comes when the organism becomes irreversibly entropic.

We might remind ourselves that Epicureanism is not a method of finding irresistibly delectable pleasures, but a religious philosophy that had a powerful intellectual appeal to Mediterranean culture for many centuries. Modern scientific theory in many obvious ways is deeply Epicurean in its theoretical approach to life and death. Life is not some special essence or even some special process. Life constitutes no exception to the lawfulness of natural phenomena. The line that marks the living from the dead is in most respects nonexistent to the scientific view. What is being observed is not a process that will come to an absolute end, but one that will only continue to undergo modification. The great concern with the precise *moment* of death does not arise from the refined Epicurean interests of the modern theoretician, but from the necessity of making certain decisions about a dying body under a variety of social pressures. The issue in this Conference is really the irreconcilable conflict of the social, and largely moral, demand to push back the dark wall of death with the scientific, and largely intellectual, interest in simply observing and describing a continuing process.

The issue is further complicated by the fact that the proclaimed moral disinterest of medical research is not altogether innocent in this connection. In one respect, the extraordinary technological capacities we have been discussing here *are* the result of the dispassionate investigation into the nature of things I have characterized as a refined Epicureanism. In another respect that investigation has been lavishly supported out of the moral impulse to vanquish the ancient enemy. To ignore this now, to stand back with palms raised in a gesture of innocence, would be too ingenuous. Medical science got itself into this dilemma, or was led into it, through moral passion; it cannot with integrity back out through the exit marked "pure science."

What I am arguing here is that there is a subtle reciprocity between society and medicine in the matter of the changing attitudes toward death. The social desire to eliminate, or at least to forestall, death has encouraged the sort of research that puts death-defying power in the hands of trained practitioners. As this power is increasingly publicized, social demand is not satisfied but only increased. In other words, because of this reciprocity the social *effects* of changing attitudes toward death in medicine become the social *causes* for continuing change in those attitudes. There is, of course, nothing problematic in the interpenetration of society and medicine as such; what is problematic is the apparent irreconcilability of the two attitudes toward death. We therefore find ourselves in the perplexing dilemma of attempting to deal with moral questions by scientific deliberation. How shall we resolve that dilemma?

As I suggested in the opening remarks of this paper, it appears to me that the dilemma arises because we have confused the order in which technology and morality are related. That is, we have assumed that the moral question is a consequence of the technology. I shall therefore propose that the dilemma be solved by reversing that order, by facing squarely the fact that the technology is itself the result of a moral decision. The moral question is not what we should do with the technology now that we have it, but whether we should even have a technology, and, if so, for what purpose.

To have a more adequate understanding of the moral question it is useful here to look more deeply into the moral tradition that has brought us to this dilemma. If it is true that our view of death is primarily a moral one, it is only partially true that it is identical to that of the ancient Greeks, Hebrews, and Christians. We recall that there was a double edge to their view: death is a damaging alteration of human existence; and it is moreover an alteration that we have freely done to ourselves. There is one crucial difference, however, between the classical and the modern view. No classical or ancient culture entertained the possibility that death could be eliminated in the present world. It always required a translation into another state, an elevation into the bosom of a divinity, or a miraculous spiritual rebirth into a transcendent mode of existence. For this reason the ancient and classical cure of death was thought to be not only moral but religious. It required a cult, a mythology, a priesthood.

There is no doubt that in certain ways medicine has taken on powerful cultic qualities in the mind of the public. Physicians speak a mysterious language; they wear spotless liturgical vestments, and they engender mythic narratives out of their heroic struggles with the unseen enemy. The drilled precision of an operating room, the presence of fresh blood, and the exchange of priceless instruments over the exposed organs of a living body are all quite like a ritual sacrifice arranged to summon the invisible forces of healing.

This is, however, a bogus cult at best. The great flow of private and public dollars into the medical profession has not been stimulated by the hope of an other-worldly, but a this-worldly, transformation. Moreover, the priests were only secondary to the gods, and who today would think of suing the gods for malpractice?

I am not, to be sure, proposing that we revive the ancient cult of the healer, but only that we look at the moral impulse out of which the cult itself arose.

The function of a priest in the cult is not primarily to alter the physical conditions of the supplicant's life (although in decayed form the cult often is used to make rain or cause the seed to germinate and the womb to be fertile), but to make life meaningful within the conditions that cannot be changed. In a very real sense the contemporary patient and physician operate in a decadent form of the cult, that is, the conditions of his or her life. The assumption here, in contrast to that of the true cult, is that *extending a life and improving its physical conditions are precisely what will make that life meaningful.*

The question we are then led to ask by this comparison with the deeper moral origin of the true cult of healing is whether we can measure the meaningfulness of life by its length or its physical comfort. I would venture to say at this point that the dilemma we have been discussing here—the conflict between the moral and scientific attitudes toward death—is falsely understood as the failure, thus far, to eliminate disease and death. Indeed, even if we should succeed in doing this, the dilemma could only escalate, for we could no longer hide from the question as to whether the meaning of life and its length are identical. We would discover that the question *What is my life for?* is altogether distinct from the question *How long shall I live?* The length of life has nothing to do with its meaningfulness.

This brings us to what may be a surprising conclusion: the struggle to eliminate death, even if it succeeds, and in spite of its moral origin, is an inherently meaningless struggle.

If a practice of medicine that takes as its supreme value the indefinite extension of life is inherently meaningless, is there a kind of medicine that is truly meaningful? I shall answer this question positively by pleading for the recovery of the sense of morality that gave rise to the cult of healing. The difference between the ancient cult of the priest and the modern cult of the physician is that in the former the supplicants were active participants in the entire process. The purpose of the cultic act was not simply the sacerdotal lifting of the burden of guilt which would cure one of death, but the moral renewal of the supplicant. The cult was not intended to give one *more* life, but to change the moral content of the life one has.

What lies behind this ancient cultic morality is not a crude belief in the power of the priest to vanquish the power of death, as it is sometimes carelessly asserted. The insistence that death originates in our own free act is equivalent to saying that we are utterly responsible for the content of our own lives. Whatever disaster, or loss, or disease might befall us, there is no one to blame. The other side of this assumption is that we are equally responsible for the joy and health that could fill our lives.

In its higher moments, therefore, the moral view of death does not require the elimination of death itself, but the restoration of personal integrity in the face of death, that is, the recognition that life is itself a choice and not a duty, and in turn the recognition that happiness comes only from within. It is this recognition that has been lost in the present reciprocal relation between medicine and society, when the question of meaning is answered quantitatively. The decadence of the modern cult of healing is most plainly seen in the belief that happiness comes from without and must therefore be bestowed by another, preferably by a professional.

It is for this reason that I have argued that it is mistaken to believe that the technology should be used simply because we have it, even if it means the extension of a life. The practice of medicine is meaningless unless it is seen that the highest value is the personal integrity of the patient. The treatment, if there is any, is always to come as the result of a free moral choice on the part of the patient. It may well occur that a morally responsible physician would recommend to a patient suffering from a potentially mortal disease that he or she consider foregoing all treatment in the interest of preserving the spiritual integrity of his or her life. A natural death might be far more consistent with one's humanity than a desperate clinging to an array of expensive and impersonal equipment, even if it adds a year or a dozen years of biological existence.

In conclusion, I will only insist that we are not then to call in moralists to solve problems raised by technologists, but to expose and critically examine the morality inherent in the technology. We are not asking physicians to *become* moralists, but to understand that they *already are* moralists and that it therefore is only fitting that they endeavor to become as proficient with moral deliberation they they are with the strategies of healing.

I am not proposing *a* morality, but only saying that it is a profound violation of the profession of healing to allow an already inherent morality to go unexamined. I noted earlier that Socrates was amused by the prospect of conversing with the departed sages to see who was really wise, and who only thought they were wise. We know, of course, how he would distinguish between them. They only think they are wise, who live an unexamined life.

DISCUSSION

MORACZEWSKI: I also recognize that the moral error in terms of death is focusing on death as disintegration, not death as transition or transformation. The transition to a different state would not be painful or involve disintegration, and there is no moral fault there.

The moral fault is associated with death as disintegration. How does that apply to us today? An attitude exists that denies the concept of death as transition. So those who hold the attitude that death is the end, and that there is nothing beyond, have a tendency to want to continue this life almost at any cost. One extreme form of this attitude is exemplified by cryogenics, in which the body is frozen. Insurance policies can be written for many thousands of dollars to pay for a person to be frozen in liquid nitrogen after death for 50 years. The idea here is that when you "wake up" at the end of 50 years the technology would have been advanced sufficiently to replace whatever organ was defective. The person would be thawed out and the organ replaced, and the person would continue to live until the next failure. This attitude denies death as transition.

CARSE: I am reminded of Woody Allen's observation that if you were to be revived after 100 or 200 years it is likely that your Volkswagen will still be there. There are a number of things that do not go through any kind of a transition. There is a subtle notion, not that of a crude terminus, but that whether or not death is an end, it arises out of a function and lends an expression to one's moral disposition to life. The way in which we approach death is morally related to the way in which we approach life. They are not metaphysically related, but we still have a choice about how we can interrelate our attitudes towards life and death.

VEATCH: Dr. Carse, I am interested in how you would relate your formulations to the specific subject of the shifting definitions of death. It seems to me that you might view them as an attempt to be more realistic in accepting the limits of man's capacity to intervene. On the other hand, you might see them as just one more example of the pressures to intervene with new technologies, to the extent that the movement for new definitions is linked to therapies such as transplantation.

CARSE: My remarks implied that the question being discussed has arisen because we have not gone through the appropriate moral deliberation. However, moral deliberation would not have entirely eliminated the necessity for this discourse on brain death and its associated problems.

Technology, no matter how complex and lavish, always requires antecedent moral decisions. And I believe that it is exceedingly foolish not to examine that morality.

In response to another aspect of your question, the paper I originally intended to present dealt with the perplexing element of what I would call the transcendental quality of personhood, and by personhood I mean that signs of consciousness and social interaction must exist. When one attempts to use certain criteria to determine whether a corpse is capable of reachieving personhood, one comes against an extreme limitation, and that is the question of the individual with personhood making a decision about personhood using his own personhood. This is not an absolute, but a transcendental activity and inherently limits any set of criteria used. Therefore I believe your questions are unanswerable in an absolute sense. To me the problem will remain a profound mystery.

I think people ought to walk around permanently with this kind of question in their minds. There is no ultimate answer to the question of what a person is, because you must be a person even to consider this question. This is, therefore, an open-ended dilemma.

VEATCH: Would you share my view then that there may not be a perfect fit between the concept of death that you hinted at and the complete destruction of the brain? This is especially apparent in patients who have some level of brain function remaining and yet have none of the capacities you have just described as associated with personhood.

CARSE: Yes. I hate to say yes, but I must.

BOSHES: I do not think the medical profession has to accept the appellation of moral blackguards. In his address to the Congress of Anesthesiologists in 1957 Pope Pius XII suggested that there was a time when death should not be opposed. The committees at the Massachusetts General Hospital handling burn patients whose condition was such that there was no precedent for recovery faced a similar moral issue. The issue involved giving the patient the choice of being treated or not, thus allowing, if the patient so desired, a rapid, dignified death. The committees that deal with the question of whether or not to resuscitate a patient face the moral issue of accepting death as a moral right of passage, if you will forgive the pun. We shouldn't castigate ourselves on this issue.

CARSE: I agree—I would be shocked if you thought my remarks were meant to castigate physicians. The point of what I was trying to say is that all of us involved in such issues are in a profoundly moral situation. The difficulty is that some individuals do not acknowledge this situation sufficiently.

RELIGIOUS CONCEPTS OF BRAIN DEATH AND ASSOCIATED PROBLEMS

Stanley Hauerwas

Department of Theology
University of Notre Dame
Notre Dame, Indiana 46556

THE LIMITS OF A THEOLOGICAL DETERMINATION OF THE MOMENT OF DEATH

Theologians are considered to be an odd lot today. They sense the public's bemusement as soon as they try to explain what they do, because they are immediately subjected to suspicious questioning. If you are fortunate, your listener misunderstands theology for geology and assumes you are engaged in an honest endeavor. However, if you go on to explain that you are not a geologist, but a theologian, you are confronted with a quizzical stare that makes you feel that an explanation, if not an apology, is in order. Generally, I assume that this means that people do not think it odd for someone to spend his or her life thinking about rocks, but that it is an aberration to spend your life thinking about God.

There is, of course, good reason for this judgment—thinking about rocks seems to have some payoff in a way that thinking about God does not. Rocks are connected to oil in an immediate and direct way, and even the best prayer will not make a car run without gas. Therefore, when theologians are invited to speak at conferences such as this on matters such as the determination of brain death, they are extremely anxious to please. Such conferences represent an opportunity to show that theology has concrete relevance.

Therefore you will understand how disappointed I am to have to tell you that there is nothing in Christian convictions that would entail preference for one definition of death over another. That is not to say that there have not been a lot of perceptive and incisive things said by theologians about the determination of the moment of death. However, it remains unclear what connection there is between their theological views and their judgments about death.

The claim that a connection must be demonstrated between Christian conviction and determination of the moment of death may seem odd. After all, you may be accustomed to dealing with people who tell you that their Christian convictions have something to do with their death. There seems to be good reason for this claim since basic Biblical texts deal with death. Thus in Paul's letter to the Romans we are told

> If we have died with Christ, we believe that we shall also live with him. For we know that Christ being raised from the dead will never die again; death no longer has dominion over him. The death he died he died to sin, once for all, but the life he lives he lives to God. So you also must consider yourselves dead to sin and alive to God in Christ.
>
> (Romans 6: 8–11)

In even more ringing terms Paul says

> Who shall separate us from the love of Christ? Shall tribulation or distress or persecution or famine, or nakedness, or peril, or sword? As it is written, "For

0077–8923/78/0315–0329 $01.75/0 © 1978, NYAS

thy sake we are being killed all the day long; we are regarded as sheep to be slaughtered." No, in all these things we are more than conquerors through him who loved us. For I am sure that neither death, nor life, nor angels, nor principalities, nor things present, nor things to come, nor powers, not height, nor depth, nor anything else in all creation, will be able to spearate us from the love of God in Christ Jesus our Lord.

(Romans 8: 35–39)

These are powerful and substantive claims. Yet Paul Ramsey, a theologian who has dealt extensively with death and dying, stated with regard to a theological definition of the moment of death that

. . . . a theologian or moralist as such knows nothing about such questions; the determination of death is a medical matter; and a theologian or moralist can offer only his reflections upon the meaning of respect for life and of care of the dying, and issue some warnings of the moral complexities surrounding such matters [6] (p. 104).

In this essay I will explain why Ramsey is right to deny that there is a theological definition of the moment of death. Christians hold some very substantive beliefs about death itself, however, and I want to suggest how those beliefs help to provide a framework for the moral and practical considerations connected with definitions of the moment of death in general. In the foregoing passages from Paul death is described theologically and morally. I will try to show that *how* one understands a moral description of death helps to set the kind of questions that should be asked about the meaning and status of any proposed definition of the moment of death.

THE MEANING AND STATUS OF BRAIN DEATH

In order to understand the reluctance of theologians to provide a "religious concept of brain death," it is necessary to be clear about what brain death means. There is no reason for me to go over the work that Veatch [8] has already done so well, but I will center my concerns around the very helpful distinctions he provides. Veatch's central point is that the concept of death should not be confused with the criteria that determine when death has occurred. He rightly argues that the concept of death involves a philosophical judgment of a significant change that has happened in a person. Thus the concept of death is a correlative of what one takes to be the necessary conditions of human life, e.g., the capacity for bodily integration or loss of consciousness.

Correlative to different concepts of death are certain loci and criteria of death. Loci are places where we look to determine whether or not the person is dead, i.e., heart, brain, neocortex. The criteria of death are those empirical measurements that can be made to determine whether a person is dead, such as cessation of respiration or a flat EEG. The subtle point in Veatch's analysis is that there is no necessary connection between certain concepts of death and the determination of the locus and criteria of death [8] (p. 51). Rather, the claim is made that certain associations of the loci and criteria of death with certain concepts of death seem more appropriate than others, but these associations are pragmatic and contingent, not conceptual and necessary. Thus it seems reasonable to identify the locus of death with the brain if one understands the concept of death to involve the irreversible loss of the capacity for bodily interaction.

It also seems appropriate to use the criteria of the Harvard report as an indication of when death has occurred. "Brain death" is an empirical standard for verifying a death, but it does not involve one and only one concept of death. So Veatch is right to suggest that "terms such as brain death or heart death should be avoided because they tend to obscure the fact that we are searching for the meaning of death of the person as a whole" [8] (p. 37).

For those dealing with dying patients this kind of analysis may seem to be question-begging. However, such an analysis is but a reminder that genuinely practical matters often raise deep theoretical issues. These issues are absolutely crucial if we are to consider questions such as how to determine the moment of death without confusing them with questions concerning the worth of prolonging life under certain circumstances. For nothing could be more dangerous than the attempt to substitute a definition of the moment of death for a moral question concerning our obligation to keep ourselves and others alive under conditions of distress. A definition of death should not preclude the question of the worth of a life. The question regarding the worth of Karen Quinlan's life should not be precluded by defining her as dead.

This distinction helps to clarify why the issue of defining the criteria of death should not be determined in terms of the need for transplant organs. Whatever the concept of death we think appropriate, the criteria of death should take into account the dying person's needs. If the phrase "right to die" makes any sense at all, it should at least mean that we should be allowed to die without the meaning of our death being determined by someone else's needs.

More important for the purpose of this paper, however, is the distinction between the concept of death and the loci and criteria of death to help make clear the role of Christian convictions about death. As I suggested, there may not be a religious concept of brain death. That does not mean, though, that Christian beliefs may not contribute to an understanding of the concept of death. This issue has been confused in the past by assuming that the use of a metaphor like the "heart" in religious discourse implied a position about the locus or criteria of death. But "heart" so used is not an empirical description of a part of the body, but rather an indication of the whole person's engagement with life. Thus the question arises of how Christian beliefs about the nature of death might make a difference in how the concept of death is understood.

SACREDNESS OF LIFE AND THE CONCEPT OF DEATH

The claim that Christian convictions make a difference in how the concept of death is understood remains ambiguous. Note how abstract such phrases as "irreversible loss of the soul from the body," or "irreversible loss of capacity for bodily integration," or "loss of consciousness" are when compared with the life plans of people. For example, I have known some "good old boys" who felt strongly that when you became too old to ride a horse you might as well be dead. If you told them that they were thereby committed to assuming death to consist of "loss of consciousness," thereby making the neocortex the locus of death and the criterion a flat EEG, they would probably tell you that they don't give a damn.

Christian beliefs about death work like "riding a horse," i.e., the beliefs shape the Christian's conceptions of death. The Christian is concerned not with life as an end in itself, but rather as the medium for service in God's kingdom.

Put differently, no one lives just to live. We each live for some purpose or purposes. These purposes set certain boundaries that determine the meaning and significance of death. Christians believe that their lives have been determined by the purproses of God as manifest in the history of Israel and Jesus' cross and resurrection. Thus for Paul the "death" that concerns him the most is the death that reigns in this life through the power of sin. The problem is that there is no clear inference that can be drawn from this sense of the purpose of life concerning which concept of death is most appropriate for the Christian.

With respect to life, however, it has recently been claimed that the basic stance of Christians toward life is that it is sacred. This obviously has been claimed in questions concerning death and dying and abortions. There is surely much about the phrase "sanctity of life" in which Christians have a stake. We believe that God has sanctified every living thing and that each of his creatures, even the most wayward, cannot escape his care—in both life and death.

This claim regarding the sacredness of life often indicates the refusal of the Christian to separate the spirit from the body. Although there is much talk about the soul in Christian discourse, Christians always maintain the Jewish sense of the body's significance. Thus Ramsey maintains that

> Just as man is sacredness in the social and political order, so he is a sacredness in the natural, biological order. He is a sacredness in bodily life. He is a person who within the ambience of the flesh claims our care. He is an embodied soul or ensouled body. He is therefore a sacredness in illness and in his dying. The sanctity of human life prevents ultimate trespass upon him even for the sake of treating his bodily life, or for the sake of others who are also only a sacredness in their bodily life, or for the sake of treating his bodily life, or for the sake of others who are also only a sacredness in their bodily lives.[6]

This at least means that Christians will be suspicious of any concept of death that associates death only with the so-called "higher forms of our life." Of course that does not mean that the neocortex is ruled out as the locus of death since it may well be the best indication that the bodily conditions necessary for our consciousness can no longer be sustained.

It is a mistake to assume that "sanctity of life" is a sufficient criterion for an appropriate concept of death. Appeals to the sanctity of life beg exactly the question at issue, namely, that you know what kind of life it is that should be treated as sacred. More troubling for me, however, is how the phrase "sanctity of life," when separated from its theological context, became an ideological slogan for a narrow individualism antithetical to the Christian way of life. Put starkly, Christians are not fundamentally concerned about living. Rather, their concern is to die for the right thing. Appeals to the sanctity of life as an ideology make it appear that Christians are committed to the proposition that there is nothing in life worth dying for.

When this happens Christians unwittingly embody the modern view that death is the one thing we can be sure about in life and that it is to be avoided as long as possible. As my colleague Reverend John Dunne has pointed out, Descartes said "I think, therefore I am," while modern man says "I am going to die, therefore I am." Our identity is no longer anchored in life, but in death. As a result, death becomes the overriding enemy. But such an attitude is antithetical to the Christian belief that our identity is anchored in God's love as revealed in the cross. Even death itself cannot separate us from that.

Thus the phrase "sanctity of life," when used as an ideology, dangerously suggests that for a Christian life is an end in itself. Our sacredness rests then on something such as rationality. But as Ramsey has suggested

> . . . . one grasps the religious outlook upon the sanctity of human life only if he sees that this life is asserted to be surrounded by sanctity that need not be in man; that the most dignity a man ever possesses is a dignity that is alien to him. . . The value of a human life is ultimately grounded in the value God is placing on it. Anyone who can himself stand imaginatively even for a moment with an outlook where everything is referred finally to God—who, from things that are not, brings into being things that are—should be able to see that God's deliberations about the man need have only begun.[7]

Therefore life for Christians is not sacred in the strict sense. Christians view life as a gift, but a gift that they must care for.[2] Thus the claim that life is sacred is not really so much a statement about ourselves as it is an indication of the kind of respect that we owe our neighbor. Our life and the lives of our neighbor are to be protected since they are not ours to dispose of. For our dying as much as our living should be determined by our conviction that we are not our own.

But what do these homiletical flourishes have to do with the concept of death? They at least make clear why Christians have an aversion to the connotation of hastened death associated with the unhappy word, euthanasia.[2] However, these considerations also help us understand why Christians, in spite of their condemnation of euthanasia, have assumed that death need not be prolonged in all cases. The distinction between ordinary and extraordinary means of prolonging life, a distinction that is probably more trouble than it is worth, was the result of Christians' attempt to balance their sense that their lives were not at their disposal with their sense that death is not to be opposed unconditionally. Veatch is right to suggest that reflection on the right to refuse treatment is a much better means to consider such questions[8] (pp. 116–163).

Moreover, Ramsey has argued that the question of "updating the criteria" of death in the context of Christian convictions is better described as an attempt to develop a criteria for when to use a respirator[6] (p. 81). I think it is useful to note why Ramsey thinks he has a theological stake in describing the issue in this manner. He fears that "brain death" might be taken to indicate that a person's primary value is determined by intelligence rather than by his or her existence as one of God's children. Thus he can argue that the criteria of "brain death" are not essentially different from "heart death" criteria, but rather denote a procedural difference that has come about because of the extensive use of life-supporting techniques[6] (p. 87). Ramsey therefore has no objection to the criteria of death suggested by the Harvard report, since he assumes that the heart and lungs can only function artificially when there is total brain death. Thus there is no moral or theological commitment to continue using a respirator in such a case.

However, it would seem that Ramsey would have difficulty approving the definition of brain death as a "dead" neocortex accompanied by a brain stem still capable of maintaining heart and lung function. I mention this because Veatch has argued that, all other things being equal, the death of the neocortex should be sufficient to indicate that death should be declared. There are, of course, empirical issues involved in this proposal (i.e., whether an EEG unfailingly predicts the irreversible loss of consciousness associated with the death of the neocortex). My concern, however, is whether or not there is any theological issue at stake in this difference between Ramsey and Veatch.

Ramsey might well suggest that Veatch assumes that the value of human life is only related to our consciousness and capacity for social interaction, and thus fails to see that the value of life should primarily be determined by God. However, this kind of argument assumes that there is a strong logical connection between the criteria of death and the concept and correlative worth of life. Veatch is not saying that the value of life is associated only with consciousness, but rather that consciousness is the necessary condition for any values. Moreover, Veatch's concern is primarily practical. His question is whether there are any indications that might help us to know when not to subject those who are dying to a mercy grown cruel through the power of our technology. While it is cruel not to try to sustain life, it may be just as cruel to extend care unconditionally. Interestingly, it is in terms of these practical issues that Christian convictions may be the most relevant.

THE CHRISTIAN WAY OF DEATH

With respect to the practical issues surrounding the care of the dying I now want to provide a slightly different perspective. Briefly, I want to suggest that we have had trouble considering how we should care for the dying, because we have not thought enough about what kind of responsibilities the one who is dying should have. In other words, the moral street here is not one way—the dying person has obligations to the living that are important for us to understand the care of the dying. The attempt to determine the moment of death may be an attempt to avoid determining when it is time to die.

Today there is much talk about learning to care for the dying. Generally this means that the patient ought to be regarded as primary, that he or she is someone to whom something terrible is happening to, and that we ought to help if we can. The assumption is that death, like a serious illness, robs persons of almost all claims to moral agency. The primary issue, then, is embodied in the question of the kind of care we ought to give someone so struck.

Also, the admonition that we must learn to care for the dying is an attempt to recover the more personal side of medicine. What the dying often need is not further medical care, especially if that care is used only to prolong the dying process; but it is claimed that the patient needs personal care. Care is not synonymous with cure and it is argued that the doctor and nurses should help the patient in a psychological and moral way. These admonitions to learn how to care for the dying are salutary, but they assume that the care of the dying is primarily concerned with the attitudes of the living toward what is essentially a passive object.

However, as Milton Mayeroff has reminded us, care must be extended in such a manner that the one cared for is given the freedom to care also:

> To care for another person, in the most significant sense, is to help him grow the actualize himself. Consider, for example, a father caring for his child. He respects the child as existing in his own right and as striving to grow. He feels needed by the child and helps him grow by responding to his need to grow. Caring is the antithesis of simply using the other person to satisfy one's own needs. Caring, as helping another grow and actualize himself, is a process, a way of relating to someone that involves development, in the same

way that friendship can only emerge in time through mutual trust and a deepening and qualitative transformation of the relationship.[5]

This sense of caring cannot help but strike us as a little odd when it comes to caring for the dying, because the dying seem to be ending their growing. Interestingly, we have recently come up with an answer to this problem. We can help the one who is dying to accept his or her death in the manner suggested by Kübler-Ross.[9] We are thus engaged in the extremely odd enterprise of encouraging people to die better than they have lived. No one can die angry or apathetically because it becomes imperative that we all die with a quiet, brave acceptance.

There are some deep problems associated with this kind of proposal. By transforming her descriptive stages into normative recommendations, Dr. Ross runs the risk of developing an extraordinarily manipulative strategy to deal with the dying. More importantly, there is nothing associated with Christian beliefs that should make us want to accept our death. More accurately, those beliefs make a great deal of difference with respect to our learning how to die.

It is clear from the passages from Paul cited at the beginning of this paper that death is not the worst thing that could happen to a Christian. But neither is it a good thing. According to Paul, a Christian may desire death in a manner which denotes lack of trust in God's triumph over death. Death is both a friend and an enemy. It is a friend in that without it we would not be forced to value one thing in life over another. Ironically, death creates the economy that makes life worthwhile. But because death is a friend it also becomes our enemy, for what we come to value and love we want to continue to value and love.[3]

Moreover, the language associated with the acceptance of death must be carefully used. If the one who is dying accepts death too well, it plays a cruel trick on the living. One who is too willing to die can make us feel that our own lack of care caused the one who died to leave life without wishing to retain anything. (Of course, we are talking here about a gradual rather than a sudden or accidental death.)

It is important, then, that the one who is dying exercise the responsibility to die well. That is, the person should die in a manner that is morally commensurate with the kind of trust that has sustained him or her in life. In terms of the language that I used earlier, it means that we should die in such a manner that others see that they are sustaining us and that correlatively due credit is given to God as the ultimate giver of life.

Thus the concern to recapture the meaning of "natural death" is salutary. Daniel Callahan has recently tried to define natural death as when (1) one's life work has been accomplished; (2) one's moral obligations to those for whom one has had responsibilities have been discharged; (3) one's death will not seem to others an offense to sense or sensibility, or will not tempt others to despair and rage at human existence; and (4) one's process of dying is not marked by unbearable and degrading pain.[1]

Callahan notes that all four points are filled with ambiguity (e.g., it makes a lot of difference how you conceive your life's work and who you think you have responsibilities to) and that it is hard to die without offending someone. However, there is much to commend Callahan's suggestion. As Eberhard Jungel has argued, the Christian conviction that we have been freed from the curse of death by Jesus Christ implies that:

. . . . human life has a natural end which comes when the time allotted to life has expired. Man has a right to die this death and no other. One of the duties of Christian faith is to see that this right is recognized. There is therefore an immediate connection between the proclamation of the death of Jesus Christ and the concern that man should have the right to die a natural death.[4]

There are a couple of qualifications that need to be made with respect to Jungel and Callahan's defense of the idea of "natural death." First, we should avoid the phrase "right to die." The term is unclear and Callahan observes that no society can guarantee that there will be no "deaths of the kind that lead people to fear their own death, or wonder about the rationality and benigness of the universe."[1] Secondly, I suspect that the phrase "natural death" is too misleading to be of much help. In a sense no death is natural, but is, as Veatch suggests, the result of some human choices. To perpetuate the fiction of "natural death" may give us the feeling that we are relieved of responsibility, but it does so at the "expense of continuing the suffering of death striking out in random and unregulated viciousness"[8] (p. 302).

It seems to me, however, that Callahan's proposal does not hinge on a notion of natural death, but is really an attempt to indicate what an acceptable or perhaps even a good death would entail. A good death is a death that we can prepare for through living because we are able to see that death is but a necessary correlative to a good life. Thus a good death is not natural in the sense that it may well occur before our natural machinery runs down, but it is good if it is commensurate with those commitments that sustained our life. For Christians this means that while we do not wish to die, we do not oppose death as if life were an end in itself. For as Augustine said, "Death is [to not] love God, and that is when we prefer anything to Him in affection and pursuit."

Finally, what do these kinds of concerns have to do with the issue of brain death? They remind us that "brain death" does not function just as a locus of death, but as a symbol of when it is time to die. But I am suggesting that if we are to die a good death, we must not allow the symbol of brain death to tyrannize us by requiring that we delay death so long that we can no longer die a good death. "Brain death" may well serve as an indication of when the living are released from certain claims having to do with care of the dying, but it should not be used as a substitute for the responsibility each of us has to die our own death. "Brain death" or "heart death" should not remove the responsibility and risk that are the necessary concomitants of our willingness to die a good death.

REFERENCES

1. CALLAHAN, DANIEL. 1977. On defining a "natural death." Hastings Center Rep. 7(3): 32–27.
2. HAUERWAS, STANLEY. 1977. Truthfulness and Tragedy: Further Investigations in Christian Ethics. : 101–115. University of Notre Dame Press. Notre Dame, Ind.
3. HAUERWAS, STANLEY. 1974. Vision and Virtue: Essays in Christian Ethical Reflection. : 166–186. Fides Press. Notre Dame, Ind.
4. JUNGEL, EBERHARD. 1974. Death: The Riddle and the Mystery. : 132. The Westminister Press. Philadelphia, Pa.
5. MAYEROFF, MILTON. 1971. On Caring. : 1. Harper and Row. New York, N. Y.
6. RAMSEY, PAUL. 1970. The Patient as Person: XIII. : 59–164. Yale University Press. New Haven, Conn.
7. RAMSEY, PAUL. 1971. The Morality of Abortion. In Moral Problems. James Rachels, Ed. : 11–12. Harper and Row. New York, N. Y.

8. VEATCH, ROBERT. 1976. Death, Dying, and the Biological Revolution: Our Last Quest for Responsibility. : 1–323. Yale University Press. New Haven, Conn.
9. KÜBLER-ROSS, E. 1969. On Death and Dying. Macmillan. New York, N.Y.

DISCUSSION

C. HENRY (*Cleveland Clinic, Cleveland, Ohio*): This subject has been considered throughout the ages by poets and playwrights and physicians who have eloquently studied and written about death as well as problems relating to the individual's right to die. Its significance is illustrated by the following quote from *King Lear*: "Vex not his ghost: O let him pass! he hates him that would upon the rack of this tough life stretch him out longer."

HAUERWAS: I do not wish to comment on the quote for in its eloquence it speaks for itself. I would like to note that the ancient Greeks had a very interesting notion. Aristotle thought that it was terrible to die before your time because he thought that life was about happiness. Happiness was considered the satisfaction that is garnered from a life well lived all the way to the end. Aristotle did not wish one to live too long, beyond the point where one could no longer enjoy the satisfaction of living. This may be contrasted to Christianity, in which the moral man is willing to die at any moment because what charges him morally is sufficient at any moment. It does not depend upon a life fully lived. This is a very serious difference.

Notice that I do not say anything about public policy issues. This is because I do not think the issue resolvable. The concepts are so immense that although there are pragmatic solutions that can help, given the pluralism of our times and in particular given the perversion of death today, I do not believe there are any particular laws that are enacted that will solve the issues satisfactorily. However, some laws may be more helpful than others.

Finally, my point is that the law is one of the ways in which society has a conversation with itself. To be good the law must be based on common fundamental convictions of what it means to die a "good" death. We do not have that, and so I fear that a set of criteria for brain death may become a symbol to be substituted for thinking and moral evaluation. And this may leave us morally deficient.

VEATCH: I would like to press you a bit more. I have recently had several encounters with people who are also questioning deeply the effort to redefine death. It has been suggested that this is a short cut or an easy way of solving the much more difficult question of the ethics of allowing patients to die. It is implied that if the patient can be simply defined as dead, the difficult ethical question of allowing the patient to die disappears. But it seems to me that this just does not work. In 99 of 100 cases where the question of allowing a patient to die arises, there is no conceivable possibility that the redefinition of death will solve the problem.

HAUERWAS: That is a very important point, and I do not wish to take that line entirely. A definition of death has the danger of being used in that manner; that is, as a way of telling you when it is no longer worthwhile to keep someone alive, but when it is all right to let someone die or to let themselves die.

Therefore it is very important to be very clear about what kind of patient we are talking about and under what circumstances such criteria should be applied. And that is because criteria often start to take on a life of their own in a manner in which they are no longer criteria but become policy. Let me give you an example.

I have a friend who was part of a covenanted Calvinist community in Grand Rapids. There are some Calvinists there who live in community, pray together, raise their families together, and who are very committed. They tend to be pacifists, and one of them was an aspiring young architect, and one of them was a doctor. The architect got cancer of the spine and was going to die relatively quickly.

He was in the hospital where he was offered all kinds of chemotherapy and radiotherapy. When his friend, the doctor, came in the patient said, "I've been talking to all these people and they say they can do all these things and give me a little more time." His friend said, "John, you are a Christian—they say they can do all that and give you six months, but you are dying. Why do you want to do all that? Why don't you just go on and get your affairs in order and die?" And so the architect did, and died in two weeks.

The wrong application of the criteria of brain death in this situation could lead to the statement, "Well, you are not dead yet, John. Your brain is still functioning, and you have got to live it out all the way somehow or other."

Now this is clearly a perversion of the use of "brain death." And we must be aware of this perversion, especially when one lives in a community where there is no sense of the perception of death; this perversion manifests itself when death is considered an overriding evil.

I wish to emphasize another point similar to that made by Dr. Veatch: There is no necessary connection between the conception of death and determination of the loci or criteria of death. The only thing that connects these factors is the practice of communities. Doctors are part of those communities; they may help the community to come to some understanding of itself through talking about how their criteria for brain death function in their practice. It becomes very important for these criteria to symbolically tie in to what the community thinks life is about in terms of its worthwhileness.

UNIDENTIFIED SPEAKER: I do not want to take the part of Kübler-Ross, but I think there's more than the idea of the hospice and getting the patients' affairs in order and just making him feel happy. . . .

HAUERWAS: Oh, absolutely. I don't mean to disparage Dr. Ross's contribution, but it seems to me to have had some dreadful consequences. For example, the development of a specialty called thanatology is surely something right out of a Vonnegut novel. There is evidence that she is right, that people fear dying. One of these fears is the sense of complete abandonment. Certainly one of the most effective ways of being abandoned is to be left to technology rather than personal presence. It is important that we learn to train ourselves to be around the dying because this is our responsibility. There is something correct in Kübler-Ross's emphasis, although her ideas have been taken up and developed in some extraordinary and bizarre ways.

VEATCH: In the last part of the discussion I sensed that we may not have focused enough on the question of the care of the dying patient. A major theme is that there is a radical difference between the ethics of allowing a patient to die and the decision that the patient is dead. Since those two situation can be clearly separated, we will not primarily address ourselves to some of the very important issues about the ethics of caring for the dying patient. That may be unfortunate in a way, but it seems to me to be the logical outcome of a very important distinction.

COGNITIVE DEATH: DIFFERENTIAL PROBLEMS AND LEGAL OVERTONES

H. Richard Beresford

Department of Neurology
North Shore University Hospital
Manhasset, New York 11030; and the
Cornell University Medical College
New York, New York 10021

THE PROBLEM OF COGNITIVE DEATH

The *Quinlan* case [1] raised the issue of when physicians may lawfully terminate care for severely brain-damaged adults. The question was not whether Karen Quinlan was dead, for the medical testimony clearly indicated that she did not meet existing criteria for brain death. Instead, the question was whether her physicians and family could take steps that the court thought would lead to her death. The New Jersey court made "cognition" the touchstone of decision-making. It formulated a procedure to permit withdrawal of a presumptively life-supporting respirator following a medical determination that cognition was irretrievably lost. The court thus established a legal precedent for terminating care of those adults who, while retaining vegetative neurologic functions, lack the capacity to interact with the external environment. But, although many seem to have applauded the decision, it has some disturbing features which bear mention.

To support its judgment, the court stated some conclusions that had limited evidentiary support. [2] For example, it flatly assumed that Miss Quinlan herself would have wished the respirator removed if only she could have perceived that there was *almost* no hope of recovery.* It concluded that she was suffering, despite extensive medical testimony that she lacked the capacity for conscious emotional experience. It suggested that her attending physicians would willingly turn off the respirator if it weren't for the fear or civil or criminal liability, despite testimony by them that this was not the basis of their reluctance. It concluded that she would not survive withdrawal of the respirator, despite medical testimony that she might survive for an indefinite period after it was removed. It assumed that the capacity of physicians to predict outcome for persons such as Miss Quinlan was well-enough developed to permit the drastic step of withdrawing life-support measures, despite the lack of systematic, statistically validated studies of prognosis in chronic vegetative states.

If this seems to be ungracious quibbling that has lost sight of the "good" the court was trying to achieve, let me move the dialogue to another level. Recall that the court was being asked to appoint Miss Quinlan's father as her guardian for the express purpose of authorizing removal of life support. To

---

* As of this date, Ms. Quinlan's condition has not improved. She has been in a persistent vegetative or noncognitive state for over three years despite the fact that she breathes spontaneously.—*J.K.*

0077–8923/78/0315–0339 $01.75/0 © 1978, NYAS

make this appointment the court had to satisfy itself that Miss Quinlan was disabled from making such a momentous decision on her own, that the father was a proper person to whom to delegate the power of decision, and that the act of removing the respirator would not violate laws punishing homicide.

It was clear that Miss Quinlan was unable to act on her behalf, and there was ample evidence that her father is a devout and moral man who wanted to do what was best for his daughter. But the next step does not come so easily. Intentionally ending the life of another, whether by act or omission, is homicide. The court obliquely conceded this, but concluded that in order to protect Miss Quinlan's constitutional right of privacy her right to refuse medical care could only be exercised by another person. The state's interest in protecting life was not believed compelling in view of the evidence that she was a permanently noncognitive person. Therefore, the reach of the criminal law does not, according to the court, extend to decisions to end the life of the noncognitive. In other words, the noncognitive are like previable human fetuses whom the state cannot protect from abortion.

While much is done in the name of the Constitution that its framers never contemplated, the *Quinlan* decision strikes me as an uncomfortably novel expansion of a constitutional right to refuse intrusions on one's person. Permitting a delegation of one's power to exercise this right to families transmutes a notion of personal autonomy into a socially protected power to hasten or accomplish another's death. Unless there is a social compact that one who has lost cognition forfeits substantial legal protections, including those afforded by the laws against homicide, then I question the notion that the Constitution requires that families of noncognitive adults be given authority to seek withdrawal of life-support measures. Less tortuous approaches seem available if society is now convinced that ending the lives of the noncognitive is a desirable goal.

THE LAW'S RESPONSE

A New Social Compact?

Suppose for the sake of argument that the public now agrees that those without cognition should be allowed to die. If so, whatever is meant by the phrase "death with dignity" may become a generalized reality, and arguably scarce medical resources can be allocated to more deserving purposes.

As of 1947 the great judge, Learned Hand, thought the public was not ready to approve the "mercy-killing" of a blind, deaf, noncognitive child. Thus, in *In re Repouille* [3] he declared:

> We can say no more than that, quite independently of what may be the current moral feeling as to legally administered euthanasia, we feel reasonably secure in holding that only a minority of virtuous persons would deem the practice morally justifiable, while it remains in private hands, even when the provocation is as overwhelming as it was in this instance . . .[4]

Now, thirty years later, the climate may have changed. Advances in technology enable physicians to support the lives of the noncognitive for weeks to months, and sometimes longer. And some apparently believe that physicians abuse the technology of life-support to keep the noncognitive alive against the wishes of their families. Also, if previable fetuses no longer enjoy legal protection, then it may not be a quantum leap to deny such protection to living but noncognitive persons.

Changes in the Physician's Role

A physician is ordinarily responsible for determining the level of a patient's care, subject to the patient's right to refuse care entirely or to refuse a particular form of treatment. If society espouses the principle that physicians now have a duty to terminate life support for the noncognitive on the request of a family, and expresses the principle in the form of a legal imperative, physicians' own value preferences will no longer affect the decision of when to stop care for those who are living but noncognitive.

Some physicians might prefer this role since it places the burden of decision squarely on the family. But other physicians either may not wish to relinquish a decision-making function or may simply recoil from the act of "pulling the plug." Dissenters may, of course, avoid the conflict by withdrawing from a case. Even if this is feasible, however, it may be an unsatisfactory resolution of an already delicate, emotionally charged problem. Since both medical knowledge and value preferences are elements of decisions to reduce care, it seems important to encourage continuing participation by the original attending physician, if for no other reason than to use his or her detailed knowledge of the relevant medical facts.

Competing Values

There is no empirical basis for doubting that physicians share the same range of values as the rest of the society with respect to the care of the severely brain-damaged. The extent to which they express these values may, however, be modified by legal, ethical and peer constraints. Assuming for the moment that a physician had complete autonomy in the care of a severely and hopelessly brain-damaged patient, he or she might elect one of several courses of action. The physician might provide maximal care (including use of respirators, transfusions, feeding tubes), thereby expressing a sense of absolute duty to preserve life. Or, the physician might prescribe modified care (e.g., antibiotics but no respirator), thus indicating a belief that it is humane and practical to reduce but not eliminate care for one whose life hardly seems worth living. Or, the physician might prescribe nothing save custodial care, reflecting a judgment that there is no moral duty to maintain a patient in a vegetative state. Rarely the physician might even actively end the patient's life, convinced that there exists a higher duty to end a futile or worthless existence.

However, it is hardly likely today that physicians believe they possess complete discretion to exercise these options. Assuming that active euthanasia is foreclosed by the strictures of criminal law, the scope of potential physician-family conflict narrows to the issue of whether or not to use life-prolonging treatment. In *Quinlan*, the physicians opted for such treatment, while the family was against it. But one can readily imagine the reverse situation where the physician prefers to withhold treatment while the family seeks maximal treatment. In both situations, it is difficult to see that either protagonist enjoys a clear advantage in the moral argument. I can see no greater wrong in either supporting life or not supporting life in this context. But I do question the merits of a rule of law that would encourage a physician to terminate life-support despite a disinclination which derives from a mixture of value preferences and skepticism about the reliability of predictions of outcome.

If there must be any bias in the law, it ought to be toward preserving life. The attending physician may be right in believing that recovery, while a remote possibility, may nevertheless occur.[5] Also, preserving life, even though expensive and of questionable value, does not seem morally offensive. An optimal legal standard might therefore assure that physicians of living but noncognitive adults retain the primary responsibility for deciding on levels of care, a responsibility that may be shared with families where there is compelling clinical evidence that cognition is permanently lost.

Legislation

General Considerations

Any legislation that expressly allows termination of care for the severely brain-damaged would reflect a social judgment that the lives of the noncognitive do not deserve full legal protection. This judgment might rest on various assumptions. One is that it is morally right to end an inhuman existence. Another is that it is a misallocation of scarce medical resources to support life in those who won't recover. Still another is that it is simply irrational to care for those whose prognosis is hopeless.

Utilizing the legislative process has several advantages. It allows extensive fact-finding with respect to prognosis after brain injury. It permits expressions of competing moral, ethical and economic arguments. It favors consideration of a variety of strategies for handling the delicate problems at hand. If it is successfully played out, it will generate standards or rules that manifest society's views about the care of the noncognitive. If there is no societal consensus about terminating life support for the noncognitive, then either no legislation would be enacted or laws might be passed that explicitly prohibit or discourage reductions in care for the noncognitive. But even if no legislation evolves, the legislative process may serve to educate legislators and the public as to the relevant moral, medical and social policy questions.

Legislative Strategies

Permissive legislation might take several forms. One approach is to declare that it is justifiable homicide to terminate life support for a person who has permanently lost cognition. Those who view "pulling the plug" from persons who are not medically and/or legally dead as something other than a homicidal act might object to such a law, for it implicitly concedes that such conduct is homicide. A less evocative approach might be to declare that no one shall be prosecuted for homicide who terminates life support for a noncognitive person. This makes no concessions about the nature of the act, but nonetheless excuses it.

A way to skirt the homicide issue is to expand the definition of death to include permanent loss of cognition. Such a law, while seemingly straightforward, would nevertheless generate substantial difficulties. What constitutes a permanent loss of cognition would require careful definition. The issue of how to handle the patient who has lost cognition, yet has intact cardiorespiratory function, would have to be faced. And, determining a precise time of death, which often has important legal and social implications, might prove even more taxing than deciding when brain death has occurred.

Legislation might effectively codify the *Quinlan* decision by providing for a determination of prognosis by a committee and, if recovery of cognition is deemed hopeless, a formalized agreement between family and physician to terminate life support. If the statutory procedures were followed, no liability would attach to the various participants in the decision. While potentially cumbersome, this approach might promote extensive dialogue and shared responsibility with respect to a hard decision. Whether it gives too much visibility to the decision-making process or may actually encourage resort to termination of care is open to debate. A variation of this mode is to mandate that family and attending physician obtain a court order to terminate care after the prognosis committee has concluded that recovery of cognition is hopeless and the family and attending physician have concurred about ending life support. Many procedural formalities could be included in such a statute.

"Living will" laws might be adapted to allow someone other than a patient to authorize termination of life support. But even if a statute like that recently enacted in California [6] were amended to allow such a delegation of authority, it would not resolve the problem posed by the *Quinlan* case. The current California law requires not only a formal written statement by a person, while competent, that he or she does not want "life sustaining procedures" if a "terminal condition" eventuates, but also evidence that death is imminent but for the life support measures. The evidence in the *Quinlan* case did not clearly establish that death was imminent but for the use of the respirator.

Removing from a "living will" statute the requirement that death occur promptly upon withdrawal of life support would permit discontinuance of respirators for those noncognitive who may survive for an appreciable period thereafter. If this approach is chosen, the statute should explicitly declare that it covers withdrawal of technological support from the noncognitive. This would reflect a legislative recognition of the fact that patients in vegetative states often retain spontaneous respiratory functions.

Nonlegislative Options

Because each of the preceding legislative changes would require an agreement among legislators that the noncognitive person is to be denied certain legal protections, it is highly doubtful that major enactments are about to occur. The difficulties of gaining acceptance of "brain death" laws in some states emphasize this.

If no legislation emerges, physicians and families—unless they reside in New Jersey—will have scant legal guidance for decisions about care of the noncognitive. Every party to such a decision may therefore allow the possibility of civil or criminal liability to affect their judgment about the rightness of withdrawing care. This may have the potentially salutary effect of generating consultations with knowledgeable medical and ethical advisers to establish a sound factual and moral basis for whatever decision is made. But it might also rigidify the conduct of the parties. They might retreat to intractable positions that are more self-protective than cognizant of the interests of the afflicted patient. This would only increase the likelihood of a legal confrontation, and bring the courts more and more into the decision-making process, I, for one, do not believe that this is a desirable role for the judiciary.

Concluding Remarks

The testimony in the *Quinlan* case reminded the public that physicians and families sometimes make value-laden decisions about care of the severely brain-damaged. Since prognosis is the most factual element of such decisions, it is the most amenable to analysis. But even prognosis is only an estimate of future probabilities based on whatever present data are available. If these data are less than conclusive, as is the case when predicting the chance of recovery of some noncognitive persons, prognostication becomes distressingly speculative. Where such imprecision exists, a restrained approach to withdrawing life support seems appropriate. Unless a physician has clearly misinterpreted factual data which compel the conclusion that maximal care is futile, I question whether society should attempt, through the courts or otherwise, to overrule his or her judgment. That the judgment might also involve an assertion of personal values or an anxiety about the reach of the law does not, in my mind, dictate that we diminish the physician's role in determining what level of care to provide.

Protecting the physician's discretionary power to prescribe care may, in the long run, provide the flexibility that is needed for informed and humane decisions about the proper level of care for noncognitive persons.[7] The physician is in the best position to assemble and evaluate, with the aid of his or her consultants, the pertinent medical data. Once the data are fully analyzed, some predictions about outcome may be possible, although the degree of certainty may vary. In some situations, particularly after current studies[8] of outcome in vegetative states are completed, the physician may be able to venture a highly certain prediction of nonrecovery. Given a great degree of certainty about prognosis and a family's clearly articulated desire to reduce care, a *Quinlan*-style disagreement should not occur. Legislation which in some way insulated such private decision-making from legal inquiry might do much to relieve the agonies of the decision-makers about the propriety of their conduct and, if properly drawn, need not bias decisions for or against reductions or withdrawal of care.

Professor Joseph Goldstein of Yale Law School has recently advocated restraining interventions by the state into parental decisions about the care of children whose lives seem not worth living or who have little prospect of growth to a normal adulthood.[9] He would deny the state any role in a life/death decision where there is no proven treatment, or the parents are faced with conflicting medical advice, or there is less than a high probability that treatment will improve the child's prospect for a normal life. In his words:

> . . . Precisely because there is no objectively wrong or right answer, the burden must be on the state to establish *wrong*, not on the parent to establish that what is right for them is necessarily right for others.[9] (p. 655)

His analysis of the *Quinlan* case suggests that he would also give families of noncognitive adults a major voice in decisions about care, because families are at least as capable of weighing the value questions as are physicians or judges.

Although he apparently would make this a principle of constitutional law, some of the legislative approaches outlined above have the advantage of both explicitly codifying a societal consensus (assuming it exists) about cognitive death and protecting joint decision-making by physicians and families. Leaving the issue as one of constitutional interpretation would probably promote continuing resort to the courts on a case-by-case basis. This would needlessly encumber already hard decisions.

REFERENCES

1. *In re Quinlan,* 70, N.J.10, 355A. 2d 647 (1976).
2. BERESFORD, H.R. 1977. The Quinlan decision: Problems and legislative alternatives. Ann. Neurol. **2:** 74–81.
3. *In re Repouille,* 165 F. 2d 152 (2d Cir. 1947).
4. *Idem.* at 153.
5. ROSENBERG, G.A., S.F. JOHNSON & R.P. BRENNER. 1977. Recovery of cognition after prolonged vegetative state. Ann. Neurol. **2:** 167–168.
6. California Statutes Annotated, Health and Safety Code, Sec. 7185–7195 (West Cum. Supp. 1976).
7. 1976. Optimum care for hopelessly ill patients: A report of the Clinical Care Committee of the Massachusetts General Hospital. New Eng. J. Med. **295:** 362–364.
8. BATES, D., J. J. CARONNA, N. E. F. CARTLIDGE et al. 1977. A prospective study of non-traumatic coma: Methods and results in 310 patients. Ann. Neurol. **2:** 211–220.
9. GOLDSTEIN, J. 1977. Medical care for the child at risk: On state superventions of parental autonomy. Yale Law J. **86:** 645–670.

DISCUSSION

J. FRAPPIER (*Jefferson City, Missouri*): I supported legislation on brain death following the suggested outlines of Capron and Kass in 1976 and the ABA in 1977. We did not make it with either one of them. We have always taken the position that Blacks' Law is our problem and interferes in relationships between doctors and the patients and families. Would you comment on the legal situation in a state with Blacks' Law in terms of making a diagnosis of brain death?

BERESFORD: Professor Capron is the authority on this. There are a number of states in which physicians have made the decision. Remember, the subject I have discussed is different from brain death. I am evaluating the next generation of problems, which involve cognitive death, so anything I say related to your question does not pertain to the issue of cognitive death but to brain death. In fact, in some states physicians have withdrawn medical care in patients in whom they deem it appropriate on medical grounds. The criteria used are related to absence of brain function and brain death. This occurs despite the lack of protection of a statutory "umbrella." This happens in New York as well as in other places, I am sure. I know of no murder prosecutions against physicians. The issue of murder has come up indirectly when a person is being

346 Annals New York Academy of Sciences

charged with the murder of the brain-dead individual. The defense has interposed that it was the physician who removed the respirator and by removing the life-support system was the actual killer. The courts have thrown out that notion as well. In practice physicians are using brain-related criteria in determinations of death, even where there are not umbrella statutes. Of course, I do not know how often they are doing this. There have been some civil suits in one form or another, all of which have been unsuccessful so far, I believe.

GRENVIK: For two and a half years at the Presbyterian University Hospital in Pittsburgh we have used a program similar to the one outlined in your presentation. In our intensive care unit, we have 900 admissions per year and about 8 or 9 percent of those patients are finally categorized as so-called "no extraordinary measures" patients. We have an agreement in all of these cases with the next of kin and the family, but we do not have formalized papers that they sign. Two things are done in each case: a progress note is entered into the medical record, indicating that discussion has taken place with the family and that agreement has been reached, and an order is written in the order sheet. Do you see any legal problem with this procedure?

BERESFORD: Are you referring to brain-dead or to noncognitive patients?

GRENVIK: I am not referring to the brain-dead patients. I mentioned the term "no extraordinary measures," which refers to the nonaware patients, the hopeless cases, not the brain-dead ones.

BERESFORD: A potential problem exists, but you have to remember that the way any legal action comes about is that the District Attorney in the jurisdiction has to decide whether this was a case that he thought merited prosecution, as a homicide or as manslaughter. This is one advantage of allowing people in responsible positions to have some discretion. However, some of those acts may technically be homicide, although one can introduce the element of moral culpability as a necessary foundation for a homicidal charge.

GRENVIK: We are aware of that risk. The question is: Do you deem it necessary to have a consent form for them to sign?

BERESFORD: I am a nonbeliever in forms as a general rule.

A. VAN TILL (*The Hague, The Netherlands*): I have one remark to make and two questions to ask concerning a proposition for legislation. If an individual with irreversible loss of cognition were declared dead, which could be possible, then one of the questions that can be asked is: why should the respirator be shut off? The irreversibly comatose person who has been labelled dead could be used for teaching, experiments, or organ transplantation. Such practices are not unthinkable. Therefore, legislators should be aware of this possibility and seek to eliminate it.

My first question is: what are the chances that the New Jersey Supreme Court decision in the Quinlan case will be accepted as legal procedure in other states? Second, how far does the legal basis go in the United States for parents or legal representatives to have or be given rights by a court to decide about life and death of their children? Could children possibly be given rights to decide about life and death of their parents in reverse situations?

BERESFORD: These are difficult questions to answer. In response to the question about the right of parents to refuse life-saving care for their children, there is a "mixed bag" of cases, which are usually related to transfusions for the children of Jehovah's Witnesses, a religious group in this country that rejects the use of blood. The courts have gone both ways in this, so the situation is a jumble. As far as children being surrogate decision-makers for parents, the issues are the same as in the Quinlan case, where there was an adult patient and an adult parent.

I think it is highly doubtful that the Quinlan case will become the law of the land. My criticisms of the Quinlan decision are relatively mild compared to the criticisms of some who believe the decision to be an artistic legal product. I believe that many people are intuitively happy with the decision. It is really a social policy question, and I could not begin to predict what gravitational effect this sort of decision will have in other states.

CAPRON: I think that the cases involving the refusal by parents of transfusion for their children on religious grounds have gone pretty much one way; that is, that parents do not have that authority. As for people who are allegedly incompetent choosing for themselves, the case lore is a complete muddle. Concerning parental decision-making, the courts have gone so far as to say if a Jehovah's Witness is pregnant and is at risk of hemorrhaging etc., during the birth process, and refuses permission to have transfusion, the doctors have to decide whether a transfusion is necessary to save the child's life. The only time a physician can overrule the parent's decision in this case is during the birth process. This is an indication that, as the court said in one famous decision, parents have the right to any beliefs they want, but they cannot make martyrs of their children for those beliefs.

BOSHES: I am particularly appreciative of Dr. Beresford's statements. For those of you who have not read it, I recommend your reviewing his commentary written some months ago in the *Annals of Neurology*. It is a careful and very scholarly analysis of the Quinlan decision, in which he points out the inherent danger of this decision.

Universal application of the results of the Quinlan decision could result in great abuse. One could go through hospitals for the mentally defective or through "coma wards" where there are patients who have been lying in a state of coma for up to 18 years. Many of these patients are in a noncognitive and nonsapient state.

None of these patients could meet Professor Joseph Fletcher's criteria of humanhood. All of these people could be "disposed of" by not feeding or not treating them, if we are to open up this Pandora's box. The question remains: Are we going to be pragmatists or are we still going to remain moral physicians?

S. VERNON: I praise Dr. Beresford for placing the burden of responsibility and decision-making on families, but I would have been even more gratified if I could have heard some plea for making a physician, no matter how competent or moral he may be, less vulnerable. Could this be done by having anyone who wants to attack him (by means of) law suits do so by the placement of a fee with a clerk of the court.

BERESFORD: I do not know if that covers the whole question of professional liability. This is one area I won't try to take on.

KEENE: How comfortable would you feel about a judicial or medical decision to remove life-support systems in a case in which a patient gave ample evidence beforehand that he desired removal of life-support systems if he should enter into a permanent noncognitive state?

BERESFORD: I would be more comfortable; and I think the Quinlan court would have been more comfortable. The query relates to the medical prognosis. The medical standard of brain death as developed by scientific investigators demands that we not make any mistakes at all. We have to be 100 percent certain. We do not want to declare somebody dead who might recover. So the same rigid scientific criteria seemed necessary to withdraw care from patients in noncognitive states, such as Karen Quinlan. The fact that the patient has said that he wants to have care withdrawn if this state of brain dysfunction eventuates would make decision-making much easier if one gets around the prognosis issue. But how good is our prognosis when it deals with noncognition as opposed to brain death? At this stage we are becoming more accurate. As more data are being produced, the prognosis in these situations is becoming more reliable. However there are few grounds for the physicians interposing himself against a rush to establish the right to die, etc.

NESBAKKEN: I enjoyed your presentation, Dr. Beresford, but I object to its title—Cognitive Death. Could you please find another word to use instead of *death,* just in this context? Death is one definite thing based on the total destruction of the brain. Cognitive death may cause difficulty in understanding the topic, at least among laymen.

BERESFORD: That opens up the philosophic conception. I accept your criticism. It is a reasonable one and it is almost by default that I use the word death because the conceptualization of this is very difficult.

LEGAL DEFINITION OF DEATH

Alexander Morgan Capron

University of Pennsylvania Law School
Philadelphia, Pennsylvania 19104

Current antagonism notwithstanding, substantive conflict between medicine and the law is minor. Basically, good medicine is still good law—that is, actions of a physician that are acceptable among his or her colleagues will seldom be deemed improper by the legal system.[1] There may, however, be times when good law does not seem like good medicine, and indeed when doctors think that the law makes no sense at all.

This can sometimes result from the law's well-known ability to engage in what are called legal fictions. To lawyers there is, for instance, nothing astonishing about the idea that a hospital is a person. This fiction has important consequences. The Fourteenth Amendment, in speaking of due process, says "Nor shall any state deprive any *person* of life, liberty or property without due process of law," rather than saying "Nor shall any state deprive any *corporation*" of due process. But a hospital is nonetheless entitled to due process because, for purposes of the Fourteenth Amendment, it is not merely a corporate entity but a "person," even though physicians may have no tools for determining whether such a "person" is "alive" or "dead." There seems to be an inherent division in analytic outlook between physicians as servants of an empirical science and lawyers as servants of society. For the latter group, if not for the former, saying something *can* make it true, if not wise.

Sometimes the divergence between the positions of law and medicine is great enough to throw into question the wisdom of a legal doctrine that draws conclusions far from those that comport with accepted medical or cultural understanding. Such was the state of the "definition of death" in the late 1960s. On the one hand, surgical procedures had been developed to take "live" organs from "dead" people (including that organ, the heart, long identified in the popular mind with life itself), and generally, medical means were increasingly employed to maintain function in the heart and lungs of patients who were otherwise deeply and irreversibly comatose. In the medical view, patients without any brain functioning (including those from whom organs were removed for transplantation) were "dead."[2] Yet on the other hand, the common law definition of death held that all patients with circulation and respiration—from whatever source—are still alive.[3]

This apparent conflict and the tale of what followed are by now familiar. The story of the litigation questioning the continued appropriateness of the common law definition and legislation updating it has been related before.[4] By 1972 it appeared as though there might be rapid adoption of statutes "defining" death. Indeed, in that year the state of Maryland[5] adopted with minor modifications the law first enacted in 1970 in Kansas,[6] and bills were pending in numerous other jurisdictions. While the Kansas statute was greeted with general approbation for its intent,[7, 8] questions were raised about its wisdom and effectiveness,[9] and Dr. Leon Kass and I undertook to set forth an alternative statute.[10]

This chapter surveys the developments since 1972 with an eye to identifying the points debated at that time on which there no longer seems to be any dis-

0077-8923/78/0315-0349 $01.75/0 © 1978, NYAS

agreement and then scrutinizes some of the issues that persist and others that have come into focus since that time and require resolution.

Areas of Agreement

It seemed in 1972 that there were many points needing to be resolved before one could conclude that a new *legal* definition of death was required or that such a definition should be adopted by legislatures rather than the courts, much less that the definition should take any particular form. Perhaps I am too sanguine, but it seems to me that at least seven of those points of disagreement are no longer seriously in contention.

Whether Medical-Legal Conflict Creates Uncertainty

The first point of agreement is that a conflict exists, at least in the verbal formulation, between the common law view that death is the total cessation of all bodily functions and the medical view that death can occur before heart and lung functioning cease if the total function of the brain is permanently destroyed, since the heart and lungs are dependent upon the brain just as the brain is dependent upon the circulation of oxygenated blood. Even those who oppose statutory change admit that a conflict exists, although some of them take the view that the common law cannot possibly mean what it says.[9] But most of those who initially took that view, such as organized groups of physicians,[11] seem to have backed off from it, and to have concluded that the law is at best uncertain and that a person acting upon any particular view of the law takes a risk of being told that the action was improper, and an even greater risk of facing litigation on the issue.[12]

Whether Such Uncertainty is Undesirable

Second, it seems agreed that conflict and the resulting uncertainty are not good for society in this situation. It is undeniable that sometimes conflict is beneficial to society or, at the very least, that it may be inevitable since it is not worth the trouble to eliminate the uncertainty or the means to eliminate it are unavailable. But uncertainty on the definition of death is not one such area. On the contrary, the cost of uncertainty is extremely great—not only may unnecessary treatment be given, resulting in a waste of financial, human and psychic resources, but also, in the absence of any agreed-upon alternative to the common law, treatment may be discontinued on patients whom society would not want to have treated as dead. Moreover, after the fact the public interest in a just and proper disposition of civil [13-16] and criminal cases [17-22] is seriously undermined by uncertainty about the dividing line between citizens and corpses.

Whether the Choice is for Professionals or the Public

These two points were never, I believe, very seriously disputed. It is more remarkable that agreement seems to have emerged on the third question:

whether the framing of a definition of death should be left to physicians as experts without involving the public. In recent writings, it seems accepted that this is not an area that can be regarded as a professional prerogative inherent in the role assigned by society to physicians.[4] Furthermore, since the framing of a definition calls for choices about the degree of certainty needed, the characteristics that make a being human, and other value questions, the standards need to be informed by medical expertise, but ultimately go beyond it, although the application of the general standards through specific criteria and tests applied to actual patients remains in medical hands. It is appropriate that as a matter of public policy the definition of death be set by society through the agencies of government because of the many consequences that society by tradition and by reason has had turn on the occurrence of death.

Whether to Wait for Judicial Updating

Fourth, the courts themselves have concluded that they are not the preferable agents for resolving the conflict and uncertainty.[13, 23] Judicial decision-making is not public enough, and it operates only when a problem has arisen and usually after the fact; until a clear rule is enunciated by a court of final jurisdiction, there is no prospective rule and the uncertainties facing decision-makers in actual practice persist. The judgments of courts are tied to the facts of the case to be decided, and the rulings may thereby take on characteristics not intended—as is illustrated by the fact that most of the judicial decisions since 1972 have involved transplantation, which might lead one to the undesirable conclusion that a special "definition of death" applies to organ donors but not to other people. As the court declared in *Tucker v. Lower*:[13]

> While it is recognized that none of the cases cited above involved transplants, to employ a different standard in this field would create chaos in other fields of the law and certainly it cannot be successfully argued that there should be one concept of death which applies to one type of litigation while an entirely different standard applies in other areas.

Court cases also tend to dichotomize issues through the adversary process, when in fact a complex question like the definition of death may be characterized by a range of opinions. Moreover, the information before the court is not typically the result of its own independent research (for indeed it does not have any public opinion or technical research capability as a legislative committee has), but is instead dependent upon the quality of the advocates appearing before it.

Nonetheless, the judicial resolution of the handful of American cases that have arisen since 1971 has shown the courts capable of departing from the common law on this subject despite the general rule of stare decisis. (In at least one criminal case, *People v. Flores*,[21] the punishment may have been affected—as it also apparently was in the unreported British case, *Reginia v. Potter*[22]—by the judge's uncertainty whether the victim died because of the defendant's act or the physician's decision.[4]) Those cases still display a central weakness in relying upon judicial updating of the definition of death, for in all of the litigation there is only one reported opinion of the highest court of a state, the Supreme Judicial Court of Massachusetts in the *Golston* murder case,[17] a ruling limited to the criminal-law aspects of death. Only through the reports of appellate opinions is the common law defined and disseminated.

Whether the "Definition" Should be Legislated

A complementary consensus has emerged that legislative action is the appropriate route to a new legal "definition of death." The legislative process permits more active public participation in decision-making and brings a wider range of data into the framing of the standards for determining death. It can guard against premature change in the law while also serving to educate the public about the benefits of change. Furthermore, in providing prospective rules, statutes thenceforth lay to rest public and professional uncertainty, and thereby reduce the likelihood of inappropriate decisions and vexatious litigation. Finally, legislation that arises from "model bills" is characterized by greater uniformity among the states than is true of judicial opinions. (Unfortunately, this additional reason for preferring the legislative route has only been partially realized regarding the "definition" of death.)

Whether a Statute Should Specify Tests and Criteria

At the time of the earlier debates, there was some disagreement about the things a statute should contain and the appropriate level of specificity. The provision adopted in France in April 1968, for example, had included a specific criterion, i.e., death could be declared on the basis of a flat electroencephalogram of ten minutes' duration.[24] The fear that such criteria would be written into law was a major concern of the opponents of statutes.[9] In response there emerged a general agreement that statutes should speak at the level of general physiologic standards for recognizing death, rather than enumerating either the criteria or the specific tests for implementing those criteria that physicians would employ to determine whether the standards have been met. At the opposite end of the continuum between specificity and generality, it seems also to be agreed that statutes ought not to speak in terms of the abstract concept of death.[4]

All the statutes in the eighteen American states that had adopted legislative definitions, as well as those that have been suggested by the commentators, follow these precepts. None contains verbiage about the basic concepts, such as the "irreversible loss of personhood" or "the departure of the animating principle." Rather, all are written at the level of a general standard such as "irreversible cessation of spontaneous respiratory and circulatory functions" and/or "irreversible loss of spontaneous brain functions." None goes on to specify operational criteria, such as deep coma or the absence of reflexes or spontaneous muscular movements, or further to enumerate tests and procedures, such as checking for pulse, blood pressure, electrical current in the brain or blood flow to the brain.

Whether the "Definition" Should be Uniform

In defending our proposal, Dr. Kass and I argued that uniformity was a desirable attribute for a statute, that is, that the statute ought to make clear that there is one phenomenon of concern—human death—which is the same in all people, although it may manifest itself in different ways depending on medical circumstances.[10] We wished particularly to overcome the popular impression that since the "brain death" standard was used with transplant donors it applied to people who were somehow "less dead" than people judged by the heart-lung standard, a misunderstanding that the Kansas statute had only made worse by setting forth two separate and unrelated definitions.[6] This point has not drawn any real dissent, so far as I know, and the medical evidence that has been developed in the past five years lends, as you know, overwhelming support to the underlying scientific premise.[25-28] The breakdown in integrated operation of the crucial trisystemic (heart-lungs-brain) functioning is equivalent whether measured by a proper diagnosis of irreversible cessation of heart and lung functions or, in medically supported comatose patients, irreversible loss of total brain function.

Another aspect of the uniformity that we sought—that there should be only one definition of death for all legal purposes—was disputed by Professor Roger Dworkin in 1973.[29] Dworkin, employing a traditional legal method, suggested that the law might want different definitions for different purposes. The plainest refutation of Professor Dworkin's position lies in the fact that no alternative definitions have been suggested as necessary by anyone, himself included. "Rather than asking the purpose for which we are defining death, we must ask what use the law should make of a 'definition of death' which has been framed not as a legal fiction, but as a reflection of social and biological reality." [30] The resounding silence with which the purpose-based argument has been received leads me to conclude that there is a consensus on the desirability of a single definition of death uniformly applicable to all.

REMAINING AREAS OF DISAGREEMENT

The remaining problems on which agreement has yet to occur are of three different sorts. First are some points on which the disputants seem simply to be misunderstanding one another, second are disagreements of form, and third are at least two disagreements of substance presenting major issues for society to resolve in "defining" death.

Misunderstandings

The first misunderstanding is that which persists between organized medicine and the proponents of statutory definitions. Despite urgings by many physicians, the American Medical Association has on several occasions gone on record as opposing any legislation on death.[31] There seem to be two points of concern to the AMA. First is the impression that a statutory definition represents the intrusion of the law into an area that should be left to the sole discretion of physicians. Whatever the merits of that position, it misperceives the current state of the law, for the absence of a statute does not mean the absence of law— and indeed physicians who have come to understand this point, perhaps through litigation occurring in their state, become very unhappy with the current common law rule. Second, as the Judicial Council of the AMA has stated, a statute is seen as leading to "confusion instead of clarification as advances in scientific capabilities occur." [32] Again, this is a misunderstanding of the effect of the statutes that have been proposed. By avoiding any statement on the criteria or tests to be employed, the statutes are not at risk of being outdated by advances in scientific capabilities.

Another misunderstanding underlies the opposition of certain "right to life" organizations. It is their perception that a neurologically-based definition of death is the same as euthanasia because treatment is ceased on a living body. The belief that a statutory definition would address the question "when should a person be allowed to die?" rather than "when is a person dead?" is understandable since the Kansas statute predicates action based on attempts at resuscitation being "hopeless,"[6] a term that often appears in discussions of passive euthanasia. A properly drafted statute need not give rise to such concern, however. If, as the scientific evidence establishes, the phenomenon called "brain death" is really no different than that of "heart and lung death," then the concern over euthanasia melts away, for it can never be euthanasia to cease treatment of a dead body.[33]

Disagreements Over Form

The central disagreement about the form of expression a statute should follow is whether the statute should only explicitly mention a neurologic standard. The Capron-Kass proposal—now adopted in five states[34-38]—says a person is dead when there is an irreversible cessation of spontaneous respiratory and circulatory functions or, in the event that artificial means of support preclude a determination that these functions have ceased, if there has been an irreversible cessation of brain functions, while the proposal put forward by the American Bar Association in 1975[39]—following the 1974 California law[40] and since adopted in five more states[41-45]—speaks solely in terms of the irreversible cessation of brain functioning. In exploring alternative formulations, Dr. Kass and I considered the possibility of a statute that spoke solely in neurologic terms, but we rejected that alternative for a number of reasons.[10] First, reliance only on brain activity would mean a sharp break with tradition, which is not only unfortunate in violating a generally agreed-upon goal of incremental change in this sensitive field but which also creates practical difficulties since most physicians customarily use cardiopulmonary tests for death and will for the forseeable future continue to do so in the vast majority of cases.[46] A single-standard statute would make physicians either go through a charade of using brain criteria and tests in every case or engage in the theoretical work, which the legislature itself should recognize, by equating the irreversible absence of cardiopulmonary functions, which physicians actually measure, with a presumed loss of brain function, which the statute requires. Recognizing these difficulties, the governments of California,[40] Georgia[41] and Idaho[42] in adopting ABA-type statutes additionally provided that physicians are not prohibited from using other customary and usual procedures as the exclusive basis for pronouncing a person dead. Regrettably, these statutes thereby repeat a central fault of the Kansas statute and create unnecessary confusion about whether there are different kinds of deaths. Accordingly, I would conclude, perhaps too immodestly, that a statute of the type suggested by Dr. Kass and myself (which by its terms relates the two standards of death, explains when each is to be employed, and thereby implies that they are two different means of measuring the same single phenomenon) is preferable to the ABA statute, which—though on its face speaking of a single phenomenon—by ignoring the traditional cardiopulmonary standard creates potential misunderstanding and abuse or invites legislative amendment.

There is a second and perhaps more minor disagreement about the form of expression. The Capron-Kass statute speaks of "an irreversible cessation of *spontaneous* brain functions" (emphasis added). This has led the noted Dutch medicolegal expert Dr. Adrienne van Till to suggest that brain functioning is not "spontaneous" when supported by heart- or lung-assisting devices.[46] It does not seem to me that the phrase "spontaneous brain functions" ought so to be read. Clearly, brain functioning is always dependent upon a source of oxygenated blood and the determination of spontaneity refers solely to the organ system itself. The underlying problem to which Dr. van Till's objection points is that there is at the moment no such thing as *nonspontaneous* brain functions, as there are nonspontaneous respiratory and circulatory functions when mechanical or other medical means are employed to replace those occurring naturally. Perhaps, then, the word spontaneous could well be dropped as a modifier of brain functions. (To keep it is merely to look forward to the day when it may be possible mechanically to replace the human brain and the question will then arise whether the result of such replacement is a living human being or not. That is one bridge we certainly need not cross until we are much further down the road toward it.)

Disagreements Over Substance

The major substantive disagreement remaining is between those who would look to the cessation of total brain functioning and those who urge that we take the opportunity presented by the need for a new definition to move the concept of death from its present state to a recognition that a person "without the capacities which are thought to reside in the higher brain (cerebral) centers should really be considered dead." [47] (It is important to distinguish this use of "cerebral death," meaning solely the higher brain centers concerned with consciousness and thought, from its use by some physicians to mean "total destruction of the brain so that both volitional and reflex evidences of responsivity are absent." [25]) Robert Veatch, a leading proponent of the concept of cerebral * death rather than whole brain death,[48] acknowledges that only a few people may turn out to be dead according to a cerebral concept but alive by a whole-brain definition and that the risk of empirical error may be greater with a cerebral definition. But he argues that these reasons are not sufficient to stand in the way of recognizing that a person with the loss of the capabilities dependent upon the higher brain, a person without the ability to interact meaningfully with other people, is no longer truly a human being.

Although patients in that category undeniably present a terrible dilemma for those around them and many people would say that such people "aren't really alive" when only the vegetative functions remain, the persistence of those functions graphically underlines the division between such a higher brain and a whole-brain "definition of death." Under the latter concept, termination of mechanical means of support following a declaration of death will lead very promptly to spontaneous cessation of the remaining artefacts of respiration and circulation. Yet the patient without cognitive functioning may—as the case of Karen Quinlan reminds us—continue to live long after the mechanical supports are withdrawn. Clearly, the removal of other, less extraordinary forms of medical assistance (such as antibiotics), or the cessation of all interventions (including food), would in time lead to the collapse of a patient such as Miss Quinlan.

---

* Also called "cognitive" death or persistent vegetative state in this context.—*J.K.*

But the time period between the withdrawal of antibiotics or intravenous feeding or the like and cessation of all major organ functions would likely be measured in hours or even days rather than in seconds or minutes. During that period the prospect of a "dead" body breathing on its own with a beating heart maintaining warm flesh and residual reflexes and spontaneous muscular movements is so far from our present biological and cultural norms of "death" as to be basically unacceptable. Clearly such patients present a question that must be answered— the question of when treatment should cease and the patient should be allowed to die. But even in the expert hands of Dr. Veatch the case for defining such patients as dead is not a convincing one, and so far as I know no legislation along this line has been introduced or acted upon in any state. Indeed, many of the statutes that have been adopted emphasize the contrary point by including the word "total" to modify "brain functions" [36, 40] (a word that is absent from our 1972 proposal, although it was explicit in our commentary and ought probably be added to the language of the statute †).

Moreover, the proponents of cerebral death must be prepared to explain why the line that they have drawn at a particular level of functioning of a particular part of the brain is the most defensible line when, given the opportunity to draft an entirely new definition, others might feel that a higher standard of functioning ought to be required before a person is considered a "living human being," a level of functioning that mentally retarded or senile people (or those who did not graduate from Harvard Medical School or what have you) may not meet.

Finally, Dr. Veatch has made another suggestion that may spawn further disagreement. As part of his suggested redefinition of death as the cessation of cerebral function, he wants to anticipate the objection of those who find such a standard unacceptable by including a "conscience clause" in the statute, permitting a patient or his or her legal guardian to preclude application of the cerebral definition. Veatch states that "individual freedom" must be limited to "the reasonable choices of a concept of death," [47] although he does not explain why this should be. Unfortunately, his proposed statute does not incorporate any such "reasonable choice" alternatives that a person could be permitted to insist upon having used in the place of the cerebral definition, which could lead to contrary results: (1) physicians acting upon such a rejection of the cerebral definition might insist that the only alternative explicitly provided in the statute is total cessation of spontaneous respiratory and circulatory functions (and hence, a comatose patient with "whole-brain death" could not be declared dead and removed from the respirator); or (2) the patient or guardian might exercise the statutory right to reject the "cerebral death" standard and instead take the view that death occurs at some point *prior* to the loss of all cerebral functions (and hence insist that steps be taken to bring about the cessation of other functions, including the cerebral function, which inconveniently have not yet disappeared from this "dead" body).

---

† The proposed model statute could be clarified in this and other regards to read: "A person will be considered dead if in the announced opinion of a physician [licensed to practice in this state], based on ordinary standards of medical practice, he has experienced an irreversible cessation of spontaneous respiratory and circulatory functions, or in the event that artificial means of support preclude a determination that these functions have ceased, he has experienced an irreversible cessation of total brain functions. Death will have occurred at the time when the relevant functions ceased."

In the enactment of statutes, none (save perhaps the recent North Carolina act [49]) incorporates anything like Dr. Veatch's conscience clause. This is all to the good in my opinion. There is certainly a place for conscience clauses in legislation authorizing treatment termination—indeed the purpose of such laws is to assure that a patient's wishes about the extent of medical treatment to which he or she is subjected will be preserved in some fashion after the patient is unable to exercise choice directly. (The appearance of something like a conscience clause in the North Carolina statute is probably explained by the fact that it combines in one statute provisions on termination of treatment and definition of death.) But the problem with a conscience clause in a "definition of death" act is that it contradicts the entire notion lying behind such statutes, which is that society has a basic interest in defining for all people a uniform basis on which to decide who is alive—and consequently subject to all the protections and benefits of the law—and who is dead. The public's interest is great enough to override individual scruples, even when based in religious beliefs, just as statutes authorize autopsies without familial consent in cases of concern to the public.

The mischief that would be worked by a conscience clause of the sort recommended by Dr. Veatch is probably not great because the underlying statute includes provisions on traditional cardiopulmonary death, which would protect against any very idiosyncratic definition on at least one end of the spectrum. But any notion that a statute should do nothing more than establish the minimum point at which death can first be said to have occurred, leaving each individual free to demand for himself or his relatives a later point, is sure to work great harm. Are we to say that a man who shoots his wife has not murdered her because he insists that the standard of death that she (or he) wishes to apply— perhaps for peculiar religious reasons—is that a body is not dead until a year and two days after respiration ceases?—thereby defeating the common law rule of a year-and-a-day for measuring the connection between a defendant's act and his victim's demise. And must the wife's retirement fund continue to send her benefit checks during this period, if her entitlement to them ends with her death?

CONCLUSION

I am tempted, then, to conclude that even these remaining points of disagreement, which have not been fully hammered out and publicly resolved, do not divide the main body of informed opinion on the subject. If the differences of form are also soluble—and I think they are—it would appear that the remaining difficulties in the completion of the movement toward defining death by statute are political ones, on which I as a mere academic have little to say. If the apathy of the general public (until it is aroused by a newsworthy case) and the last vestiges of medical misunderstanding and distrust can be removed, I see no substantial technical or policy impediments to satisfactory definition of death laws along the lines of the model bill.

REFERENCES

1. But see *Helling* v. *Carey,* 83 Wash.2d 514, 519 P.2d 981 (1974).
2. AD HOC COMMITTEE OF THE HARVARD MEDICAL SCHOOL TO EXAMINE THE DEFINITION OF BRAIN DEATH. 1968. A definition of irreversible coma. JAMA **206**(6): 337–340.

3. 1968. Black's Law Dictionary. 4th ed. : 488. West Publishing Co. St. Paul, Minn.

4. VEITH, F. J., J. M. FEIN, M. D. TENDLER, R. M. VEATCH, M. A. KLEIMAN & G. KALKINES. 1977. Brain death: II. A status report of legal considerations. JAMA 238(16): 1744–1748.

5. Md. Code Ann., Art. 43, § 54F (Cum. Supp. 1976).

6. Kan. Stat. Ann. § 77-202 (Supp. 1974).

7. CURRAN, W. J. 1971. Legal and medical death—Kansas takes the first step. New Engl. J. Med. 284(5): 260–261.

8. MILLS, D. H. 1971. The Kansas death statute: Bold and innovative. New Engl. J. Med. 285(17): 968–969.

9. KENNEDY, J. M. 1971. The Kansas statute on death—An appraisal. New Engl. J. Med. 285(17): 946–950.

10. CAPRON, A. M. & L. R. KASS. 1972. A statutory definition of the standards for determining human death: An appraisal and a proposal. Univ. Pa. Law Rev. 121(1): 87–118.

11. NATIONAL CONFERENCE OF COMMISSIONERS ON UNIFORM STATE LAWS. 1976. Handbook and Proceedings of the Annual Conference. National Conference, Headquarters Office. Chicago, Illinois.

12. 1972. Drug Research Report 15(123): 1–5.

13. *Tucker* v. *Lower,* No. 2831 (Richmond, Va., L. & Eq. Ct., 1972).

14. *United Trust Co.* v. *Pyke,* 427 P.2d 67 (Kansas 1967).

15. *In re Estate of Schmidt,* 261 Cal. App.2d 262, 67 Cal. Rptr. 847 (1968).

16. *In re Karen Miller,* a minor, J. V. Docket No. 19049 (Delaware Co., Pa., Ct. Common Pleas, 1977).

17. *Commonwealth* v. *Golston,* 366 N.E.2d 744 (Mass. 1977).

18. *State* v. *Brown,* 8 Ore. App. 72 (1971).

19. *People* v. *Saldana,* 47 Cal. App. 3d 954, 121 Cal. Rptr. 243 (1975).

20. *People* v. *Lyons,* 15 Crim. L. Pptr. 2240 (Alameda County, Cal. Super. 1974).

21. *People* v. *Flores,* No. 7246-C (Sonoma County, Cal., Super. Ct., 1974).

22. *Regina* v. *Porter* (unreported British case). 1963. Med.-Leg. J. **31:** 195.

23. *New York City Health & Hospitals Corp.* v. *Sulsona,* 81 Misc.2d 1002 (Sup. Ct. 1975).

24. MEYERS, D. W. 1970. The Human Body and the Law. : 113–114. Aldine Publishing Co. Chicago, Ill.

25. An appraisal of the criteria of cerebral death: A summary statement. 1977. JAMA. 237(10): 982–986.

26. VEITH, F. J., J. M. FEIN, M. D. TENDLER, R. M. VEATCH, M. A. KLEIMAN & G. KALKINES. 1977. Brain death: I. A status report of medical and ethical considerations. JAMA 238(15): 1651–1655.

27. KOREIN, J., P. BRAUNSTEIN, A. GEORGE, M. WICHTER, I. KRICHEFF, A. LIEBERMAN & J. PEARSON. 1977. Brain death: I. Angiographic correlation with the radioisotopic bolus technique for evaluation of critical deficit of cerebral blood flow. Ann. Neurol. 2(3): 195–205.

28. PEARSON, J., J. KOREIN, J. H. HARRIS, M. WICHTER & P. BRAUNSTEIN. 1977. Brain death: II. Neuropathological correlation with the radioisotopic bolus technique for evaluation of critical deficit of cerebral blood flow. Ann. Neurol. 2(3): 206–210.

29. DWORKIN, R. B. 1973. Death in context. Indiana Law J. 48(4): 623–639.

30. CAPRON, A. M. 1973. The purpose of death: A reply to Professor Dworkin. Indiana Law J. 48(4): 640–646.

31. Definition of death. 1974. JAMA 227(6): 728.

32. 1977. Opinions and Reports of the Judicial Council, § 515. : 23. American Medical Association. Chicago, Ill.

33. RAMSEY, P. 1970. The Patient as Person: Explorations in Medical Ethics. : 101–112. Yale University Press. New Haven, Conn.

34. Alaska Stat. § 09.65.120 (Supp. 1977).

35. Iowa Code Ann. ch. 1, § 208 (Spec. Pamphlet, Crim. Laws 1977).
36. La. Rev. Stat. Ann. § 9:111 (West Cum. Supp. 1977).
37. Mich. Comp. Laws Ann. § 326.8b (Cum. Supp. 1977).
38. W. Va. Code § 16-19-1(c) (Cum. Supp. 1977).
39. AMERICAN BAR ASSOCIATION. 1978. Annual Report, February 1975 Midyear Meeting. Vol. 100. American Bar Association, Chicago, Ill.
40. Cal. Health & Safety Code § 7180 (West. Ann. Cum. Supp. 1977).
41. Ga. Code Ann. § 88-1715.1 (Cum. Supp. 1977).
42. 1977 Idaho Sess. Laws ch. 130, § 1.
43. Ill. Ann Stat. ch. 3, § 552(b) (Smith-Hurd Cum. Supp. 1977).
44. Mont. Rev. Code Ann. § 69-7201 (Cum. Supp. 1977).
45. Tenn. Code Ann. § 53-459 (1977).
46. VAN TILL-D'AULNIS DE BOUROUILL, H. A. H. 1976. Legal aspects of the definition and diagnosis of death. In Handbook of Clinical Neurology. P. J. Vinken & G. W. Bruyn, Eds. Vol. 24: 787–828. Injuries of the Brain and Skull. Part II. R. Braakman, Collab. Ed. North-Holland Publishing Company. Amsterdam, The Netherlands.
47. VEATCH, R. M. 1976. Death, Dying and the Biological Revolution. : 71–76. Yale University Press. New Haven, Conn.
48. VEATCH, R. M. 1975. The whole-brain-oriented concept of death: An outmoded philosophical formulation. J. Thanatol. 3(1): 13–30.
49. 1977 N.C. Adv. Legis. Serv. ch. 815, § 90–320.

DISCUSSION

LEAFFER: Do you have any specific recommendations on legal guidelines, Mr. Capron, in instances in which there is no living will or no statement of a donor gift for authorization to do research on persons in noncognitive states? This is especially pertinent when there is no next of kin or when a member of the family or legal guardian gives consent for research.

CAPRON: That topic extends far beyond any question that has to be raised on either brain or cognitive death.

Generally the rule about experimentation is that it is undertaken only with the informed voluntary consent of the subject. If you are speaking of persons whose mental deterioration is so great that they cannot be participants in that decision there is very little legal authority for making any use of such subjects.

Clearly there are instances in which therapeutic intent is mixed with an experimental desire on the part of the physician. In that case the so-called "double effect" takes place. The physician, after getting both proper approval from an institutional review committee of the quality of the experiment and its benefit and permission from the guardian of the patient, can proceed to engage in the treatment and derive useful experimental knowledge from that treatment. There is no problem provided that one is confident there is not a terrible conflict of interest and the physician is not deceiving himself in that there is an attempt to help the patient.

In a case in which the patient is going to be used solely for experimental purposes, it would be worthwhile to differentiate between interactive experimentation that may affect the patient's illness and simply collection of baseline data. In the former circumstances, we are concerned with the deterioration of the patient's medical condition and the experimental means to change it. In the latter, we are concerned with observations on the nature of the state. These situations raise some problems, but I think plainly fewer ones than are implicit in an experiment unconnected with a person's condition.

The starkest example of the latter is the case that occurred in 1963 at the Jewish Hospital for Chronic Diseases in New York. At that time mentally confused patients in that hospital who were debilitated and in whom no informed consent was obtained were injected with live cultured cancer cells to see whether the rejection rate of the cells was similar to that of cancer patients. The investigators wanted to determine what caused a difference between the two groups with respect to rejection time for the cancer cells. Of course difficulties of language existed, even in those who could communicate. The doctors involved were severely censured and rightly so. Here is an example of an experiment that is unconnected to the patient's status performed on patients who were incapable of consenting. This illustrates the worst type of experiment.

I do not know whether there are yet any good legal guidelines on the question. If I were legal counsel to a hospital that proposed to do this kind of experiment, I would advise against it. There is no one who can give legal permission to do a completely unrelated study on patients who cannot consent, anymore than such procedures could be carried out on other nonconsenting groups.

A procedure may be established based on the NIH guidelines. How these affect the common law of the states' damage actions has yet to be determined. Just because the federal government allows a certain procedure does not make it clear that the same applies to state law.

Therefore, the issue you pose is an extremely difficult one. It is a little outside the scope of most of what we are talking about here. I cannot do more than to try and define it and break it down the way I have.

LEAFFER: To just get back to the question of therapeutic versus experimental procedures, the National Commission for the Protection of Human Subjects of Biological and Behavioral Research has attempted to do away with this distinction. This is because their definition of research is intended to produce generalizable knowledge and it is not required to directly benefit individuals. It is focused on groups. For example, in cases of Alzheimer's disease, which is different from total brain death, institutional review boards (IRBs) are having trouble in determining whether the research would directly benefit that individual patient since we know so little about this condition. Creating obstacles to ever doing research on this problem would not be advantageous, and yet some guidelines need to be set up. I think these IRBs are in a particularly difficult state when these grant applications come through and they have to make a judgment. A number of the procedures that are used for diagnostic purposes alone involve a high degree of risk ‡ and are just related to collecting data. The funding agency must then determine whether this is ethical or legal before it passes on a grant in which these procedures are used. Although we cannot predict whether the findings are going to directly benefit this individual, they may benefit patients with this disease in years to come.

CAPRON: All the concerns that you raise are very valid. I am reminded, however, of a remark of Professor Hans Jonas of the New School some years age in which he was talking about human experimentation generally. He stated a proposition that I think most people in our society would agree with, which is that progress is an optional goal and that the desire to learn things and to move ahead is not the highest value in our society. There are other values, such as

‡ For example, brain biopsy.—*J.K.*

the protection of individuals from harm by others, that have a much greater standing in our pantheon of values.

That is not to say that I would not try to find means that would both protect those higher values and permit research. I am not arguing for throwing up additional barriers, but I am saying that the law now gives no warrant to an investigator who would take a person merely because he or she was comatose and say, "I have gotten permission from X, Y, or Z, their son, mother, wife, or whoever, to go ahead and do some experiments on this person." I do not think that this permission should be the basis for that kind of authority.

The whole field of what is called, quite inappropriately, proxy consent is a very troubled one. I wish I could shed further illumination on it but I cannot.

R. M. WOOLSEY (*St. Louis University, St. Louis, Mo.*): You referred several times to the law that you have proposed. How exactly is that stated?

CAPRON: I paraphrased it at one point. It says that persons are considered dead when there has been an irreversible cessation of spontaneous cardiorespiratory and circulatory functions or, if artificial maintenance of these functions precludes a determination that they have ceased, when there has been an irreversible cessation of brain functioning.

VAN TILL: I would still prefer the word "spontaneous" to be scratched from your proposal, but otherwise I fully agree with you.

Have lawyers in these trials ever attacked the accuracy or the lack of accuracy and arguments derived from the Harvard criteria for death? I find them markedly inconsistent and therefore open to attack.

Also, I believe that there is a difference between the signs and the condition of brain function. There is a difference between evidence of lack of brain function and indisputable proof of absent brain function. In order to irrefutably prove brain death the physician has to prove the *impossibility* of the existence of brain function. He can do this by demonstrating that one or more requisites for brain function are missing.

Impossibility could be proved, for instance, by proof of total cessation of intracranial blood circulation during a long enough period for all neurons in the brain to be destroyed. This can be done by four-vessel angiography or other methods. Impossibility of brain function can also reliably be proved by something other than cessation of intracranial blood circulation. That is a technical problem for physicians to decide.

I have described these things more elaborately in a contribution to the *Handbook of Clinical Neurology* in 1976, and in an article in the *American Journal of Law and Medicine*. I have made specific suggestions that might be incorporated into a statute or law. Do you think that would be useful or not?

CAPRON: To answer your first question, the lawyers in cases in which there has been a dispute about the application of the so-called Harvard criteria being brain-death criteria or irreversible coma did indeed try to show that those were not reliable enough. However, they did not have the benefit at that time of your very illuminating articles. I do not think that they attacked it on the sophisticated level that you have in suggesting that there is a difference between the *signs* of brain functioning and the *preconditions* of brain functioning. I disagree with you somewhat on the question of whether there is a difference in kind or in degree because in effect the so-called conditions of brain functioning are also merely probabilistic statements. That is, insofar as we know, patients without intracranial blood flow, etc., cannot have a living brain. Cases have occurred that indicate that there is at least some variation in human response to that. With respect to your broader point about whether this is compatible with changes in the law, I believe that certainly these kinds of changes, such as those described by Dr. Korein and his colleagues, indicate that the American physicians are moving toward a standard, a set of criteria, which in practice would be much closer to the ones that you endorse.

The result, I believe, will be highly consistent with the current model statute precisely because by *not* specifying criteria room is left open for development of greater scientific understanding about the most accurate, precise and conclusive way of determining that death has occurred in the brain. So, in response to your last comment, I do not see any need to change the statute. The changes in diagnostic method you recommend would be legally acceptable if they become a part of "standard medical practice" in statutory terms.

EUTHANASIA AND BRAIN DEATH: ETHICAL AND LEGAL CONSIDERATIONS

Dennis J. Horan

Hinshaw, Culbertson, Moelmann, Hoban & Fuller
69 West Washington Street
Chicago, Illinois 60602

I

For many years the problem of defining death was basically one of a simple medical judgment, a diagnosis, made by a physician at the deathbed in a home or in a hospital.[1] The criteria for determining when death occurred were medical criteria easily applied by physicians and seldom, if ever, questioned by the public. There existed no statutory definitions of death, and the common law considered the issue only in relation to the distribution of property or in determining whether a person who had been the victim of an assault died within a year and a day.[2] The common law defined death as a moment when life had ceased, "defined by physicians as a total stoppage of the circulation of the blood and a cessation of the animal and vital functions consequent therein, such as respiration, pulsation, etc."[3] Any more was not necessary, and so no more was undertaken.

Then two advancing areas of medicine converged on the deathbed to create one of our current problems. The first of these was the increasing ability of medicine to resuscitate dying patients and to maintain those patients on sophisticated machinery. The second was the ability of medicine to transplant organs from one person to another. Both of these advances depended upon a myriad of factors too complicated to discuss here, but were related to the tremendous growth in medical technology of recent years.

In response to the problems of resuscitation and the modern use of respirators, several states passed new laws redefining death in two ways.[4] One definition is used when the death occurred in the hospital where resuscitative methods were being used. This definition brought in the relatively recent requirement of "brain death." The other definition of death was applicable when resuscitative means were not involved. This definition continued to reply on the traditional grounds of cessation of heartbeat and respiration.

My concern here is the ethical and legal considerations for society in adopting brain death as a basis for a diagnosis of death. I did not say *the* basis for such a diagnosis since I presume that no one intends but that brain death should be an additional way—albeit, the "sole" way—of determining death in a given case.* That is, where mechanical support is not in use or transplantation is not in issue, we would not have the problem since the diagnosis would be a matter of clinical judgment by the attending physician. Obviously, brain death is also a matter of clinical judgment, but is only too seldom discussed in those terms. We are not per se discussing a statutory definition of death, but rather two other questions: one, a broad philosophical moral, ethical and legal ques-

---

* Almost all the statutes add brain death as a separate but new criterion for determining death.

0077-8923/78/0315-0363 $01.75/0 © 1978, NYAS

tion; and the other, a narrow technical medical problem. These questions are: (1) Is a person who is brain dead really dead? If the answer is yes, then (2) What means of proof is acceptable to society that brain death has occurred?

Many of the parts of this volume are concerned with the second question. Even though I have labeled that a technical medical question, there indeed can be ethical-legal problems associated with that question also, but those problems are not my concern here. My concern is with the first question—is a person who is brain-dead really dead? This is similar to the question we ask when we ask whether brain death may be a statutory criterion for defining death. However, to say we are defining death is really incorrect. What we mean to ask is: What are the criteria on which the medical diagnosis of death may be made. We cannot really define death since it is the absence of life that we can only describe.

II

If the determination of death is a diagnosis made by a physician and a person is dead when his or her brain is dead, then why can't a physician make such a diagnosis and declare the brain-dead person to be dead? Why does he need a statute? In short, what are we doing here? Why are statutes being created to give a physician a "right" (to declare a brain-dead person dead) he presumptively has?

In my opinion, the answer to those questions is twofold: (1) The public and public-policy makers lag behind the physician in understanding these concepts; and (2) some persons, indeed some physicians, have used the concept of brain death in a socially unacceptable way. The first answer means that more and better ways to reach the public and to inform public opinion on these issues must be found, which is, presumably, the purpose of this volume. The second point must be discussed further to illustrate my point.

I do not wish to set up a straw man, but the nature of the legal-ethical problem I am about to discuss can be clearly delineated by an article published in the *Baylor Law Review* entitled "Medical Death." [5] In that article Sheff D. Olinger, M.D., who is the Director of the Department of Neurology and the Director of the Stroke Unit and EEG Department of the Baylor University Medical School in Dallas, took great care in discussing the issue of brain death to make a distinction that is at the heart of the problem as to why some public-policy makers have refused (and rightly so) to accept brain death as an alternative means of defining death. In that paper Dr. Olinger stated:

> I would like to distinguish the term cerebral death from brain death. The brain is composed of several parts, including the medulla, cerebellum, mid-brain, and cerebrum. We are concerned here with the cerebrum. The other portions of the brain may function to produce spontaneous circulation and respiration in the absence of the cerebrum without consciousness or awareness. When all the brain has lost its function, there is no spontaneous respiration, and usually no effective circulation. I would emphasize again that cerebral death and brain death are different things and that the term cerebral death expresses the medical concept which is equated with death of the individual person.[5] (p. 24)

After discussing the Harvard criteria and criticizing them because they are highly technical and incapable of understanding by the layman and, more importantly, because they "do not recognize the cerebral quality of human life, [since] the cerebrum might be totally destroyed without hope of recovery, although circulation and respiration could persist or be supported indefinitely," [5] (p. 25) Dr. Olinger then proceeds to the heart of the matter:

> Having defined medical or scientific death as death of the cerebrum, it must be pointed out that this definition is not usually used in ascertainment of death by physicians.[5] (p. 25)

Dr. Olinger's last statement presents two problems that are important to discuss: (1) Is that definition (death of the cerebrum) not used because there is a lag in the knowledge necessary to make a determination of death based on brain death? Or (2) is it not used because the concept of brain death as cerebral death is not (as I asked previously) really death?

Death of the cerebrum alone has not been accepted as real death in our society.[6] Those who push this definition of death, whether they realize it or not, are asking for a change in the current homicide laws and asking for the introduction of euthanasia, which creates for each of us substantial ethical problems as well.

Although the American Medical Association has not opted for any definition of death, a two-part article recently published in the *Journal of the American Medical Association* has reviewed the concept of brain death and has reported on the current status of these medical and ethical considerations. Throughout this two-part article continued reference is made to brain death as the *complete* destruction of brain function or the irreversible cessation of *all* brain function. The authors review the current ethical positions and conclude that only destruction of the *entire* brain constitutes an acceptable definition of death. Consistently throughout this article such language is used as this: "Patients with irreversible total destruction of the brain fulfill this definition, even if heart action and circulation are artificially maintained." [6] (p. 1654)

The American Bar Association (ABA) in its Resolution, voted and approved by the House of Delegates on February 24, 1975, accepted as a definition of brain death the irreversible cessation of total brain function. However, it is important in considering that definition that the thrust of the entire Resolution be understood. The preamble to that Resolution recites that the concern of the medicine and law committee, which formulated the Resolution after extensive research and investigation, was the necessity to cease all artificial means of life support when someone has died and to maintain the best cellular condition of a donor's organs. The Resolution in full reads as follows:

> WHEREAS, it is to the well being of the public to cease all artificial life supports, respiratory and circulatory, after a human body is dead; and
>
> WHEREAS, it is currently medically established that irreversible cessation of brain function is determinative of death; and
>
> WHEREAS, in the current technology of organ transplants it is vital that the donor's gift be in the best cellular condition,
>
> THEREFORE, be it resolved: that the American Bar Association offers a Current Definition of Death as follows:
>
> For all legal purposes, a human body with irreversible cessation of total brain function, according to usual and customary standards of medical practice, shall be considered dead.

The preamble is important to keep in mind because it limits and explains the applicability of the resolution. The ABA definition is intended for those occasions when artificial means of life support are in use or organ donation is contemplated. Even though the definition includes the words "for all legal purposes," the definition is not intended to supplant a physician's use of clinical judgment when he or she declares a person dead. The intent of the resolution is to aid the physician in the specific area of artificial life supports where clinical judgment, it is said, has become tentative and confused.

Consequently the ABA definition does not mean that a person who has spontaneous respiration and circulation, but who has a brain lesion that makes him comatose, can be declared dead. So too, the hydranencephalic child cannot be declared brain-dead under the ABA test because he probably has a thalamus and upper brain stem. The anencephalic child is another question, but even this child, if it has voluntary respiration or circulation, is not brain-dead under the ABA definition. In any event, anencephaly is incompatible with life and such a child will not normally live more than a few hours.† However, even that child is a person under our law and is protected by the full panoply of legal and constitutional rights.

In addition to the preamble to that Resolution, which is frequently forgotten in discussing the nature of the ABA's position on brain death, the advantages of such a definition, as published in the American Bar Association's report when it accepted this definition, are the following reasons in support of or as "advantages of the definition." It:

1. Permits judicial determination of the *ultimate* fact of death;
2. Permits medical determination of the *evidentiary* fact of death;
3. Avoids religious determination of *any* facts;
4. Avoids *prescribing* the medical criteria;
5. Enhances *changing* medical criteria;
6. Enhances *local* medical practice tests;
7. Covers the *three known tests* (brain, beat and breath deaths);
8. Covers death as a *process* (medical preference);
9. Covers death as a *point in time* (legal preference);
10. Avoids *passive* euthanasia;
11. Avoids *active* euthanasia;
12. Covers current American and European *medical practices*;
13. Covers both *civil* law and *criminal* law;
14. Covers current American *judicial decisions*;
15. Avoids *nonphysical* sciences.

A fair reading of the articles concerning the medical, legal and ethical aspects of brain death which appeared in the October issue of the *Journal of the American Medical Association* clearly indicates support of the American Bar Association Resolution on brain death. The importance of that resolution for our discussion is its explicit rejection of the notion that cerebral or partial brain death are satisfactory definitions. As one author stated: "Thus, destruction of the entire brain, or brain death, and only that is consonant with biblical pronouncements on what constitutes an acceptable definition of death . . ."[6] (p. 1655). The article concluded that total brain death is acceptable as a

---

† A child with anencephaly with no evidence of congitive function is still living, under the total care of the mother, at the age of 17 years and has been observed by Dr. C. Suter.—*J.K.*

definition of death to most Jewish, Roman Catholic and Protestant scholars. I would agree.

So, also, in a recent review of European practices concerning brain death it was said:

> The term "cerebral death" is too ambiguous to be adequate for use in any serious discussion of death because linguistically and medically the term means the death of only the cerebrum and not of the entire brain, even though colloquially it encompasses both senses of the word. The author knows of no proof nor unanimous opinion that the total and irreversible cessation of function of only the cerebrum guarantees or proves total and irreversible cessation of all perceptions. Therefore, proof of the death of the cerebrum does not prove that the person is dead (as person is defined in this article).[7]

This article states that there is no general agreement or proof that all levels and forms of psychic activity are produced exclusively by the cortex.[7] (pp. 8–9) A number of German doctors state that brain-stem activity may be able to produce primitive psychic activity. Consequently only the *total* and irreversible cessation of all brain function guarantees that all perception has totally and irreversibly ceased and that the person is medically and legally dead. This author then defines death as: ". . . [occurring] exclusively if and when brain death occurs, that is, when total and irreversible cessation of all neuronal function in all parts of the brain occurs." [7] (p. 9)

In my opinion, the irreversible cessation of total brain function is an ethically acceptable, as well as adequate legal and medical definition of death. However, death of only the cerebrum is not.

III

What then are the legal and ethical implications of the distinction between cerebral brain death and total brain death? In discussing this question we should first indicate that we are not speaking about when it may be proper to cease treatment in a terminal case, even if that treatment is a Bennett respirator, such as was involved in the Quinlan case. My own position on that issue is that a physician is authorized under the standards of medical practice to discontinue a form of therapy which in his medical judgment is useless. He is not mandated by the law to render useless treatment, nor does the standard of medical care require useless treatment. Under those circumstances, if the treating physicians have determined that continued use of a respirator is useless, then they may decide to discontinue it without fear of civil or criminal liability. By useless is meant that the continued use of the therapy cannot and does not improve the prognosis for recovery. Even if the therapy is necessary to maintain stability, such therapy should not be mandatory where the ultimate prognosis is hopeless. This does not mean that ordinary means of life support, such as food and drink, can be discontinued merely because the ultimate prognosis is hopeless. In addition, we will reserve for some other time the discussion of whether or not the intravenous drip may be discontinued even under those circumstances. My own position is that they may not. By hopeless is meant that the prognosis for life (not meaningful life) is very poor. The fact that someone may or may not return to "sapient or cognitive life" may or may not fulfill the requirement depending upon other medical factors, but in and of itself it does not.[8] The

Supreme Court of West Germany put this idea very succinctly in its recent opinion on the abortion issue: "Where human life exists, human dignity is present to it; it is not decisive that the bearer of this dignity himself be conscious of it and knows personally how to preserve it." [9]

Nor are we discussing the equally difficult legal-ethical question of whether (and, if so, when) orders not to resuscitate may be given. Such orders, in my opinion, should be given only when based on good medical judgment that the ultimate prognosis for recovery is hopeless and when informed consents have been obtained from the patient and/or the patient's family (if the patient cannot consent). The order should be in writing and signed by the attending physician. Some hospitals, as has been recently suggested, may want this done by a committee. Some physicians are willing to give such an order, but balk at writing it in the record. This attitude solves little, but perhaps as an accommodation to this problem the physician's order could be a separate record, such as a sterilization consent form, that does not become a part of the patient's bedside record.

As is typical when discussing these emerging issues concerning death and dying, I have spent considerable time telling you what the issue is not. What then is the issue? The issue in the problem of brain death is that the occurrence of total brain death is an acceptable legal and medical criterion for declaring persons dead. The fact of cerebral death is not an acceptable legal, ethical, medical or moral criterion for declaring persons dead. The acceptance of cerebral death as a criterion for death paves the way for euthanasia, which is morally and legally unacceptable.

IV

Percy Foreman has said that euthanasia is a highfalutin word for murder.[10] Under our law euthanasia is a homicide.[11] Even though the one who commits euthanasia bears no ill will towards his victim and believes his act to be morally justified, he nonetheless acts with malice in the eyes of the law if he is able to comprehend that society prohibits this act regardless of his personal belief. The motive of the perpetrator of euthanasia is rejected as an ameliorative fact in American law. If the facts establish that the killing was done willfully, that is with intent and as a result of premeditation and deliberation, our law calls it murder in the first degree regardless of what the defendant's motive may have been.[12]

Even if the homicide is committed at the request of the decedent it still constitutes a homicide since, as our courts have indicated, murder is no less murder because it is committed at the desire of the victim. "He who kills another upon the other's desire or command is in the judgment of the law as much a murderer as if he had done it merely from his own volition." [13]

All nations consider euthanasia the crime of homicide, although it is frequently indicated that Uruguay may be the one exception.[11] (p. 407) In a number of countries, such as Germany, Norway, and Switzerland, a compassionate motive or homicide on request will operate to reduce the penalty, but the crime remains the same—homicide. Homicide is no less homicide because the victim is aged, senile or near death. The criminal law has as great a respect for the young and hearty as for the aged. The law teaches that mankind has not supported euthanasia. It is considered homicide by all nations and societies.

For the medical profession our discussion of euthanasia has particular importance. Already our society has legalized abortion and has made the killing of the unborn an option between the mother and her physician. It is significant that that decision—to abort—must be a matter of medical judgment as well as the mother's wish. At least it was such in the eyes of the United States Supreme Court, but, as we have all seen, in the majority of cases, if not well in excess of 98 percent of the cases, no medical reasons exist to support the abortion.[15]

From the point of view of the physician who has been trained to preserve life, the legalization of homicide at the request of the actor is of very great significance primarily because the actor would be the physician. To understand euthanasia you must understand that we are focusing not on the conduct of the person dying, but on the conduct of the person who will participate in the act of killing that person either voluntarily or involuntarily. Make no mistake about it, that person would be a physician.

Suicide is not considered a crime and assisting at suicide is a crime in only a small number of jurisdictions.[16] Although euthanasia is frequently equated with assisted suicide,[17] it is really something very different from the point of view of the physician.[16] The legalization of euthanasia is always sought on the basis that the physician would be the one who would assist in the killing. Under current arguments for legalization, it is the physician who is being asked to kill the person involved. In determining whether or not euthanasia should be legalized, society must focus on the act of the physician or the person administering the euthanasia to understand the nature of euthanasia under both our law and our medical-ethical concepts of what euthanasia is. Do we wish to legalize killing? In his famous article [11] Professor Yale Kamisar answered that question "no," arguing from purely nonreligious grounds against mercy-killing legislation that for the good of society there should be no exception to our universal societal expectations that we will not kill nor will be killed. Kamisar regards any breach in that absolute as the beginning of a slippery slope, the danger of which is the creation of "legal machinery initially designed to kill those who are a nuisance to themselves [that] may someday engulf those who are a nuisance to others."

Those who would legalize euthanasia want it to be legalized so that a physician can kill someone who desires euthanasia. This fact should not be glossed over or eliminated from any discussion of this important issue, especially by physicians. The legalization of euthanasia will make death an option or a treatment of choice in some circumstances. Will the ideology of cost containment one day make it mandatory? Before answering these questions we must understand that there is a vital distinction between killing and letting die.‡

All men are ultimately helpless before the face of death. Any thing we say or do at this Conference is not going to alter that fact. We shall all die. The vital distinction is whether we shall die as a result of being allowed to die, or whether we shall die as a result of the actions of ourselves or others.

Where there is no obligation to treat because treatment is not beneficial and is therefore useless, treatment may be ceased and the patient may be allowed to die. Whether or not such a state has been reached by the patient is a medical judgment to be made by the attending physician. Direct intervention to end life is never licit. It is neither legal nor ethical. The use of drugs to alleviate pain and suffering in terminal patients is not only licit, but is a desired medical intervention to avoid unnecessary suffering. The distinction, however, between

‡ For an excellent discussion of this distinction see the article by Louisell [18] in *Death, Dying and Euthanasia.*

the positive act of killing and allowing a patient to die as a result of the natural disease which is killing him is of vital importance and should be understood by all.

The distinction is really no different in the law than in moral or ethical matters. Where there is no duty to act, there is no mandate to act, and the physician and health personnel are excused from acting under those circumstances. The law only requires that a physician or nurse possess and exercise the skill and judgment of an ordinarily well-qualified physician or nurse in the same locale and under similar circumstances. Neither the means nor the ability are required to be extraordinary or heroic. It is not necessary that all available means be used to prolong life to its ultimate. Good medical judgment can be the basis for termination of treatment when that treatment is no longer beneficial to the patient.

So too the patient may reject medical treatment.[16] The cessation of medical treatment because it is useless or the rejection of medical treatment by a competent adult has never been considered to be suicide or assisted suicide, either medically, legally or ethically.[19]

Those who would opt for the legalization of euthanasia are very prone to confuse these necessary ethical and legal distinctions. For example, Joseph Fletcher is fond of saying that the omission of extraordinary or heroic means is just as much a decision to kill as is the positive act of euthanasia.[20] True, the distinction between killing and letting die may be fine "but so are many other lines that men must draw in their fallible perception and limited wisdom." [18] The kinds of distinction and judgment that a physician makes when he determines that heroic means are no longer proper and necessary are the same kinds of distinctions and judgments that he makes daily during the course of his medical practice. The fact that he is making these decisions with regard to a terminal patient should not deter him from making such judgments. There is nothing more mysterious or extraordinary happening in treating a terminal patient than any other type of patient. Obviously this distinction between extraordinary and ordinary means of medical practice is difficult to ascertain and is changing from day to day. In my opinion, a physician is better guided by determining whether or not the treatment will be beneficial to life, rather than in trying to determine whether it is heroic or extraordinary. The importance of the heroic or extraordinary aspect is that consideration of the problem in those terms allows consideration of familial difficulties, such as inability to pay for the proffered treatment.

If cerebral death is not really death, then the use of cerebral death as a criterion for letting die would be legally unjustified. There are few cases to guide us in this area. In the California case of *People* v. *Lyons* [21] the jury had to determine whether the bullet from a defendant's gun caused the death of the victim, or whether the death occurred as a result of the removal of organs from the decreased's body by the physicians. This case was not appealed and consequently there is no opinion of precedential value. However, the trial court used the following instruction to the jury:

> Death is the cessation of life. A person may be pronounced dead if, based on the usual and customary standards of medical practice, it has been determined that the person has suffered an irreversible cessation of brain function . . . and since that the deceased, Samuel Moore, was dead before the removal of his heart there was no issue of fact as to the cause of death.[2]

The trial court relied on the medical testimony of two physicians of the California Medical Transplant Center. I am unable to determine whether or not the words "brain function" as understood by the physicians and the court meant only cerebral function or total brain function. In another *nisi prius* case, *Tucker* v. *Lower*,[22] similar issues were involved and the court instructed the jury on both the traditional definition of death as contained in *Black's Law Dictionary* and as an alternative "the loss of brain function test." The Tucker case was not appealed and consequently no written opinion of precedential value exists.

There is an issue concerning medical judgment that must be faced. If physicians agree that total brain death is equivalent to being really dead, then society will eventually come to that position also. However, the concept of cerebral death is objectionable because traditionally it has not been accepted, either medically, ethically or legally. In addition, it cannot properly be applied to otherwise comatose persons who have spontaneous respiration and circulation, but who are in some stage of deep coma. Ceasing to treat these persons because the treatment is extraordinary does not resolve the question as to whether or not they are alive or dead. I think that no one disagrees that those persons are alive as we understand it. They are neither dead nor brain-dead.

Ethically our understanding of this problem must be based upon our understanding of respect for the person. Each person is a unique entity not only in the eyes of God, but also in the eyes of the United States Constitution and the criminal law of all our states. A dying person is no less a person in the eyes of the law. Ethically he not only continues to be a person of infinite moral worth and humanity, but also he now has a greater claim on us and on our humanity because he is ill and helpless. Even more so, his claim upon the practitioner of the healing arts is raised to a higher level because of his illness. Indeed, some courts have found the relationship between a physician and his patient to be of the highest legal relationship—that of a fiduciary.

Each one of us deserves from each other the respect we all feel is due ourselves. That respect for a person means that we should be treated as an end in ourselves and never as a means towards an end. In addition, as each of us exists in this society we depend upon the covenant that each one of us has with each other, that certain rules of the game—certain unspoken promises we have made to one another—will be followed by all of us. One of those rules or promises is that we will not kill one another.

Such a burden rests even more heavily on the shoulders of the physician, who, in addition to his moral role as an individual in this covenantial society, has elected to heal the sick. He, therefore, has a double duty to respect the individuality of those he is treating and to accord those persons the same degree of respect he would wish for himself were he in a similar circumstance. He must, in short, see persons as an end in themselves and never as a means towards an end. Acting thus he will do no harm.

Arthur Dyck, Saltonstall Professor of Population Ethics at Harvard, has coined a new word to clarify the ethical debate about euthanasia.[23] Those who favor euthanasia in our society, such as Marvin Kohl,[24] use terminology such as beneficent euthanasia. Dyck, in order to distinguish a true death with dignity from mercy killing, uses the term "benemortasia." Confining the definition of mercy killing and euthanasia to mean only the deliberate inducement of a quick painless death, Dyck coins the word benemortasia to signify an ethic that rests on certain presuppositions about human dignity. Those who support mercy killing justify it when it is done out of a sense of kindness to obtain relief of suffering.[24] They wish to uphold the general prohibition against killing and limit its use only to relieve suffering in instances where suffering serves no useful purpose. Dyck argues that the desire and obligation to be merciful or kind does not commit us to a policy of euthanasia and that, indeed, such a policy has widespread effects that are not intended, but are foreseeable. Although there are deep philosophical and religious differences that divide people on this issue, the injunction not to kill and the promise we have made one to the other that we will not kill does not invite that type of division. For doctors that sense of divisiveness between themselves and their patients should be a crucial factor in determining whether or not they would opt for mercy killing as an alternative treatment of choice. In my opinion, that option undermines the relationship between physician and patient and would create a sense of distrust that would undermine not only the patient's rapport with his physician, but the physician's rapport with his professionalism and his profession.

Dyck argues compellingly that the point of the wedge argument is very simple when applied to the euthanasia debate. Killing is generally wrong and should be kept to as narrow a range of exceptions as possible. But beneficent euthanasia or mercy killing applies logically to a wide range of cases depending upon who is making the application and, in particular, depending upon the ideology of cost containment over the ever-escalating health costs that loom in the horizon. There is no way to limit the application of beneficent euthanasia or mercy killing to a narrow range of cases definitely circumscribed and carefully controlled. As in the case of abortion, to open the door and legalize mercy killing in one case is to legalize it in a full range of cases that are never contemplated by the progenitors of the policy. For these reasons even what appears as a small inroad into the creation of this policy, namely, the use of cerebral death as a criterion of death itself, must be opposed. However, if the irreversible cessation of total brain function is really death, as it appears to me and to most observers to be, then such a concept can be supported without creating the dangers of which I have spoken.

REFERENCES

1. CAPRON, A. M. & L. R. KASS. 1972. A statutory definition of the standards for determining human death: An appraisal and a proposal. Univ. Penn. Law Rev. **121:** 87–118.
2. FRILOUX, C. A. 1975. Death: When does it occur?. Baylor Law Rev., **27:** 10–21.
3. Black's Law Dictionary 4th ed. (1959). : 488.
4. Sec. 77-202, Kan. Stat. Anon. (1973); Ch. 19.2, Sec. 32-364, 3:1 Vir. Ann. Code (1974); Ark. 43, Sec. 54 F; Md. Ann Code (1974), Ch 3.7; Ca. Code, Sec. 7180, *et seq.* (1974).
5. OLINGER, S. D. 1975. Medical death. Baylor Law Rev. **1:** 22–26. (The entire issue of this law review is devoted to the issue of euthanasia.)
6. VEITH, F. *et al.* 1977. Brain death. JAMA **238** (15): 1651–1655.
7. VAN TILL, A. 1976. Diagnosis of death in comatose patients under resuscitation treatment: A critical review of the Harvard Report. Am. J. Law & Med. **2:** 1–40. 1976, No. 1, pp. 1–40 at p. 10.
8. HORAN, D. 1976. The Quinlan case. Linacre Quarterly **44**(2): 168–176. (Published also *in* Death, Dying and Euthanasia. 1977. D. Horan & D. Mall, Eds. University Publications of America. Washington, D.C.)
9. GORBY, 1976. West German abortion decision: A contrast to *Roe* v. *Wade*. John Marshall J. Pract. & Proc., **9**(3): 551–684.

10. FOREMAN, P. 1975. The physician's criminal liability for the practise of euthanasia. Baylor Law Rev. **27:** 54–61.
11. KAMISAR, Y. 1977. Some non-religious views against proposed mercy killing legislation. *In* Death, Dying and Euthanasia.[8] : 406–479.
12. *People* v. *Conley,* 49 Cal. Rptr. 815, 822, 411 P.2d 911, 918 (1966).
13. *State* v. *Ehler,* 98 N.J.L. 236, 240, (1922).
14. HORAN, D. 1977. Euthanasia as medical management. *In* Death, Dying and Euthanasia.[8] : 209.
15. Testimony of plaintiff's expert witness in *McCrae* v. *Matthews,* U.S. District Court, Eastern District of New York, No. 76-C-1804 and 76-C-1805.
16. BYRN, 1977. Compulsory life saving treatment for the competent adult. *In* Death, Dying and Euthanasia.[8] : 706–741.
17. LEBACQZ, K. & ENGELHARDT. 1977. Suicide. *In* Death, Dying and Euthanasia.[8] : 669–705.
18. LOUISELL, D. 1977. Euthanasia & biathanasia: On dying & killing. *In* Death, Dying and Euthanasia.[8] : 383–405.
19. GRISEZ, 1977. Suicide and euthanasia. *In* Death, Dying and Euthanasia.[8] : 742–817.
20. FLETCHER, J. 1977. Ethics and euthanasia. *In* Death, Dying and Euthanasia.[8] : 293–304.
21. *People* v. *Lyons* Cal. Sup. Ct., Oakland, Cal., 5-21-74.
22. San Diego Law Rev. 1975. **12**(2): 424–435.
23. DYCK, A. J. 1977. Beneficient euthanasia and benemortasia: Alternative views of mercy. *In* Death, Dying and Euthanasia.[8] : 348–361.
24. KOHL, M., Ed. 1975. Beneficient Euthanasia. Prometheus Books. Buffalo, N.Y.

DISCUSSION

A. VAN TILL: You have mentioned several times the word euthanasia, which, as you said, can be used to camouflage homicide among other things. On the other hand, many people desire to die with dignity when they themselves think the time has come. This raises the demand for voluntary euthanasia to be openly and legally possible. Whether there is legislation to cover the situation depends on the differences in a government's policy.

In order to meet such demands, if required, I think that euthanasia should be redefined to include the words "the benefit of the patient." In the Netherlands, which is my native country, the word euthanasia, by common agreement, is only used if there is omission or cessation of life-preserving treatment, or the performance of a life-terminating act in the interests and based on the wishes of an incurable patient. I believe that the practive of euthanasia should be applied by the attending physician or someone acting directly under his instructions and responsibility. This results inevitably from the fact that the physician is the only one who can decide whether the patient is incurable or not.

CAPRON: Do you care to reply to Dr. Van Till's description of the situation in the Netherlands?

HORAN: I do not know if it needs comment, although I would say that if I were a physician who had been trained to preserve life, I would object if society tried to impose such laws. In these debates, I have often run into problems involving the physician's attitude which I cannot condone. For example, neurosurgeons dealing with newborn who has a myelomeningocele will say to the parent, "I am a technician, I will do what you desire." Another example is the surgeon's refusal to repair an esophageal atresia or duodenal atresia in a mongoloid child.

A physician has a multiplicity of moral and ethical as well as legal problems. He is *not* a technician. He is a person in our society and because society opts for him to be a technician does not mean he has to become one. Indeed, Pellegrino, who is the President of Yale-New Haven Medical Center, recently said that if abortion were a mandated policy under national health insurance, he would refuse to practice medicine. That's a moral commitment to life. The physician's position, make no mistake about it, will be the perpetrator of euthanasia. I say this in a pejorative sense. I do not think the physician desires to be the individual to perform euthanasia. If I were a physician and our society were asking for the acceptance of euthanasia, I would say, "Good, go create yourself a new group of people who wear different clothes, take different oaths and do different things, and let them be the perpetrators of euthanasia. My job is to preserve life. If society wants to kill people, it's not my job. I do not intend to do it. I will not do it. That is not the way I practice medicine."

VAN TILL: I do agree with you that no physician or anyone else should be obliged to apply euthanasia if it's against his conscience or religion. The practice of euthanasia that I refer to only means that one can ask for active euthanasia without being certain of getting it. However, one can obtain active euthanasia for oneself by refusing treatment.

HORAN: This is part of the confusion. One more point: a physician is not only a person in our society who has his own moral and ethical concerns; he is also a member of a profession. He has those professional, moral and ethical concerns and he might, as I would, take the position that he does not want to be a part of a profession that kills life. This is a policy position that physicians are going to have to take in future years as we move on in all these areas of bioethical concerns. Some do not care, which is their prerogative.

S. BACHBACH (*Worcester, Mass.*): As you pointed out, there are situations in which intravenous administration of medication or use of the respirator cannot be discontinued without endangering the patient, regardless of how hopeless his condition is. Currently, medical care is being evaluated by the Peer Service Review Organization, utilization review and government groups. These agencies may cut off payments to hospitals after certain lengths of stay, even in these instances. Do you feel from what you have stated that this is illegal and that hospitals should bring suit to recover for the care that they rendered the patient?

HORAN: I assume the question refers to, for example, the refusal of a third party to reimburse the costs that are attributable to maintaining a patient or a group of patients on a respirator over an extended period of time. I would say they have very little, under the current status of the law, to support that position unless those patients are dead and are being supported because the insurance policy has not run out yet. In the circumstances of the brain-dead patients, the third-party payer might have a legitimate legal and moral complaint because everything has two sides. Maintaining patients on respirators in an ICU at $750 or $900 a day until the policy runs out, even though they are brain-dead, is just as morally wrong as the reverse of the coin, which we have just discussed. As suggested in my paper cost containment is an ideology that will loom even larger in the future, and will impose these decisions upon us by a faceless bureaucracy. Since we have representatives here it's nothing personal.

Cost containment, in my opinion, has a legitimate use, just as when General Motors or Standard Oil tries to contain costs. It also has an ideological use in some areas to attain societal ends without legislation, and without public-policy makers being involved. A good example of this is the Commission on Experimentation's involving human patients but, more appropriately, involving the unborn. These are areas of public policy that have been usurped from the people because our traditional way of addressing ourselves to those matters and policies through the legislature may not be effective. Only the rare lawyer knows when a public instrument comes out in CFR (Code of Federal Regulation) discussion leading to new rule-making. Therefore, it is ludicrous to say that the public has access to making public-policy decisions in that manner.

QUESTION: Could I ask about the problem in using the words "curable" and "terminal?" I am particularly interested in the situation concerning the patient who is in the vegetative state. This patient may be incurable, but is not terminal since he may live 15 years. Could we clarify whether or not withholding treatment such as antibiotics for an infection in such a patient would be legal?

HORAN: One of the problems of the medical profession is that it imposes standards upon itself. There is no malpractice unless the standard that the medical profession has imposed upon itself is breached. That standard has been proven in a myriad of fashions by oral testimony of other experts and by written evidence of maintenance of these standards. If you have created a standard that, in a given case, treatment for that infection is standard care in the community, then it must be done under those circumstances; otherwise you have violated the standards that you yourself created.

My quarrel with the Quinlan case is that the court can create that standard even if it is a standard contrary to prevailing medical practice. That is very wrong. Only trained physicians can determine what the medical standards can be. When one criticizes the lawyers about medical malpractice, remember there is no medical malpractice unless it is proved that, in a given case, there is a factual determination that the physician involved violated accepted standards. These standards are made by doctors, not words. I personally defend doctors and hospitals; I do not sue them.

THE NATURAL DEATH ACT: A WELL-BABY CHECK-UP ON ITS FIRST BIRTHDAY

Barry Keene

Chairman, Assembly Committee on Health
California Legislature
Sacramento, California 95814

The California Natural Death Act, the first "Right to Die" legislation enacted in the United States, will soon celebrate its first birthday. Conceived in the belief that the judiciary does not guarantee a timely and convenient forum to protect the rights of the dying at the time when they are systematically and deliberately stripped of their autonomy, the Act offers a procedure to enable the terminally ill patient to exercise control over decision-making relating to his medical treatment. Although the Act was partially disabled by the imperfections of the "high risk" legislative process and the reluctant acceptance by professionals of this unique stepchild of the law, the Natural Death Act has progressed beyond infancy towards restoring individual dignity and security to the terminally ill.

In 1923, Robert Frost said in one of his poems:

> I met a Californian who would
> talk California—
> A state so blessed,
> He said, in climate, none had
> ever died there
> A natural death.[1]

As of 1976, many Californians were still not dying natural deaths.

The enactment of the California Natural Death Act [2] must be viewed in the context of our changing attitudes on death.

The Act is the product of a generation that demands that death be openly discussed and that is searching for ways to re-humanize the dying process. The Act is also the product of a generation that views with horror the confrontation between modern technology and the human needs of the dying. Empirically, it seems that many terminally ill patients say they view the dying process as more threatening than death itself. Medically, there is questioning of the sterile and complex physical apparatus that has sometimes divorced itself from reference to the underlying human element it is purportedly designed to serve. Legally, there is a desire to give practical application to both traditional and expanding doctrines of informed consent and the right to privacy. Theologically, there are moral judgments that the sanctity of life can be jeopardized by extraordinary efforts to maintain it beyond natural limits. Politically, there is a growing public demand that the terminally ill be allowed to control their own medical destiny.

My commitment to the terminally ill predates my election to public office (in November 1972). It began with a neighbor, a 40-year-old mother of two teenage children, who had terminal cancer. She was called upon to come to grips with the finality of her situation and she did. She was called upon to endure a period of agonizing pain and she did. What she could not bear was an almost perverse medical determination to artificially elongate the dying process,

0077-8923/78/0315-0376 $01.75/0 © 1978, NYAS

dehumanize her precious remaining days, and sustain the physiologic being long after the human being had expired.

When my mother-in-law developed cancer, and the outcome was questionable, I discovered that the legal machinery did not recognize a document directing the cessation of medical treatment when death is imminent.

The meaning of these two events was clear. Out of some misplaced benevolent custodialism, the dying have been systematically and deliberately stripped of their autonomy at a time when psychologically they are desperately in need of it. To their condition of hopelessness there has been added, almost ironically, a thoughtlessly inflicted helplessness.

I

The development of institutionalized medicine, the emphasis on specialization and subspecialization, and the evolution of advanced therapeutic technology are antagonistic to the human needs of the terminally ill. At times, this "cure" orientation of modern medicine is fundamentally inconsistent with the "care" needed by the terminally ill.

At the beginning of the twentieth century, most Americans attained the measure of their days in a familiar setting, usually at home, surrounded by their family, friends, and clergy.[3] Today, nearly 80 percent of the terminally ill, especially those suffering degenerative diseases, are consigned to institutional settings.[4, 5]

While the facilities of the contemporary hospital reflect the marvels of modern science, the architectural design and daily routine are often oppressive and demeaning to human dignity. Prior to his death, Stewart Alsop described the solid-tumor ward at the National Institutes of Health as a place resembling a prison more than a hospital. Hospital windows were always locked shut despite poor ventilation or near-suffocation. On the 14th floor, the solarium was surrounded by heavy wire mesh "like a pheasant run," the purpose of which was to prevent patients from jumping.[6]

In addition to the sterility of the physical environment, the orderliness of the hospital routine fosters loneliness and forces separation from family and loved ones. In some facilities, terminally ill patients are bounced from room to room and from ward to ward in order to avoid contact with other patients.[7] Children and personal friends are often excluded. The dying discover that while they are abandoned when they cry out for companionship, their privacy is invaded when they seek solitude.

The reluctance of our medical schools to impact psychological preparation for physicians leaves many professionals unequipped to adequately serve the terminally ill.[8, 9] Studies have shown that physicians and nurses routinely avoid making rounds to the rooms of the terminal patient.[10]

The unfortunate misdirection in medical education which places a "preponderant emphasis on preserving life at all costs,"[11] causes many physicians, particularly specialists, to focus on a specific disease or illness rather than on the whole needs of the patient.[12, 13] Death is often perceived by the medical staff not as a perfectly natural event, but as a technological failure to effectively utilize the armamentaria at their disposal.[14]

The treatment delivered to the dying often raises a question as to whether its continuation is really for the benefit of the patient or to distract us from our own inability to accept the hopeless condition of the patient.[15] Ironically, at the time when the acceleration of the medical regimen accentuates loss of control and isolation, the terminally ill are increasingly preoccupied with preserving autonomy and resisting separation.[12, 16-18]

When the patient most desperately seeks human contact, his ties to a "community of men," as Dr. Leon Kass described, are medically replaced by an attachment to a "community of machines." [19]

As Paul Ramsey so eloquently states, "Desertion is more choking than death, and more feared. The chief problem of the dying is how not to die alone." [20]

Thus, the real terror for the institutionalized dying is not death, but mechanical maintenance without medical purpose, wrists restrained by leather bonds so that tubes cannot be removed, potentially continuous pain, and the ultimate indignity of having one's remaining days controlled by strangers.[21, 22]

This denial of autonomy does not emanate from the law. While medical jurisprudence guarantees a well-established right to control the decisions relating to medical treatment,[23] the law has not provided an effective mechanism for exercising these rights.

During the twentieth century, the judiciary has expounded, and expanded, the doctrine of informed consent as the cornerstone of the physician-patient relationship.[24-29] Whether expressed in terms of assault, battery, trespass, negligence, or malpractice,[30] the courts have proclaimed man to be the master of his own body. They have admonished the physician that he may not substitute his own judgment for that of the patient.[31] Although there are exceptions for the incompetent patient, children, and emergencies,[32] the doctrine of informed consent, and its corollary, the right to refuse, have been invoked even when treatment may be life-saving.[33-36]

More recently, the Supreme Court has enunciated a constitutional right to privacy which exists in the penumbra of specific guarantees of the Bill of Rights.[37] The concept has been found sufficient to encompass a patient's decision to decline medical treatment.[38]

While these doctrines and declarations purport to guarantee a right to control one's medical destiny, they do not form an adequate framework for exercising that right or for guiding day-to-day decisions.[39] Each opinion is invariably limited by construction to its particular set of facts. The judicial reluctance to devise a practical mechanism for exercising these rights is reflected in a recent decision by a Florida circuit court. In ordering the cessation of a respirator sustaining a patient without brain waves, the judge specifically stated that his ruling was not an attempt to set "blanket criteria or guidelines for future cases." [40]

So, despite theoretical guarantees, no matter how constitutionally fundamental, there is no way to provide assurance to the terminally ill person that anyone will pay attention. Having a right without power to exercise it leaves him in spirit at the mercy of his worst imaginings and in fact at the mercy of a chaotic, ill-defined, ad hoc decision-making process that will decide for him when enough is enough.

When the patient does try to exercise his rights, orally or in writing, even if the physician indicates a willingness to comply with instructions, the patient's wishes may be denied because the family has countermanded his instructions with threats of personal discomfort or legal reprisal against the physician.

The absence of a defined process for asserting the right to refuse thoughtlessly prescribed or medically meaningless treatment reinforces the pre-existing dependency relationship that society has created between patient and physician. Added to the sterile physical environment, the enforced separation and the frequent invasions of privacy, a degree of helplessness is created that will over-whelm even the most strong-willed patient.

Thus, while the legal principles are clear, the public does not perceive that those rights exist, or if they exist, that they can really be exercised.[41] If it did, the Natural Death Act would not have passed.

II

The purpose of the Natural Death Act was to set forth in statute one method for the assertion of these fundamental rights.[42] The Act established in law a legally sanctioned mechanism through which a person could exercise some measure of control over his final days even though he might no longer be able to communicate effectively his right to refuse treatment.[43]

In assessing the design and draftsmanship of the Act, let me begin by acknowledging that the Natural Death Act is not perfect legislation.[44] It was not perfect before its subjection to one of the most difficult political processes imaginable. It never will be perfect because professionals, patients and politicians cannot always agree as to what constitutes legislative perfection in this sensitive area.

The decision to pursue a legislative solution was arrived at only following great soul-searching.[45] After carefully examining the formidable arguments against legislation, including the problems of assuring an informed consent,[46-48] drafting reasonably clear definitions,[47] and precluding interpretation of any intent to cheapen human life,[49-54] I concluded that the Legislature is the proper forum to address the controversial issues surrounding care of the terminally ill.

As the embodiment of societal diversity, the Legislature is well suited to balance the sensitive legal questions, the potential stress on the medical relationship, the theologian's ethical concerns, and the public's clear concern about the dying process.

At the commencement of the legislative process, my personal preference, as the earlier drafts of the Natural Death Act reflected,[55] was to construct a statute that would not distinguish between binding and nonbinding directives, and that would not impose unnecessary obstacles that could frustrate patients and physicians in utilizing the statutory procedures.

Unfortunately, the political climate in Sacramento did not permit the full realization of my objectives. In pursuing the passage of the Natural Death Act, critics and supporters were coming from vastly different directions. One must include in the legislative equation the desires of overzealous supporters, which at times approached advocacy of active euthanasia, the dire warnings of a determined, emotional opposition, which equated the Act with Nazism and me with Adolf Hitler,[56] and the reluctance of well-intentioned but nearsighted legislators who felt uncomfortable in tackling this sensitive issue.

At times, the need to enact legislation had to be balanced with the demand for crippling amendments.[57] In view of the uncertainty of this first venture into legislating the "right to die," is it any surprise that these forces coalesced to lower our expectations?

III

Prior to commenting on the benefits of the Act, a review of the critical commentary might be helpful.

1. The Act is too narrow.[58]

In drafting the Act, it was clear that a measure that went too far would only validate the fears of a determined opposition and render useless any likelihood that the medical and legal professions would honor the law. In addition, the broader the Act, the greater the chance it might undercut the solid legal foundation and perhaps invite abuse and confusion.

As a result, the measure could not serve as a vehicle to solve all the dilemmas of caring for the terminally ill. Unfortunately, in my view—because at the time of passage the necessary consensus had not yet developed—the Act did not create a statutory framework for the patient who might lapse into a persistent and irreversible vegetative or permanently noncognitive state.[59] It did not address the problems of treating the terminally ill newborn or child.[60, 61] To avoid discussing the collateral issue of abortion, the law specifically excluded the pregnant mother from its coverage.[62]

On the other hand, there were, and still are, some "twilight states" that should not be dealt with legislatively. Why? Because of the potential for slippage into active or involuntary euthanasia based on external subjective judgments about the quality of life and without regard to well defined medical states. Thus, the Natural Death Act purposely did not apply to quadriplegia, retardation, senility, or other conditions of diminished brain or motor capacity. It was likewise inapplicable to cases of reversible coma where the patient may recover although with severe mental or physical deficiencies.

Where there is a total and irreversible cessation of brain function (the Harvard definition of "brain death") the Act augmented previously enacted legislation in California permitting the withdrawal of treatment.[63]

2. The Act does not permit discretion in drafting the directive,[64] nor does it validate the living will.[65-68]

Although individually drafted documents may be more consistent with individual freedom, it was believed that a statutorily worded directive would be more practical in the everyday medical world and avoid the subjectivity inherent in interpreting variations in written instructions.[69]

Without a prescribed form, the person could state his instructions in ambiguous language: for example, to discontinue "heroic measures" or to instruct the doctor to act in a manner beyond the scope of the legislation, thereby requiring the physician to sort out the permissible from the impermissible. The possibilities of confusion are endless and would often require either a refusal to honor a directive or a judicial construction of each individual document. Needless to say, neither option would be acceptable public policy.

If the law was to impose an obligation to honor the directive, only a uniform document could satisfy the need for certainty.[70]

3. The Act creates a confusing dichotomy between binding and nonbinding directives and lacks civil sanctions against physicians who refuse to honor a directive.

In determining the weight to be accorded the directive, extensive discussions with legislators, supporters, and opposition made it clear that the chief assumption of the Natural Death Act should be that the wishes of the terminally ill declarant should be paramount. The directive of a terminally ill person who notified of his condition, soberly weighed and accepted his situation should be conclusively presumed, unless revoked, to represent the final expression of his instructions.

Thus, if the patient has been diagnosed as having a terminal condition and he or she signed or re-executed a directive at least 14 days after notification, the directive is binding.[71] If the physician does not wish to honor the directive, then he must transfer the patient to a second physician who will effectuate it.[71]

On the other hand, many legislators and constituent organizations believed that a person who had prepared a directive while in good health may have done so without adequate appreciation of a future condition or contemplation of death. In these cases, the Act afforded the physician discretion to review the case with the family to determine whether the totality of circumstances justifies effectuation of the directive.[72]

Irrespective of whether the declarant was terminally ill or in good health at the time the directive was prepared, the Act incorporated a critical judgment that although failure to honor the directive when it is binding may constitute unprofessional conduct (a violation of the State Medical Practice Act),[73] the attending physician should not be held criminally or civilly liable for failure to effectuate the directive.[74] Should the physician have any doubt as to the purpose of using life-sustaining procedures or the imminence of death, the Act removed the threat of civil liability from the physician in determining whether the patient's condition has deteriorated to an extent justifying the effectuation of the directive. In this respect, the Act permitted the physician to decide in favor of life where a reasonable doubt exists.

4. The Act is the first step towards public acceptance of mercy killing.[75]

The most intense objection to the Natural Death Act has been the concern that such a law must inevitably open the door to mercy killing and involuntary euthanasia. Although written 19 years ago, the words of Professor Kamisar remain the foundation of the right-to-life attack on right-to-die legislation: "Whether or not the first step is precarious, is perilous, is worth taking, rests in part on what the second step is likely to be." [76]

As supportive evidence, Kamisar pointed to the parade of horrors and atrocities which the Nazis perpetrated in the name of killing "incurables" and the "useless." [76] He concluded that the only way we could prevent a recurrence of the Nazi mentality is "by adamantly holding the line, by swiftly snuffing out what are or might be small beginnings of what we do not want to happen here." [77] Joseph Fletcher offers one succinct reply: the Nazis never engaged in euthanasia or mercy killing; what they did was merciless killing, either genocidal or for ruthless experimental purposes.[78]

As Kamisar's critics have also responded, the "wedge argument" fails to consider the voluntariness of the patient's request [79] or the fact that you have a medically well-defined category of individuals who are going to die shortly. We do not determine for someone; they determine for themselves. The decision is not even whether someone should die, but how.

To buttress this position, the Natural Death Act contains a provision declaring that the Act shall not be construed to condone, authorize, or approve mercy killing or to permit any affirmative act or omission to end life other than to permit the natural process of dying.[80] As far as can be determined, this was the first statutory pronouncement in this country explicitly rejecting the concept of active and involuntary euthanasia. It serves as a reminder to physicians, patients, and the public of the narrow purpose of the Act and the reverence that we all share for life.

IV

On January 1, 1978 the Natural Death Act will celebrate its first birthday.[81] During this year, we have had to adjust to this unique legislative stepchild. The Act's most fervent supporters would probably assert that the law has not been utilized to its full extent. The Act's detractors would probably agree that their deepest fears of mercy killing have not been realized. Most of us are pleased that the Act has remained in the private sector and has not come within the province of the judiciary.

The experience with the Act since its passage indicates that the initial judgment to proceed with legislation was a sound one. Notwithstanding the political obstacles and the Act's weaknesses, the very fact that the Natural Death Act survived the legislative process, the Governor's critical examination,[82] and one year of operation, indicates that a legislative solution is not only possible, but also desirable.

1. For the terminally ill, the Natural Death Act has clarified their right to refuse treatment and has offered protection to several classes of persons:

(a) The person who is heavily sedated or comatose and thus cannot communicate his right to decline continuing medical intervention.[83]

(b) The physically disabled person, who, though fully conscious, is treated, or feels as if he is treated, in a custodial situation. This includes the case where the nature of treatment—both medical and personal—causes the patient to wonder whether he has any rights left to exercise.

(c) The person who communicates to his physician that he wishes life-supporting procedures terminated and the physician is in doubt as to whether the patient is at that point sufficiently lucid. If the patient had previously prepared a directive, the physician could rely on the document and act upon the patient's request.

(d) The person whose physician finds himself either caught between conflicting pressures of family, hospital policy, or colleagues, or whose physician refuses to pay attention to his wishes. Here, the directive invokes a legal procedure that accords validity to the written record of the patient's instructions, and may, if the patient was terminally ill when the directive was prepared, subject the physician who fails to honor the document to a finding of unprofessional conduct.

(e) The person who finds it difficult to communicate with his physician. In many cases, the physician or the patient, or both, may feel awkward in discussing the patient's condition and the hopeless prognosis. Here, the directive may serve a most useful purpose—to initiate dialogue between the physician and the patient.

(f) The person who never bothered to consider the appropriate limits of life-sustaining medical treatment and communicate his personal instructions in advance of an unexpected illness or accident.

2. For the physician, the Natural Death Act has clarified the state of the law regarding terminating life-supporting systems in dying patients.[84] It has allayed fears of malpractice litigation from families whose agenda for the patient differ from the patient's own directions.

Significantly, it appears that the Act may be strengthening the physician-patient relationship. A recent survey by the California Medical Association found that although most physicians had not utilized the directive in withdrawing or withholding life-sustaining treatment, more than half stated that the Act had been useful to them in their practice.[85] Quoting from the survey, "Several respondents mentioned that the Act provided a mechanism for patients to communicate with their physicians and also has served to bring the subject 'out of the closet,' making possible open discussion between patients and their families." [85]

I am encouraged by the survey results because they reflect a shift in the attitudes of physicians toward their patients. From the questions and comments I received from health providers, I have often noticed that the professional perspective may preclude a complete understanding of the patient's frustration in exercising fundamental rights.

Legislation cannot alter overnight deep-rooted behavioral patterns. Developing greater sensitivity may take another generation. However, the incentives in the Natural Death Act which clarify liability [86] and express a clear statutory policy in favor of honoring a patient's rights [87] impose at least a moral obligation on professionals to bring a change in their method of practice. The legal recognition of the directive, even if it is not always binding, positively reinforces the statutory incentives and offers a framework within which physicians and patients can communicate.

3. For society, the greatest impact of the law has been the triggering of an awareness of the need for public education and a perception that legislative activity in this area is possible. The Act has drawn attention to the need to treat the terminally ill as persons, not patients. It has focused attention on the appropriate and inappropriate application of our medical technology.

The passage of the Natural Death Act has encouraged seven other states to enact similar legislation.[88] Throughout the State of California, the nation, and even abroad, the Natural Death Act and its progeny have generated public and professional dialogue to discuss the legislation and how it can be applied to humanize the treatment of the dying.

The Act has been on the agenda at the conventions of the American [89] and state Bar associations,[90] the National Conference of State Legislatures,[91] the American College of Surgeons,[92] and at colloquia sponsored by the National Conference of Christians and Jews [93] and the Hastings Center.[94] The Act has been the subject of hospital grand rounds, including those at the University of California, San Francisco, School of Medicine,[95] courses in medical and nursing continuing education, a national moot court competition,[96] and law review commentary.[97–101]

4. What is most important is how the Act affects the tens of thousands of Californians who have come in contact with the Act or have requested copies of the directive. At this most personal level, the Act forces us to project ourselves into the world of the terminally ill, and brings us more into touch with a feared part of ourselves—a strained relationship with death that we now know begins in the earliest stages of life.

V

The patient's protection, the professional response, the public reaction, and our personal reflection on the Natural Death Act are evidence in the growing recognition that we must offer a more humane, caring system for the dying person. Many communities are turning towards the hospice concept, where professionals and volunteers can offer a multidisciplinary treatment approach to the terminally ill and their families. Some physicians are re-examining the legal impediments that restrict doctors from offering optimal drug therapy for ameliorating the intractable pain associated with some terminal diseases.[102]

In my judgment, there are too many problems in our society that are simply not approached because they seem too complicated, or because they are politically risky, or because proposed solutions come from so many different places that there is only a very tiny area of consensus.

The Natural Death Act represents symbolically—and symbols are important —that legislative bodies can achieve progress in an area which most thought impossible. It signifies that we should continue to move forward in solving some of the problems. It reminds us that it is impossible to travel from the land of "what is" to the land of "what ought to be" until we at least step onto the path between them.

ACKNOWLEDGMENT

Without the tireless efforts and creative energy of Steve Lipton, the Natural Death Act, and this paper, would not have been possible.

NOTES AND REFERENCES

1. FROST, R. 1923. "New Hampshire."
2. California Health and Safety Code Sections 7185–7195 (Chapter 1437, Statutes of 1976); for a derivation of the short title, see "Statement of Melvin J. Krant" *in* Hearings on Death with Dignity, Special Committee on Aging, U.S. Senate, August 9, 1972. : 114; *see also* CALLAHAN, D. June 1977. On defining a "natural death." Hastings Center Rep. **7**: 32.
3. BOK, S. 1973. Euthanasia and the care of the dying. Bioscience **23**: 416, 463.
4. KRANT, M. 1973. The other dimensions of death. Prism **1**: 54, 56.
5. BOK, S. 1976. Personal directions for care at the end of life. N. Engl. J. Med. **295**: 367.
6. ALSOP, S. 1974. The right to die with dignity. Good Housekeeping, August : 130.
7. In a seminar on death and dying, Dr. Elizabeth Kübler-Ross referred to this phenomenon as the "ping-pong syndrome." Seminar on Death and Dying, Red Lion Inn, Sacramento, November, 1975.
8. HEIFETZ, M. 1975. The Right to Die. : 144. Putnams. New York, N.Y.
9. See also KRANT, M.[2] : 115: "Where death is unwelcome, the enemy, the evil, the dying individual has little opportunity to be assisted in worning out meaningful details of the dying experience. He is often treated as a leper, rather than as a man or woman reaching the end of a personal life." See also KRANT, M.[4] : 55: "In his dying, the individual patient is often denied his unique individuality, and is, in fact, forced to become a common amalgam of complaints, symptoms, and physical findings, so that an orderly pathophysiologic explanation of his demise can be construed."
10. BOK, S.[3] : 463–464.
11. MORISON, R. S. 1973. Dying. Scientific American **229**: 55.
12. BOK, S.[3] : 464.
13. CASSELL, E. J. 1975. Dying in a technological society. *In* Death Inside Act. P. Steinfels & R. M. Veatch, Eds. : 42–46. Harper & Row. New York, N.Y.

14. CASSELL, E. J.[13] : 42–43.
15. KÜBLER-ROSS, E. 1976. Prolongation of life. *In* Life or Death—Who Controls? N. C. Ostheimer & J. M. Ostheimer, Eds. : 216. Springer. New York, N.Y.
16. The terminally ill patient may even develop a new disease—the "intensive care syndrome"—which has been characterized as an acute psychological and behavioral disturbance caused by deprivation of sleep, unfamiliar surroundings, mechanization, and uncertainty.
17. MCKEGNEY, F. 1966. Intensive Care Syndrome. Conn. Med. **30:** 633–644.
18. HACKETT, T. N., N. CASSELL & H. WISHNIE. 1968. The coronary care unit: An appraisal of its psychological hazards. 279 N. Engl. J. Med. **279:** 1365–1370.
19. KASS, L. 1972. Man's right to die. Pharos **35:** 73, 77.
20. RAMSEY, P. 1970. The Patient as Person. : 134. Yale University Press. New Haven and London.
21. Ernlé W. D. Young, Chaplain at Stanford University, eloquently expressed this thought: "To be reduced to the level of a puppet, moved only by strings is tantamount to a denial of what we, in our culture, reckon to be an essential constituent of the humanum."
22. YOUNG, E. W. D. An experiental viewpoint of the needs of the dying patient. California Dept. of Health Seminar, Sacramento, California, June 9, 1976 (p. 2).
23. *Union Pacific Railway* v. *Botsford*, 141 U.S. 250, 251 (1891): "No right is held more sacred, or is more carefully guarded, by the common law, than the right of every individual to the possession and control of his own person, free from all restraint or interference by others, unless by clear and unquestionable authority of law."
24. *Schloendorff* v. *Society of New York Hospital*, 211 N.Y. 125, 129–130, 105 N.E. 92, 93 (1914) ("Every human being of adult years and sound mind has a right to determine what shall be done with his own body . . .").
25. *Natanson* v. *Kline*, 186 Kan. 393, 350 P.2d 1093, rehearing denied, 187 Kan. 186, 354 P.2d 670 (1960).
26. *Canterbury* v. *Spence*, 464 F.2d 772, cert. denied, 409 U.S. 1064 (1972).
27. *Cobbs* v. *Grant*, 8 Cal. 3d 229, 502 P.2d 1, 104 Cal. Rptr. 505 (1972).
28. Informed Consent and the Dying Patient. Yale Law. J. **83:** 1032.
29. CANTOR, N. 1972. A patient's decision to decline life-saving medical treatment: Bodily integrity versus the preservation of life. Rutgers Law Rev. **26:** 228.
30. CANTOR, N. **29:** 237.
31. *Natanson* v. *Kline*, 186 Kan. : 406–7, 350 P.2d : 1104.
32. *Cobbs* v. *Grant*, 8 Cal.3d : 243.
33. *Erickson* v. *Dilgard*, 44 Misc.2d 27, 252 N.Y.S.2d 705 (1962).
34. *In Re Brook's Estate*, 32 Ill.2d 361, 205 N.E.2d (1965).
35. *In Re Raasch*, No. 455–996 (Prob. Div., Milwaukee County Ct., January 21, 1972).
36. 1977. When the Patient Says No. Time Magazine January 24 : 77.
37. *Griswold* v. *Connecticut*, 381 U.S. 479, 85 S. Ct. 1678, 14 L.Ed.2d 510 (1965).
38. *In Re Quinlan*, 70 N.J. 10, 355 A.2d 647 (1976).
39. For one reaction to the *Quinlan* decision, see : 1976. Life or death—A committee decision?" San Francisco Chronicle July 21 : 14.
40. *In Re Cain* (Florida Circuit Ct., 1976), quoted in Lawson, H. 1976. California's "Natural Death Act." Wall Street Journal December **28:** 14.
41. HEIFETZ, M.,[8] : 39.
42. The Natural Death Act is not intended to be the exclusive means to assert these rights. California Health and Safety Code Section 7193 states: "Nothing in this chapter shall impair or supersede any legal right or legal responsibility which any person may have to effect the withholding or withdrawal of life-supporting procedures in any lawful manner." In such respect the provisions of this chapter are cumulative.
43. California Health and Safety Code Section 7186.

44. There were other models to choose from, each imperfect in their own way. See KRAUSS, R. 1976. The tragic choice: Termination of care for patients in a permanent vegetative state. N.Y.U. Law Rev. **51:** 285; KAPLAN, R. 1976. Euthanasia legislation. Am. J. Law Med. **2:** 41; STEELE, W. & B. HILL. 1976. A Legislative Proposal For a Legal Right to Die. Crim. Law Bull. **12:** 140.
45. This included heeding the admonition of Ian Kennedy that such an issue should not find its way into the statute books as a result of sustained lobbying or a Friday afternoon session : KENNEDY, I. 1975. A legal perspective on determining death. The Month February : 48, quoted in HUMMELL, R. 1976. Death With dignity legislation : A foot in the door?" Hosp. Progr. June : 55.

The precedent for the Natural Death Act was Assembly Bill 4444, which I introduced in the 1974 Legislative Session. This measure resulted in an interim hearing of the California State Assembly Committee on Health in San Francisco, October 8, 1974.

46. HUMMELL, R. **45:** 54.
47. SULLIVAN, W. F. 1975. Death with dignity: Ministry not legislation (a pastoral letter). Richmond, Va. : 5.
48. MORRIS, A. 1970. Voluntary euthanasia. Wash. Law Rev. **45**, **239:** 256–259.
49. SULLIVAN, W. F. **47:** 6–7.
50. HUMMELL, R.[45] : 55–56.
51. MORRIS, A.[48] : 256, 264–265.
52. KAMISAR, Y. 1958. Some non-religious views against proposed "mercy-killing" legislation. Minn. Law Rev. **42:** 969, 1030–1041.
53. CASSEM, N. H. 1976. Controversies surrounding the hopelessly ill patient. *In* Death, Dying and the Law. J. T. McHugh, Ed. : 42. Our Sunday Visitor. Huntington, Ind.
54. LOUISELL, D. W. 1973. Euthanasia and biathanasia: On death and killing. Cath. Univ. Law Rev. **22:** 723, 729–730.
55. See Assembly Bill 3060 as introduced, February 13, 1976, as amended in Assembly, April 8, 1976, May 3, 1976, May 24, 1976, and May 27, 1976.
56. One handbill signed by A. Saqueton, M.D., and dated August 2, 1976, contained the inscription: "Long Live Hitler! Kill the Aged, the Weak, the Poor." Above the inscription, someone had penned in "(Amer. Version Barry Keene)." The handbill also stated: "Support Assembly Bill No. 3060 . . . or the Legal Murder Act" superimposed over a man and a woman hanging from a gallows, and "One nation under God, but with California under Hitler, divisible with liberty to kill and justice not for all!" At the Committee hearing of the Senate Judiciary Committee on August 17, 1976, opponents of the Act placed a copy of W. Shirer's *The Rise and Fall of the Third Reich* at the front of the witness table.
57. Assembly Bill 3060 was amended nine times: April 8, 1976, May 3, 1976, May 24, 1976, May 27, 1976, June 16, 1976, June 24, 1976, August 13, 1976, August 18, 1976, and August 24, 1976.
58. VEATCH, R. 1977. Death and dying: The legislative options. Hastings Center Rep. **7:** 5, 6.
59. Pursuant to California Health and Safety Code Section 7187(e) defining "life-sustaining procedure," death must be imminent whether or not life-sustaining procedures are utilized. For our definition of "imminent," see RABKIN, M. G. GILLERMAN & N. RICE. 1976. Orders not to resuscitate. N. Engl. J. Med. **295:** 364, 365; see also KRAUSS, R.[44] note 31.
60. JONSEN, A. R. & M. J. GARLAND, Eds. 1976. Ethics of Newborn Intensive Care. University of California Press. Berkeley, Calif.
61. HEIFETZ, M.[8] : 43–73.
62. California Health and Safety Code Section 7188. Paragraph 3 of the directive states: "If I have been diagnosed as pregnant and that diagnosis is known to my physician, this directive shall have no force or effect during the course of

my pregnancy;" See also A. Etzioni, "Life or Death for a Baby: The Next Karen Quinlan Case," Parade Magazine (November 7, 1976) at 24.

63. California Health and Safety Code Sections 7180–7182.
64. *Idem.,* Section 7188.
65. KUTNER, L. 1969. Due process of euthanasia: The Living Will, a proposal. Ind. Law J. **44:** 539.
66. KUTNER, L. 1975. The Living Will: Coping with the historical event of death. Baylor L. Rev. **27:** 39.
67. STRAND, J. 1976. The "Living Will:" The right to death with dignity. Case West. Law R. **26:** 485.
68. Christian Affirmation of Life. Catholic Hospital Association.
69. BOK, S.[5] : 367–368.
70. VEATCH, R.[58] : 6.
71. California Health and Safety Code Section 7191(b).
72. *Idem.,* Section 7191 (c).
73. *Idem.,* Section 7191 (b).
74. *Idem.,* Sections 7191 (b) and (c).
75. See References 49–54. See also LAWSON, H.[40] and for a contrary view Curley, J. 1977. CACH calls Natural Death Act imperfect, but not immoral. Hosp. Progr. **58:** 6; for a collection of "mercy-killing" cases, see VAUGHAN, N. L. 1974. The right to die. Cal. West. Law R. **10:** 613, 614–615.
76. KAMISAR, Y.[52] : 1031.
77. KAMISAR, Y.[52] : 1038.
78. FLETCHER, J. 1973. Ethics and euthanasia. *In* To Live and to Die. R. H. Williams, Ed. Springer, Verlag. New York, N.Y.
79. MORRIS, A.[48] : 264–265.
80. California Health and Safety Code Section 7195.
81. For a view of the Act at birth, see LAWSON, H.[40]; HOLLES, E. 1977. Law goes into effect in California giving the terminally ill the right to die by barring medical aid. *New York Times* January 2 : 33; and GARLAND, M. 1976. Politics, legislation, and natural death. Hastings Center Rep. **6:** 5.
82. The bill was opposed by the State Director of Health, Dr. Jerome Lackner (see Lawson, H.[40]) and by Karen Lebacqz of the Office of Health, Law and Values, California State Department of Health. (See LEBACQZ, K. 1977. Commentary on natural death. Hastings Center Rep. **7:** 2, 14.
83. California Health and Safety Code Section 7188. Paragraph 2 of directive states: *"In the absence of my ability to give directions* regarding the use of such life-sustaining procedures, it is my intention that this directive shall be honored by family and physician(s) . . ." (emphasis added).
84. *Idem.,* Section 7190.
85. 1977. Survey Results Following One Year's Experience With the Natural Death Act. California Medical Association October **28:** 2.
86. California Health and Safety Code Section 7190.
87. *Idem.,* Section 7186.
88. Arkansas, Idaho, Nevada, New Mexico, North Carolina, Oregon, and Texas.
89. ROTHENBERG, L. The California Natural Death Act. Submitted at the Annual Meeting of the American Bar Association, Chicago, Illinois, August 9, 1977.
90. GUITIERREZ, M., JR. The Natural Death Act—Passive euthanasia in California. Submitted at Convention of the California State Bar, San Diego, California, September 26, 1977.
91. National Conference of State Legislatures, Detroit, Michigan, August 4, 1977.
92. Forum on Death and Dying, Northern California Chapter of American College of Surgeons, May 7, 1977.
93. In conjunction with University of Santa Clara, February 7, 1977 and in conjunction with University of Southern California, October 4, 1977.
94. Workshop in Medical and Biological Ethics, Institute of Society, Ethics, and the Life Sciences, June 19–26, 1977.

95. January 19, 1977.
96. 1977 James Patterson McBaine Moot Court Honors Competition.
97. RANDALL, M. W. 1977. The right to die a natural death: A discussion of *In Re Quinlan* and The Natural Death Act. Cincinnati Law Rev. **46:** 197.
98. FLANNERY, E. J. 1977. Statutory recognition of the right to die: The California Natural Death Act. Boston Univ. Law Rev. **57:** 148.
99. 1977. Natural Death Act. Pacific Law J. **8:** 487.
100. MILLS, D. H. 1977. California's Natural Death Act. J. Legal Med. **5:** 22.
101. MEYERS, D. W. 1977. The California Natural Death Act: A Critical Appraisal. Calif. State Bar J. July/August : 326.
102. SATCHELL, M. 1977. How to enjoy life up to the last minute. Parade Magazine, October 10.

Chronology of the Natural Death Act (1976)

January 1976

1/17—Assemblyman Keene announces intent to introduce the Natural Death Act; speech before the American Cancer Society, California Division.

February 1976

2/13—Assembly Bill 3060 introduced, assigned to Assembly Committee on Health.
18—*San Francisco Chronicle* editorially endorses AB 3060.
19—*Oakland Tribune* editorially endorses AB 3060.
25—*Sacramento Bee* runs a feature story on AB 3060.

March 1976

3/1—California Pro-Life Council communicates its opposition to AB 3060.
3—Assemblyman Keene sends copies of AB 3060 to all Catholic Bishops in California.
7—*Sacramento Bee* editorially endorses AB 3060.
9—Assemblyman Keene concurs with Dr. Milton Heifetz.
11—*Catholic Herald* editorially opposes AB 3060.
12—Assemblyman Keene responds to letter of California Pro-Life Council of March 1.
19—California Association of District Attorneys requests amendment of criminal provisions of AB 3060.
21—*Catholic Voice* editorially opposes AB 3060.
30—Rt. Rev. Clarence Haden, Jr., Bishop, Episcopal Diocese of Northern California, communicates his endorsement of AB 3060.
31—*In Re Quinlan* decision.

April 1976

4/8—AB 3060 amended.
14—Humanist Society communicates its endorsement of AB 3060.
16—California Pro-Life Council responds to Assemblyman Keene's letter of March 12.
21—AB 3060 approved by the Assembly Health Committee on a 9–2 vote.
23—KFI radio (Los Angeles) editorially endorses AB 3060.
24—*Eureka Times-Standard* editorially endorses AB 3060.
26—California Association of Catholic Hospitals distributes statement of opposition to all legislators; *San Francisco Examiner* runs page of letters to the editor on AB 3060.
29—AB 3060 amended, re-referred to Assembly Committee on Revenue and Taxation.

May 1976

  5/5—California Pro-Life Council communicates additional objections to AB 3060.
  12—National Council of Jewish Women endorses AB 3060.
  13—California Conference of Local Health Officers and American Civil Liberties Union endorse AB 3060.
  15—National Conference of Senior Citizens and Retiree's Action Coalition endorse AB 3060.
  17—Assemblyman Keene responds to May 5 letter of California Pro-Life Council; California Pro-Life Council announces formation of medical-legal coalition to oppose AB 3060.
  19—AB 3060 approved without recommendation by Assembly Committee on Revenue and Taxation; State Commission on Aging endorses AB 3060.
  20—Assemblyman Keene sends copies of AB 3060 to 37 senior organizaitons asking for their comments.
  24—AB 3060 amended; Sonoma County Board of Supervisors endorses AB 3060; California Pro-Life Council responds to Assemblyman Keene's letter of May 17.
  25—Right-to-Life organizations picket State Capitol.
  27—AB 3060 amended.

June 1976

  6/7—Assemblyman Keene meets with representatives of the California Pro-Life Council; *Catholic Voice* repeats opposition to AB 3060.
  8—Assemblyman Keene sends letter to California Pro-Life Council outlining agreed-upon amendments to AB 3060; *Long Beach Press-Telegram* editorially endorses AB 3060.
  9—California Department of Health conducts seminar on the Natural Death Act.
  16—AB 3060 amended.
  17—AB 3060 passes Assembly on 47–27 vote; California Association of Catholic Hospitals formally removes opposition to AB 3060.
  23—AB 3060 assigned to Senate Judiciary Committee.
  24—AB 3060 amended; *Sacramento Bee* editorially endorses AB 3060.
  30—*Modesto Bee* editorially endorses AB 3060.

July 1976

  7/1—Assemblyman Keene sends letter to California Pro-Life Council requesting a clarification of their position on AB 3060.
  5—*Santa Rosa Press-Democrat* editorially endorses AB 3060.
  7—KCBS radio (San Francisco) editorially endorses AB 3060.
  8—Right-to-Life organizations picket three legislators who voted in favor of AB 3060.
  19—California Pro-Life Council responds to Assemblyman Keene's letter of July 1.
  21—Assemblyman Keene responds to California Pro-Life Council's letter of July 19.
  27—California Medical Association requests amendments to AB 3060.

August 1976

  8/2—California Pro-Life Council responds to Assemblyman Keene's letter of July 21; Right-to-Life organizations distribute handbills equating AB 3060 with Nazism.
  6—National Organization for Women announce opposition to AB 3060.
  12—California Catholic Conference removes opposition and switches to a "watch" position.
  13—AB 3060 amended.
  17—AB 3060 approved by Senate Judiciary Committee on a 6–2 vote.

18—AB 3060 amended; re-referred to Senate Committee on Revenue and Taxation.
20—AB 3060 referred to Senate floor by Senate Committee on Revenue and Taxation.
23—*Los Angeles Times* editorially endorses AB 3060; Right-to-Life organizations picket State Capitol.
24—AB 3060 amended; *San Francisco Chronicle* editorially endorses AB 3060.
25—California Pro-Life Council distributes amendments to AB 3060; Dr. Jerome Lackner, State Director of Health communicates opposition to AB 3060.
26—AB 3060 passes Senate on 22–14 vote.
27—California Pro-Life Council requests eight Assemblymen to reverse their votes on AB 3060.
30—Assembly concurs in amendments of State Senate on a 43–31 vote.

September 1976

9/1—*San Francisco Chronicle* editorially endorses AB 3060.
3—*Simi Valley Enterprise* editorially endorses AB 3060.
5—*Bakersfield Californian* editorially endorses AB 3060; American Civil Liberties Union publishes feature article on *Sacramento Bee* editorial page.
7—American Civil Liberties Union article republished in *Los Angeles Times.*
8—*Los Angeles Times* and KCST radio (San Diego) editorially endorse AB 3060; Legislative Counsel issues formal opinion #15466 on AB 3060.
9—California Medical Association and Friends Committee request Governor Brown to sign AB 3060.
13—Legislative Counsel issues formal opinion #15437 on AB 3060; *Newsweek* runs article on AB 3060.
19—*Los Angeles Times* runs letter to editor on AB 3060.
22—*San Louis Post-Dispatch* editorially endorses AB 3060.
24—Legislative Counsel issues formal opinion #15261 on AB 3060; California Nurses Association requests Governor Brown to sign AB 3060.
30—Governor Brown signs AB 3060 (Chapter 1439, Statutes of 1976).

October 1976

10/5—*New York Times* editorially endorses the Natural Death Act.

January 1977

1/1—AB 3060 goes into effect.

DISCUSSION

CAPRON: From the accomplishments that Mr. Keene has claimed for his "child," it is hard to believe that this youngster is only one year old. I guess proud fathers have a way of picturing their offspring as doing so many things.

J. L. BATEMAN: My compliments to Mr. Keene for a brilliant and lucid presentation. I am a practicing clinician who is involved with cancer chemotherapy. My patients do not normally see the inside of intensive care units and frequently or generally do not have treatment for terminal infections unless they are causing physical discomfort. In essence I agree completely with what Mr. Keene has so beautifully stated. However, in Massachusetts a few years ago, I proposed the idea of a living will, possibly as a paper tiger. I would like to raise the possibility of the backlash effect on a person who has not signed such a living will. Will it be more likely that he would then be subject to more heroic procedures?

KEENE: The Natural Death Act contains a very explicit provision that it is a parallel procedure for removal of life-support systems. This does not preclude the law, as ill-defined as it may have been, prior to enactment of the Natural Death Act. It is simply one mechanism of the law that a person may choose to avail him- or herself of. It does not restrict a physician in any other way from engaging in his practice as he would have prior to the passage of the Natural Death Act, except in directives required to effectuate the law when applied. Should he apply the law, it frees the physician from both civil and criminal liability.

The hope, of course, is that physicians will become acquainted with that aspect of the Act. There was a concern expressed that they might not. I believe that physicians, as intelligent people with the ability to communicate among themselves, can be reached and can understand the components of the Act.

YOUNGSTEIN: I question our ability to protect the rights or wishes of the persons who wish to take advantage of your law. I say this because of the consequences observed after the passage of the Anatomical Gift Act. The Anatomical Gift Act was created largely to give the individual the right to donate his organs after death or to indicate what he wants done with his body. We created the donor card, which has been distributed to millions of individuals throughout the United States. More than 40 states now have it on their driver's licenses in some form, and yet we are constantly faced with the situation where families who oppose the donor card are the ones that are listened to and the wishes of the person who signed it are ignored. In other words, who protects the rights of the person who signed the card? If the family is opposing it and the physician is ambivalent or nervous about the entire episode, how are you going to insure that the person who is taking advantage of either your law or the Anatomical Gift Act is having his rights upheld?

KEENE: There is no way to assure that people, including professionals, will obey the law except to catch them at disobedience. In this case, if a physician, by virtue of personal ideology, refuses to obey the directive of a patient, then, under the terms of the Act, he could lose his license over it. Unless he is discovered it is not known whether he has obeyed or disobeyed the law. I believe that if the physician intends to disobey the Act in any individual case he could do so simply by actions of subjective judgment. I think that physicians are basically moral people and that if the law tells them to do something they pretty much abide by it. I assume that patterns will develop and that, over a period of years, physicians will be guided by the law. However, there is no absolute assurance that the law will be obeyed.

CAPRON: I assume that the answer to the question would be the same if it were taken the way that I understood it initially. This is similar to the situation of transplants when the family wishes to revoke what has been written on the consent card of the patient. The doctor may think, "I could go ahead on the basis of the permission granted on the card, and then if the family takes me into court, I can litigate and say there was no clear revocation." This is also true with the Act. The Act provides that revocation by verbal expression of a declarer shall be effective upon communication to the attending physician by the declarant or by a person acting on behalf of the declarant. It is my understanding, reading the words, that the expression "one would be speaking or acting on behalf" is not defined in the statute. There may be someone who has some apparent authority or relationship to the declarant or who simply represents that they were present when the declarant said to them, "I don't want you to do that; I want you to keep my treatment up." If that individual now states, after the patient has gone into coma, that this was what the patient told him when no one else was present, the physician would have no option but to treat, invalidating the purpose of the Act. I would take your answer to be satisfactory, which is you cannot stop people from doing wrong things such as lying when they want to do it. There is not, however, the protection that you suggest. It is in this case in which the physician is involved, where one is not subject to control by disciplinary procedures.

KEENE: No, but they are subject to civil liability under the Act. It is a misdemeanor to fraudulently suggest that there has been a . . . .

CAPRON: Is it then your serious suggestion that this is unlike a situation where you have a family who has a physician who they think will insist on stopping treatment despite their statements of revocation? In this situation, the physician has decided not to cease treatment based upon the statement of revocation. The physician would then take this person into court and suggest to the prosecutor that the person be prosecuted if the doctor concluded that the statement of revocation was doubtful.

It does not seem to me that physicians in our society are likely to take that step. They would be subject to headlines such as "Physician Asks Relative to be Sued for Misleading Statement about Revocation."

KEENE: I do not think that is likely to happen. Although we felt that the concealment of a revocation was a very serious matter and constitutes unlawful homicide under the Act, we believe that the communication of a false revocation ought to constitute something less than that, probably a misdemeanor. It may be unlikely, although not entirely improbable, that the physician might bring that to the attention of the law. It might be more likely that some relative who was concerned about the final days of the terminal illness and the condition of the patient under the kind of medical treatment that was being rendered might take another relative into court or threaten to do so. That would probably constitute the maximal enforcement that you can expect. We have come a long way from believing that laws are the absolute command of an imperial sovereign and you get your head chopped off if you do not obey them, or that you get caught every time and stricken by lightning. Laws are norms and it is hoped that behavior in accordance with the laws that we pass is going to occur, particularly in this area in which all the parties involved are likely to be very sincere in their concerns about the terminally ill patient.

VERNON: It's a serious defect of our society that lawyers take with such great aplomb the readiness to involve someone just practicing his profession to be put in the toils of the law to test our principles. I would like to have you recognize that putting someone in the toils of the law for every little thing he does is a punishment.

BERESFORD: I wish to make a technical distinction concerning the standards of proof in prognosis. I was talking about a high standard of proof in a situation of surrogate decisionmaking, where the patient is not able to state an opinion or desire with respect to treatment. The issue is allocating the responsibility for decisionmaking to someone else. In that situation you have to demand the highest possible standard of proof. Whether it is 100 percent or not I do not know. In the situation where the patient is competent and understands that he has a terminal condition and is so informed by his physician, it may not be 100 percent. The patient can comprehend that, and in this situation one could deal with a lesser standard of proof. I was really concerned about the problem of surrogate decisionmaking that we are faced with in the brain-death issue as well.

KEENE: What about prospective decisionmaking through the use of some sort of paper or document by an individual who wishes not to be subject to extraordinary treatment?

BERESFORD: That would be a very difficult document to draft. I suppose it is possible if the medical data base becomes adequate for prognosis and determinations for irreversibility in conditions other than brain death. Then one might be able to do something. However, it would be difficult.

P. M. HARDY: Mr. Horan presupposes that the fundamental underlying duty of a physician is to preserve life. This view needs to be examined further at philosophical and ethical levels. It is certainly not held by all physicians and was not true in Hellenistic times. It appeared to arise during the Scientific Revolution, when man felt that he had dominion over and could conquer nature.

HORAN: I do not know what comment one can make to that. I just took it on the basis of what most physicians say their job in society is. I do not know what it means to preserve life. Were you speaking about it in a pejorative sense that you wanted one to prolong life? Are you speaking about it in a sense that the job of a physician is to heal, as I have assumed? If that is wrong I will have to make another presentation some other date.

S. BACHRACH: Assemblyman Keene, you gave a very eloquent argument for the care of the terminally ill. Is there any procedure in California for getting the number of people that have taken advantage of the law? I would like also to note that since it took a decision of the Utah Supreme Court to follow out the wishes of Gilmore, it should also be a judicial decision to determine the right of a person who wants to have all treatment stopped. It takes more than one physician to commit a person to certain state institutions, so why is so much responsibility placed in the hands of a single physician under the Act that you have sponsored?

KEENE: As far as the first question is concerned, we will attempt to gather data at some appropriate time. The California Medical Association has done a limited survey, as previously indicated. In addition, there are some law students who are actively gathering data, and we will probably have a better idea in the years to come how well the Act is working.

I suspect that while its operational impact would be limited its orientational impact may be rather wide. It may be possible to expand the Act into other areas if that is a desirable social goal. Society will have time to evaluate that.

In answer to your second question pertaining to vesting authority for effectuation of the directive with the physician, it is a directive to a physician. If there is a problem of legal interpretation, or a problem of application of the directive, presuambly it could wind up in court and might be resolved there. If there is not, then this is simply in line with all of the other practices that enable an individual to determine the course of his own medical treatment, or at least to refuse certain modalities that are not consistent with his wishes.

CESSATION OF BRAIN FUNCTION: ETHICAL IMPLICATIONS IN TERMINAL CARE AND ORGAN TRANSPLANT

Rabbi M. D. Tendler

Department of Biology
Yeshiva University
New York, New York 10033

The moral and ethical dilemmas that the biomedical sciences are posing to society at large are necessitating a review of basic axioms and definitions. Confused concepts and fuzzy constructs cannot stand up to the test of real life-and-death decisions that must be made daily. When life begins and ends has been a favorite theological problem avidly discussed by the religious mentors of all faiths. It is now a fact of life for every intern in a hospital intensive care unit. He cannot hide under vague definitions of death based on the invisible soul leaving the body, but must have anatomic or physiologic end points that can be quantitated so as to permit ethical behavior.

The problem of accurate definitions is further complicated by the absence of social machinery to make such a definition. Who decides? Who defines life and death, right and wrong, truth and falsehood? Is it the expertise of the medical scientist that established the fact of death based on criteria approved by society, or is he also the source of the criteria? Can even the collective conscience of society serve as the yardstick for defining life and death? Is not social conscience the result or effect and not the cause or source of an ethical system? The concurrence of social behavior with the principles of an ethical system is a test of the ethics of society, not of the ethical system, unless we stoop to situation ethics.

Western civilization developed an ethical system based strongly on a Judaeo-Biblical heritage. Biblical law and ethics, as developed over the last 2,500 years, served to mold the conscience of our society and still command the respect of the vast majority of our people. When total cessation of brain function was proposed as a new definition of death, the terminology struck a discordant note. It somehow clashed with the accepted definition hallowed by centuries of use. It smacked of modernity and was "antitheological." The inertia sensed by all who have tried to introduce brain-death legislation in the New York State Legislature is a direct result of this reliance by society on biblical sources for the critical definitions that affect our lives. A confidence gap that has widened rapidly between the physician and his patients made for an increased resistance to change.

How does biblical law evaluate brain death? Can it be accepted along with the more traditional indices of cessation of respiration and circulation? By brain death here is meant total cessation of brain function, not just cerebral death.

A status report on the ethical, legal, and medical considerations of brain death appeared last month.[1, 2] In the section written by me it is shown that earliest biblical authorities fully appreciated the distinction between cellular and

0077–8923/78/0315–0394 $01.75/0 © 1978, NYAS

organismal death. The decapitated individual is considered to have died immediately upon severance of the spinal cord although cardiac function had not ceased. The residual life is considered to be without ethical import "like the twitching of a lizard's amputated tail." [3] It should follow logically that irreversible loss of spontaneous respiration due to interruption of blood flow to the brain stem is tantamount to a physiologic decapitation. In this presentation I will not review the material contained in this recently published definitive study on brain death, but rather analyze nuances that deserve our attention.

It is not the definition of death but the delineation of death from the near-death state that presents the greatest ethical concern. This concern can best be summarized by focusing on two aspects: evaluation or certitude, and erosion or prognostication.

EVALUATION OF THE COMATOSE PATIENT

How accurate is the test? How benign is the test? An ethical society is one based on the axiom of the infinite worth of man. How infinite is this worth if there is a reluctance on the part of society to use the most valid test system available because it is troublesome? Those medical and legal experts who are drafting statutes to legalize neurologic criteria for defining death are most reluctant to include specific details of the testing protocol. Their reluctance is based on two concerns. They fear "freezing" the definition of death at this point in the development of biomedical science, precluding further technological advances. Statute revision is a long and tedious process. They hope to avoid it by keeping the present statute intentionally vague and all-inclusive. Their second concern is for the interprofessional rivalry that dictates a protective stance lest the legal profession be allowed to "practice medicine" by legislating medical practice.*

These concerns are not consequential when balanced against ethical considerations. If failure to specify in detail the Harvard criteria, the use of EEG, the length of time that the coma state must persist, the need to test for the absence of barbiturates or hypothermia, or to specify that criteria for adults may not be applicable to those fourteen years old or younger, may lead to a mistaken diagnosis by some less sophisticated physician, then it is an unethical statute. If angiographic or radioisotopic bolus techniques give a greater measure of confidence in the diagnosis of brain death, failure to require this technique is a flaw in the ethical structure of our society. It speaks of neglect of the patient rather than concern for "man created in God's image who is of infinite worth!" Indeed, smaller hospitals may not be equipped to do the angiography or radio-isotope evaluations. But an ethical society must be willing to sacrifice time, money, convenience, or even the potentially life-saving organs of a brain-dead patient, rather than infringe on the integrity of its ethical imperatives.

A second ethical concern in the evaluation process is the fear that the evaluation protocol may itself be stressful and therefore harmful to the dying

---

* The enormous restrictions imposed by detailed specifications of "criteria" in a law on brain death are noted elsewhere in this volume. I would only mention that should such specifications be included in the legislation, the limitations would not only preclude refinement of "criteria," but also prevent the application of clinical judgment in applying accepted guidelines. Medicine cannot be practiced by recipe.—*J. K.*

patient. There is a biblical prohibition against unnecessarily manipulating a patient *in extremis*. "A dying patient is like a flickering candle. If you but reach out to adjust it, the flame can be extinguished." [4] Angiography or even transport to the EEG room with manual respirator substituting for the automatic respirator may indeed be a physiologic stress to be avoided. Bedside radio-isotope measuring of brain perfusion may be the best evaluative technique for two reasons: its physiologic determinations and its benign protocol.

EROSION OR PROGNOSTICATION

The problem of erosion or ethical prognostication is a valid ethical concern of society. Like metabolic pathways, ethical behaviors mesh in gear-like fashion with other social patterns, ultimately transmitting direction to the entire machinery of society. Is a neurologic definition of death a "slippery slope" or wobbly domino that will bring down the whole house? Surely there must be a common denominator between liberalized abortion laws, Living Wills, God-squads, and liberalized or at least modified definitions of death. Will this new definition slowly erode the ethical foundation of our society and "eat its way" into "Quinlan" or sapient death, social-interaction death, or even social-utility death, so that whole races of mankind or religions may declare each other "brain dead!" Society must be concerned with the Domino Theory in social ethics. Not to do so is to live hand-to-mouth without any long-range planning. It is the right and privilege of our society to insist on safeguards for itself and for generations yet unborn. The rapidly maturing field of organ transplantation has increased this need for safeguards. The possibility of saving lives by transplanting kidneys, liver, lungs, cornea, pancreas, etc., adds a positive aspect to brain death—one that can sometimes be used to rationalize or justify a questionable decision. Will terminal care become more quickly terminal and much less caring because of the empathy for the young handsome teenager in need of a kidney or liver? There is both comfort and concern in the hospital protocol that requires the use of physicians other than those of the transplant team to declare the donor dead. The safeguard is provided but so is the nightmare. Does the profession really think so poorly of itself that it is prepared to cast suspicion on the integrity of the transplant team? Will they really grab the kidney before the patient is ready to let go? Surely not! Nevertheless hospital protocol must contain this safeguard if for no other reason than a reaffirmation of the ethical imperatives. Failure to continuously reaffirm our principles inevitably leads to neglect and abuse. Legislation by society must also reflect, in the very text of the law, the values and concerns that comprise the ethical substructure of our society. Only the insignificant can be taken for granted. Not to reflect these concerns in the repository of social values—our law—is to declare lack of concern.

There is another erosion possibility that is of ethical import. Will a patient without hope of recovery be subjected to vigorous, invasive therapy so as to maintain his organs until histocompatability studies can be completed on donor and recipient, or until the recipient can be located? Not too long ago the battle cry was "dying with dignity," a slogan for euthanasia. It is a bad slogan. The only way to die with dignity is to live with dignity. The dying process itself is fundamentally undignified. The new battle cry is "Don't waste a lifesaving potential." Harvest every organ and tissue that can be of value to someone in need. But at what price? Will "organ farms" lead to a bigger, richer, better society or will it be a dehumanizing influence that ultimately can destroy our society and our civilization. Every patient has a right of privacy which extends to his body even after death. If, when alive, he expressed his willingness to donate organs to someone in critical need, this expressed wish, with its magninimity of spirit and heart, is adequate reason for maintaining a brain-dead patient on a respirator until a recipient can be located. But if this wish was not expressed, then the protection of the patient's right of privacy and of proprietary ownership over his body—and to avoid dehumanizing our social conscience—demands that we even supersede the commitment to save lives. It is the "pushing of the button" to start the respirator that deserves ethical evaluation as well as the now famous concern for "pulling the plug" to discontinue the respiratory support. Surely if the patient is yet conscious but all available therapeutic modalities have been exhausted, any treatment that prolongs a life of pain and discomfort without offering the hope of cure or amelioration is an immoral treatment.[5] Any treatment for the benefit of another patient is likewise immoral. Man is not in man's servitude. The desire to serve our fellow man is the necessary outcome of our commitment to serve God, "Who made this world and all that is contained therein." It requires desire and intent to be of service, not helplessness and dependency on others. To treat the untreatable merely for the sake of organ preservation is but an early manifestation of man's enslavement to the more powerful members of society. This enslavement of the helpless and defenseless is the beginning of the end of moral social structure and ethical behavior.

The contributions of the medical sciences to social welfare are of inestimable value. There is no excuse for an adversary relationship between society and the medical practitioner. Yet such a relationship is a distinct possibility if the present climate continues. The willingness of the medical profession to enter into dialogue with society to jointly resolve the great ethical dilemmas can do much to resolve these dilemmas and re-establish a relationship of mutual trust and consideration.

REFERENCES

1. VEITH, F. J. et al. 1977. Brain death. I. A status report of medical and ethical considerations. JAMA **238:** 1651.
2. VEITH, F. J. et al. 1977. Brain death. II. A status report of legal considerations. JAMA **238:** 1744.
3. Babylonian Talmud. Mishneh Ohaloth **1:** 6.
4. Code of Laws. Yoreh Deah **339:** 1.
5. Talmud Bavli. Avoda Zara 18a and Ketuboth 104a.

CLINICAL PROBLEMS OF BRAIN DEATH AND COMA IN INTENSIVE CARE UNITS

Cary Suter and John Brush

Department of Neurology
Medical College of Virginia
Virginia Commonwealth University
Richmond, Virginia 23298

Given the proper physical facilities (ICUs), modern equipment (CT scan, portable EEG, cerebral arteriography), and properly trained personnel (physicians, nurses, and technicians), on duty for twenty-four hours, the major clinical problems concerning patients with coma and possible brain death can be solved. In such a situation, data can be obtained rapidly at the time of admission, and clinical decisions based on such data can be made with confidence and without fear of legal repercussions. If moral problems are involved, the presence of adequate data allows the alternatives to be more clearly defined. The major concerns of the physician should be: first, effective representation of the need for such resources to the community, institution, and government so that proper facilities, equipment and personnel may be made available; and, second, the use of these resources at a consistent level of medical excellence.

FACILITIES—INTENSIVE CARE UNITS

The intensive care unit is a recent development. It grew out of experience with recovery rooms where patients rendered comatose by anesthesia and suffering the recent trauma of surgery could be watched carefully and their vital signs monitored until they awoke and were ready to be transferred to regular hospital rooms. Now ICUs have proliferated and include coronary, respiratory, trauma, cardiac surgery, neurosurgery, neurology, general medical, general surgery, general pediatric, and high-risk infant units. Despite the frequent problem of coma and possible brain death, neurology ICUs have not been common. A number of years ago a neurology ICU was established at the Medical College of Virginia. It was located on the same floor as the neurosurgery ICU, which was nearly identical. As shown in FIGURE 1, this neurology intensive care unit also had access to nearby clinical neurophysiology laboratories which served both this unit and the neurosurgery intensive care unit. Recently, however, a new hospital at the Medical College of Virginia has been under construction, in which all the intensive care units will be placed on one floor, with radiology on the floor below and the operating rooms on the floor above. As shown in FIGURE 2, the neurosurgery and neurology intensive care units will have seven beds for neurology and seven beds for neurosurgery in the same unit, with immediately adjacent labs for neurophysiology and cerebral blood flow studies. This same neurophysiology laboratory will serve the entire intensive care floor and we will be able to record EEGs, cerebral evoked potentials, and EMGs in any of the intensive care units.

398

0077-8923/78/0315-0398 $01.75/0 © 1978, NYAS

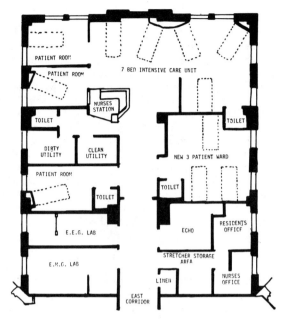

FIGURE 1. Present neurology intensive care unit at the Medical College of Virginia with adjacent neurophysiologic laboratories.

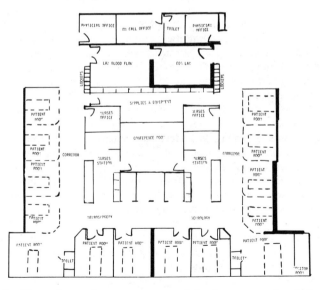

FIGURE 2. Planned neurology-neurosurgery intensive care units at the Medical College of Virginia with adjacent neurophysiologic and cerebral blood flow laboratories.

EQUIPMENT

Any hospital that undertakes to treat comatose patients must be persuaded also to provide adequate equipment for their care and study. Such equipment cannot be justified simply by the need for determination of brain death, but must be justified by its more important use, which is the rapid evaluation and care of the comatose patient. Adequate clinical pathology laboratories, toxicology laboratories, EEG equipment, and radiologic facilities must all be available, and consideration should be given to technological innovations such, for example, as the CT scanner, which is a rapid and noninvasive means of evaluating structural central nervous system lesions. At the Medical College of Virginia such equipment has been available round the clock for three years, but radioisotope equipment is not used for bedside bolus evaluation of cerebral circulation since its chief usefulness has been to determine brain death.[1] It is planned to combine this with other means of cerebral blood flow study in our new hospital. Portable equipment for EEG, EMG, cerebral evoked response, and ECHO is available.

PERSONNEL ON DUTY TWENTY-FOUR HOURS A DAY

Perhaps the most important element in the proper care of the comatose patient and in the determination of brain death is the availability of proper personnel on a twenty-four-hour basis. For more than ten years our EEG laboratories have been operating round the clock, chiefly because the Medical College of Virginia has been a large transplant center. Obviously, intensive care units must operate on a twenty-four-hour basis. It has been a perennially difficult problem to get adequately trained personnel for this type of medical work. It is difficult to convince communities, institutions, and government that such medical workers deserve special considerations as to salary. As far as twenty-four-hour operation of the EEG laboratory is concerned, one important element has been twenty-four-hour coverage by electroencephalographers. In the first place, we have a clear understanding with our EEG technologists that they will not be called in to do an EEG recording except by the neurology faculty or house staff. Second, an electroencephalographer is on call and must be called while the portable or emergency electroencephalogram is being recorded. If there is a question of brain death, the electroencephalographer comes to the hospital and aids in the completion of the EEG recording as well as in its interpretation. If there is any problem concerning the interpretation of the record of the patient in coma, the electroencephalographer also comes to the hospital. Such support for the technologist is an essential factor in job satisfaction.

It has also been very hard to get and keep nurses for our intensive care neurology unit—harder, in fact, for this unit than for the neurosurgery unit. Part of the reason is that patients admitted to the neurology unit are less often treated with quick and dramatic therapy. Ideally, from our experience, it appears that although neurology and neurosurgery intensive care units should be closely related, the actual nursing on the units should be carried out by separate teams.

RAPID EVALUATION OF THE PATIENT UPON ADMISSION

Given an intensive care unit with equipment and personnel as outlined above, complete baseline studies of the patient with coma or possible brain death can be carried out rapidly at the time of admission. In our neurology unit, it has been our aim with most comatose patients to have the blood drawn in the emergency room for the baseline blood chemistry, blood gas, and toxicology studies. Routine chest, skull, and possible cervical spine x-rays are done next, after, of course, resuscitation of the patient and institution of life-support measures, such as insertion of an intratracheal tube and use of respirator, as needed. Most patients in coma are then taken for a CT scan and admitted to the neurology intensive care unit. The availability of a CT scan for all patients either in coma or presenting the problem of possible brain death is tremendously helpful. The CT scan assures that 90 percent or better of possible intracranial mass lesions have been screened out at the time of admission. In our neurology unit we next obtain an electroencephalogram. At this point the clinical baseline has been established and clinical neurologic changes can be checked either hourly, or at three-hour intervals. This is done on a special neuroscience progress sheet which is used in both neurology and neurosurgery ICUs (FIGURE 3). Obviously, if particular metabolic or respiratory problems are found, the patient may be admitted to the appropriate medical ICU, and if particular intracranial mass lesions are found, the patient may be admitted directly to the neurosurgical ICU.

In our management of patients, particularly those with cerebral vascular disease, we have instituted a study in which the time sequence of the patient's care is diagrammed, with the patient's complete baseline data shown as having been obtained in the first two or three hours. An example of this is shown in FIGURE 4. FIGURE 5 shows the patient's CT scans. The rapid diagnosis of hypertensive intracerebral hemorrhage allowed better management of the patient, control of his blood pressure, and treatment with steroids and anticonvulsant drugs. As shown in FIGURE 4, this patient did well. Serial CT scans as seen in FIGURE 5 show the resolution of his cerebral hemorrhage.

At the Medical College of Virginia over the past three and a half years, the neurosurgical service under the direction of Dr. Donald Becker has instituted a policy of rapid study of all patients with head trauma who are not responsive to spoken command.[2] In this type of study, all patients had either an immediate twist drill air ventriculogram or, as at the present time, a CT scan. Special emphasis was put on regulation of respiration and blood gases, and on the treatment of mass lesions. In a number of patients, monitoring of intracranial pressure was carried out, and steroids and intravenous mannitol administered to prevent excessive intracranial pressure.[3] As a result of such aggressive management, 36 percent of these patients made a good recovery, 24 percent were moderately disabled, 8 percent were severely disabled, 2 percent were vegetative, and 30 percent died. The mortality rate compares favorably with outcomes in similar patients as reported from other centers, and there has been no increase in the number of severely disabled or vegetative patients.

THE USE OF THE CT SCAN IN COMA AND POSSIBLE BRAIN DEATH

As outlined above, it is our opinion that any patient in coma, and particularly any patient suspected of having brain death, should have a CT scan. The

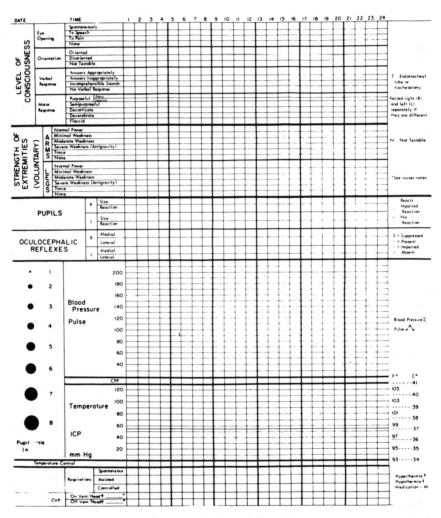

FIGURE 3. Neurologic evaluation and progress sheet for intensive care unit adapted from one that was developed by Dr. Graham Teasdale at the University of Glasgow, Scotland. (Fluid balance chart is on reverse side of the original sheet.)

simplest method is to obtain this scan at the time of admission. As shown in FIGURE 6, the CT scan obtained on an elderly patient at the time of admission shows a pontine hemorrhage. This scan allowed us to inform the family early of the desperate prognosis. In this particular case, the patient was the mother of an attorney and the family wished no unusual measures carried out. The patient was cared for in our intensive care unit, however, with ordinary respirator support. Even with this support she died within the first twenty-four hours.

FIGURE 6 shows the CT scan of a forty-year-old patient recently admitted in status epilepticus. This patient also had a history of hypertension. In this case we see a very large intracerebral hemorrhage and interventricular blood. The patient was treated with anticonvulsants, steroids, and antibiotics for pneumonia. This patient actually survived nine days. Neurosurgical consultation was obtained, but the decision was made not to intervene and also not to monitor the intracranial pressure.

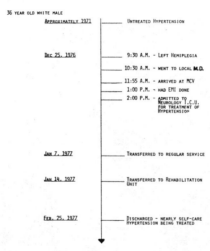

FIGURE 4. Time flow diagram showing the rapid evaluation of a patient with an intracerebral hemorrhage.

Artefact induced by movement of the patient can sometimes create considerable problems in performance and interpretation of CT scans. Such a situation is often seen in certain patients with acute brain lesions who have altered mental status. In this circumstance, a CT scan done after intubation and administration of short-acting barbiturates by an anesthesiologist allows clear delineation of any intracranial mass lesion. This is demonstrated in FIGURE 7.

USE OF THE ELECTROENCEPHALOGRAM IN PATIENTS WITH COMA AND POSSIBLE BRAIN DEATH

As outlined by Drs. Pampiglione and Bennett in their previous papers in this volume, the EEG can be of great value in evaluating the patient with coma and possible brain death. Even so, as a practical matter, the use of the EEG in

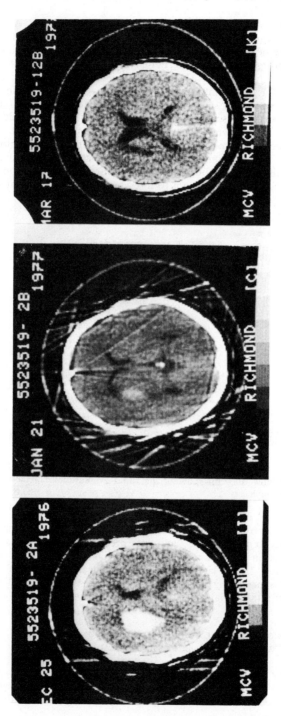

FIGURE 5. Serial CT scans in a patient with intracerebral hemorrhage and good recovery. (Left scan taken December 25, 1976; middle scan, January 2, 1977; right scan, March 17, 1977.)

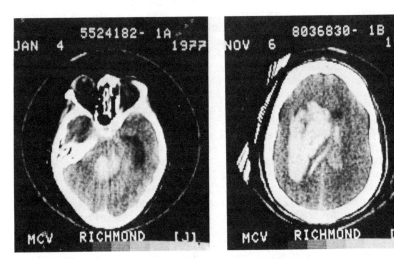

FIGURE 6. (*Left*) CT scan showing pontine hemorrhage in patient who survived 24 hours. (*Right*) CT scan showing intracerebral and intraventricular hemorrhage in a patient who survived 9 days.

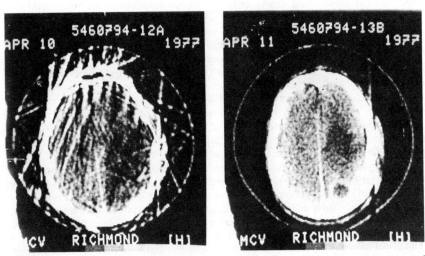

FIGURE 7. (*Left*) Movement artefact on CT scan done on patient who presented with headache, confusion and focal status epilepticus. (*Right*) Repeat CT scan six hours later on same patient after intubation and administration of short-acting barbiturate. No movement artefact is present and diagnosis of brain abscess was made.

some hospitals is limited because of the lack of a twenty-four-hour on-call system and because of the lack of experience on the part of technicians and electroencephalographers in performing frequent bedside recordings on comatose patients. As noted previously, location of the EEG laboratory close to the intensive care unit is a decided advantage. Experienced EEG technologists and electroencephalographers are a second necessary ingredient.

As far as the actual recording of the EEG is concerned, adherence to the criteria outlined by the American EEG Society is essential.[4] In addition to this, the most common problem has to do with artefacts from the confused and "unfriendly" environment of the acute care unit. A complete review of such artefacts has been presented in the *Atlas of Electroencephalography in Coma and Cerebral Death* published as a result of the NIH collaborative study.[5]

Of all the possible artefacts making an interpretation of the EEG difficult the most common is that of the muscle. At the Medical College of Virginia we have had an opportunity to study the effectiveness of succinylcholine in the control of muscle artefact.[6] Prior to 1972 succinylcholine was seldom used in our laboratory despite a large volume of records on patients in deep coma. Since 1972 we have used it frequently. Within the past eight years we have carried out approximately 800 portable EEG records, many of them in patients in deep coma. Such recordings were often for the purpose of helping to determine brain death since we have a large and active transplant program. A number of these recordings were done as part of the NIH collaborative study on cerebral survival. A study of our records for the years prior to 1972 shows that nearly 10 percent were considered inadequate for interpretation (usually because of muscle artefact) or were interpreted as showing slight cerebral activity, which on review appears most likely to be muscle artefact. On the other hand, a review of our EEG records since 1972 shows only 2 percent inadequate for interpretation, and in none of these was the question that of low-amplitude fast activity.

One case in particular illustrated this problem. This patient was studied in 1971 and five EEGs were recorded, one of these three hours prior to death. All of these records were interpreted as showing low-amplitude fast activity and not electrocerebral silence. Despite this fact, an autopsy performed three hours after death showed a so-called respirator brain. Almost certainly the brain was dead when the last EEG was made and almost certainly the low voltage activity seen in this record was due to muscle artefact and not to cerebral activity.

The use of succinylcholine is of equal importance to reveal the actual nature of cerebral activity of patients in deep coma where the activity present is otherwise obscured by muscle artefact (FIGURE 8).

Succinylcholine has universally been considered a relatively safe drug and is used every day in thousands of patients during anesthesia with very few serious side effects.[7] Nevertheless, succinylcholine may, on occasion, have adverse effects. Such effects include cardiac arrhythmias or cardiac standstill, prolonged paralysis in patients with genetic abnormality of pseudocholinesterase, and so-called malignant hyperpyrexia in patients with muscular dystrophy.[8-10] The effect of succinylcholine on the heart and circulatory system is complicated. It has been reported to produce tachycardia and increase blood pressure, particularly in anesthetized patients. Since it has almost never produced cardiac slowing or standstill in anesthetized patients, their occurrence is somewhat surprising. Nevertheless, in unanesthetized persons or animals, succinylcholine given rapidly, and particularly in repeated injections, has on occasion produced definite brachycardia and cardiac standstill. This has been proved secondary

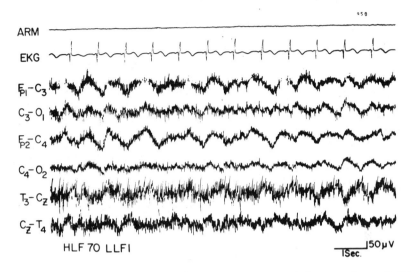

FIGURE 8A. Diffuse muscle artefact seen in electroencephalogram of a comatose patient.

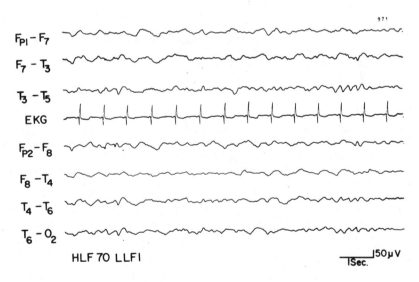

FIGURE 8B. Disappearance of muscle artefact following administration of succinylcholine.

to vagal stimulation and can be counteracted in animals by cutting the vagas nerve and in humans and animals by administering atropine.[11] At the Medical College of Virginia, we have seen only two untoward reactions to the use of succinylcholine. Both of these occurred after rapid injection of 40 to 100 mg of succinylcholine and consisted of brachycardia followed by cardiac standstill.

As a result of this experience, however, and because of the information from animal and human experiments, it is evident that succinylcholine can be given quite safely if it is given in a relatively slow intravenous infusion. Increased safety can be obtained by premedicating the patient with atropine or, if any brachycardia is seen, by giving an immediate injection of atropine. Using this technique we have not experienced this or other adverse effects of succinylcholine in the past three years. It has been reported that succinylcholine may cause cardiac arrest by producing hyperkalemia in patients with massive trauma or burns, but we have not had such a case.[12, 13]

From our experience with succinylcholine at the Medical College of Virginia we consider it a very safe and useful agent in recording of EEG in deep coma

TABLE 1

GUIDELINES FOR USE OF SUCCINYLCHOLINE IN EEG RECORDING

1. An adequate and definite reason for such a test.
2. Permission from attending physician and/or family.
3. Patient maintained on respirator.
4. Cardiac monitor (can be on EEG channel).
5. One EEG channel with observable muscle activity if possible.
6. Open, functioning intravenous infusion in place.
7. Premedicate with atropine or have atropine ready for injection if bradycardia occurs.
8. Succinylcholine in 1 to 4 mg/cc intravenous infusion given at a rate of not more than 4 mg per minute.
9. After succinylcholine continue EEG recording until muscle activity returns.
10. If test is repeated, wait at least 15 minutes.

and in the determination of electrocerebral silence. From this experience we have drawn up a list of guidelines (TABLE 1) and we believe that if these are followed, succinylcholine can be used with confidence.

At times we use pancuronium bromide instead of succinylcholine, but this takes longer to act and recovery is longer.[14]

In many institutions the electroencephalographers are not experienced in interpretation of electroencephalograms of patients in coma. As an example, for years alpha-frequency coma records were called normal. In our experience with more than 25 cases of such recordings it is obvious that diffuse brain damage is present as a cause of this type of recording.[15, 16] Although some diffuse damage is present, nearly a third of such patients may return to normal or nearly normal function. Other patterns, such as continuous state of theta-frequency coma, may seem only mildly abnormal, but are often associated with both diffuse and brain-stem damage of a severe degree [17, 18] (FIGURE 9). On the other hand, a record with diffuse large delta waves or a record with diffuse symmetrical spindle activity, although indeed abnormal, may be associated with a good outcome and

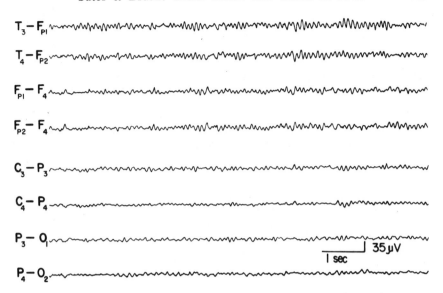

FIGURE 9A. This record shows so-called alpha-frequency coma in a patient comatose after cardiorespiratory arrest from a severe electric shock. He achieves nearly complete recovery. Some slight memory defect remains.

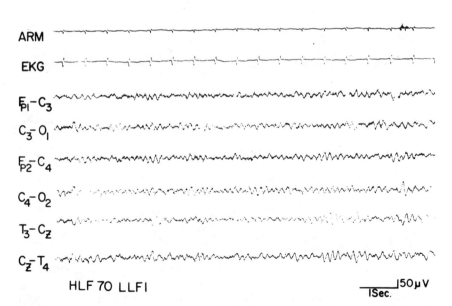

FIGURE 9B. This record shows so-called theta-frequency coma in a patient comatose after an acute brain-stem lesion.

recovery (FIGURE 10). Other patterns, such as burst suppression records and records showing only brief myoclonic jerks with electrocerebral silence between, are distinctly abnormal and almost always associated with a poor prognosis.

Not only are individual records important in understanding coma, but the direction of change may be quite important as well. In the study of patients with Reye's syndrome the electroencephalogram often gives the best indication of the direction the case is taking.[19]

Recently, cerebral evoked potential measurements have become available. The far-field auditory responses give a measure of brain-stem function [20] and the visual evoked potentials give a measure of optic nerve and occipital lobe function.[21] These tests have usually been most useful in uncovering minimal damage in patients who may appear clinically well. In patients with coma they are often clearly abnormal in accordance with what one would expect from a clinical examination. In a study at the Medical College of Virginia by Greenberg and Becker cerebral evoked potentials are shown to be of some usefulness in head injury cases.[22, 23] Even so, they give no measure of the anterior half of the cerebral hemispheres. Fortunately, practical and movable equipment is available for the carrying out of these tests, so if they are useful in a study of patients with coma and possible brain death, the tests can be made readily available.

SEIZURES AND COMATOSE PATIENTS

Many patients with severe brain damage have severe and repeated seizures. In cerebral anoxia the occurrence of repeated myoclonic seizures is an ominous sign. In patients with other lesions, such as cerebral hemorrhage or trauma,

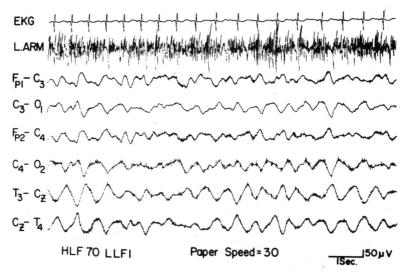

FIGURE 10A. This record shows diffuse delta activity in a comatose patient with encephalitis. After a four-week period of coma the patient awoke and achieved good recovery.

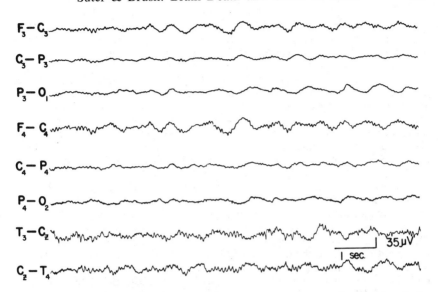

FIGURE 10B. This record shows diffuse delta activity intermixed with spindle activity in a comatose patient with a cerebellar hematoma and compression of the brain stem. Removal of the hematoma resulted in nearly complete recovery of the patient.

uncontrolled seizures may cause the underlying lesion to produce more swelling, pressure, and deterioration of the patient.

At the present time it has been our experience that the ideal treatment is immediate intravenous use of diazepam (Valium®) which frequently will give a quick control of seizures, followed by a loading dose of phenytoin given intra-veniously.[24] Usually phenobarbital is not used because of its depressant effect and the possible increase in degree of coma. However, because of its known protection of the brain in the presence of decreased blood flow, at some point a trial of reasonably large doses of phenobarbital might be considered in certain types of coma.

PROBLEMS RELATED TO ORGAN TRANSPLANT

Obviously, the desire to use organs for transplantation is a major impetus in establishing criteria for brain death. In a large transplant center such as the Medical College of Virginia patients may actually be sent to the emergency room or to the hospital for the sole purpose of being a donor of organs. Also, patients with severe gunshot wounds or head injury may be resuscitated and maintained in the emergency rooms for this reason. Ideally, all such patients should be officially admitted to an intensive care unit and the usual routine for determining brain death carried out. It is very hard to carry out proper testing in the emergency room.

Since transplantation of organs is indeed a life-saving measure for certain patients it is proper that physicians other than those on the transplant team should be concerned with providing such organs. It is for this reason that for more than a decade our EEG laboratory has been operated on a twenty-four-hour basis and we have been particularly anxious to record electroencephalograms early so that if the criteria for brain death are present, determination can be made quickly and the transplantation of organs carried out. For a number of years we have taken as criteria of brain death the usual clinical findings plus an electroencephalogram showing a 30-minute period of electrocerebral silence recorded six hours or more after the event that caused loss of spontaneous respiration and brain-stem function. In other cases where the event cannot be clearly identified we have insisted on a period of six hours between two EEG recordings, both of which show electrocerebral silence. We have recently outlined our criteria for brain death (APPENDIX I).

In relation to patients with possible brain death it is important that the physician keep a clear idea of his role. If one is requested to see the patient as an electroencephalographer, then the only opinion requested and the only opinion to be put on the chart has to do with a determination of electrocerebral silence. If, however, the physician is asked to see the patient as a neurologic consultant concerning the question of brain death, the whole case must then be reviewed in detail, the patient examined meticulously, and an opinion rendered outlining the criteria upon which it is based. Fortunately, the state of Virginia was one of the first to pass a law recognizing "brain death" as one criterion used to declare a patient medically and legally dead (APPENDIX II).

EVALUATION OF THE PATIENT WITH LONG-STANDING COMA

On several occasions we have been persuaded to admit patients to an intensive care unit for evaluation of a comatose state that has been in existence for a period of two weeks to three or four months. In general, this has not been a rewarding experience. This length of coma alone makes the possibility of recovery unlikely. If, indeed, any evidence of recovery occurs then the family is insistent upon continued care of the patient in the hope of further recovery. In one of our patients admitted after more than two weeks of coma with little or no responsiveness but with spontaneous respiration the electroencephalogram showed a rather typical theta coma (FIGURES 8 and 9). Over a period of six weeks this patient did gain some responsiveness to the spoken word and eventually was able to speak one or two words. Even so, now a year later, this patient remains essentially quadraplegic and with very limited language function. This patient's family still views our predictions of a poor outcome as misguided, while we are inclined to feel the predictions were correct. This would suggest the view that an intensive care unit should not be used for prolonged periods for evaluation of the patient with chronic coma.

PROBLEMS RELATED TO CONSULTANTS

Any extremely ill patient often requires numerous consultants. The patient may need an infectious disease consultation, cardiac consultation, pulmonary consultation, and a variety of surgical consultations, particularly a neurosurgical opinion. If all of these consultants agree this is fine, but when there is disagreement, there must be a strong primary physician who directs the management of the case. Sometimes in intensive care units it may not be clear who that physician is. For each patient, however, this should be clarified, if at all possible.

If there is a real problem of management or difference of opinion among consultants or if the family appears to be unhappy with the patient's management, it is essential that additional consultation be obtained. At this point it is often useful to bring in a consultant from outside the particular hospital. Ideally, two or three outstanding authorities may be mentioned and the family allowed to choose among them. The family should also be asked if there is any physician in whom they have unusual confidence and this physician might be contacted, either as a consultant or simply to give information about the case.

TESTING FOR SPONTANEOUS RESPIRATION

In the determination of brain death, tests of whether or not the patient has spontaneous respiration need to be carried out. In past times removing the patient from the respirator for two, three or four minutes was a common practice. Obviously, this had implications of possible further anoxic damage to the patient. Fortunately, we have now learned that this test can be carried out safely, as described previously in this symposium. This has also been described by other authors,[25] and this or some modification of such testing can now become a standard procedure when indicated.

PSYCHOLOGICAL PROBLEMS RELATED TO COMA AND POSSIBLE BRAIN DEATH

A great deal has been written recently about rational attitudes towards death, particularly in terminally ill patients. Most of this, however, has concerned patients who are themselves conscious and capable of being aware of their predicament. In comatose patients the burden falls primarily upon family and friends, often suddenly and unexpectedly. In the context of acute illness or trauma, shock, denial, guilt, and a great variety of emotions are manifest. These are, of course, in considerable contrast to the emotional reactions of the physicians, nurses, and other hospital personnel, who, by their daily work, are schooled and conditioned to deal in a controlled and matter-of-fact manner with comatose and dying patients. In this situation physicians and other medical personnel must strive to show compassion. Although the physician should deal honestly with the patient and his family, there should be a constant recognition of the uncertainty of any situation so long as life remains. The physician should also be sensitive to the family's religious orientation and be willing to talk to the family's minister, rabbi, priest, or religious advisor if the family so desires.

SUMMARY

Present knowledge and technology allow us to make an unequivocal determination of brain death, at least in adults. These same medical resources can also be life-saving and should be applied rapidly and efficiently to all patients admitted in coma. At the present time the means are available to make precise diagnoses concerning the cause and possible outcome of coma in most cases. The development of the CT scan and the aggressive use of electroencephalography are most important in these capacities.

It is the responsibility of the physician to aid in the development and planning of up-to-date ICUs with their associated laboratories and equipment and in providing rewarding salaries and positions for the hosts of nurses, technologists, and others necessary to operate these on a twenty-four-hour basis.

Although the problems of coma and of brain death can be dealt with by the physician given these resources, the problem of the person severely brain-damaged and in a so-called vegetative state remains. This is a problem for the society, the law, and religion.

REFERENCES

1. BRAUNSTEIN, P., J. KOREIN, I. KRICHEFF, K. COREY & N. CHASE. 1973. A simple bedside evaluation of cerebral blood flow in the study of cerebral death: A prospective study on 34 deeply comatose patients. Am. J. Roentgenol. **118:** 757.
2. BECKER, D. P., J. D. MILLER, J. D. WARD, R. P. GREENBERG, H. F. YOUNG & R. SAKALAS. 1977. The outcome from severe head injury with early diagnosis and intensive management. J. Neurosurg. **47:** 491–502.
3. MILLER, J. D., D. P. BECKER, J. D. WARD, H. G. SULLIVAN, W. E. ADAMS & M. J. ROSNER. 1977. Significance of intracranial hypertension in severe head injury. J. Neurosurg. **47:** 503–516.
4. 1976. American Electroencephalographic Society: Guidelines in EEG. American Electroencephalographic Society.
5. BENNETT, D. R., J. R. HUGHES & J. KOREIN, et al. 1976. Atlas of Electroencephalography in Coma and Cerebral Death. Raven Press. New York, N.Y.
6. SUTER, C. 1975. The use of succinylcholine in the determination of electrocerebral silence. Electroencephalogr. Clin. Neurophysiol. **38:** 553.
7. WOOD-SMITH, F. G., H. C. STEWART & M. D. VICKERS. 1968. Muscle Relaxants. Drugs in Anesthetic Practice, 3rd. ed. : 243–267. Appleton-Century-Crofts. New York, N.Y.
8. WILLIAMS, C. H., S. DEUTSCH, H. W. LINDE, J. W. BULLOUGH & R. D. DRIPPS. 1961. Effects of intravenously administered succinyldicholine on cardiac rate, rhythm, and arterial blood pressure in anesthetized man. Anesthesiology **22:** 947–954.
9. SCHEONSTADT, D. A. & C. E. WHITCHER. 1963. Observations on the mechanism of succinyldicholine-induced cardiac arrhythmias. Anesthesiology **24:** 358–362.
10. KALOW, W. 1965. Genetic factors in relation to drugs. Ann. Rev. Pharmacol. **5:** 9–26.
11. BERETERVIDE, K. V. 1965. Actions of succinylcholine chloride on the circulation. Brit. J. Pharmacol. Chemother. **10:** 265–269.
12. BAKER, B. B., J. A. WAGNER & W. G. HEMENWAY. 1972. Succinylcholine-induced hyperkalemia and cardiac arrest. Arch. Otolaryng. **96:** 464–465.
13. VIBY-MOGENSEN, J., H. K. HANEL, E. HANSEN & J. GRAAE. 1975. Serum cholinesterase activity in burned patients. II: Anaesthesia, suxamethonium and hyperkalaemia. Acta Anaesth. Scand. **19:** 169–179.
14. SPEIGHT, T. M. & G. S. AVERY. 1972. Pancuronium bromide: A review of its pharmacological properties and clinical application. Drugs **4:** 163–226.
15. GRINDAL, A. B. & C. SUTER. 1975. Alpha-pattern coma in high voltage electrical injury. Electroencephalogr. Clin. Neurophysiol. **38:** 521–526.
16. GRINDAL, A. B., C. SUTER & A. J. MARTINEZ. 1977. Alpha-pattern coma: 24 cases with 9 survivors. Ann. Neurol. **1:** 371–377.
17. SUTER, C. 1973. Theta coma (abstract). Neurology **23:** 445.
18. SUTER, C. 1974. Clinical advances in the evaluation of deep coma. MCV Quart. **10**(3): 152–162.

19. AOKI, Y. & C. T. LOMBROSO. 1973. Prognostic value of electroencephalography in Reye's syndrome. Neurology 23: 333–343.

20. STARR, A. & L. J. ACHIR. 1975. Auditory brain stem responses in neurological disease. Arch. Neurol. 32.

21. ASSELMAN, P. et al. 1975. Visual evoked responses in the diagnosis and management of patients suspected of multiple sclerosis. Brain 98: 91–100.

22. GREENBERG, R. P., D. J. MAUER, D. P. BECKER & D. J. MILLER. 1977. Evaluation of brain function in severe human head trauma with multimodality evoked potentials. I. Evoked brain-injury potentials, methods and analysis. J. Neurosurg. 47: 150–177.

23. GREENBERG, R. P., D. P. BECKER, J. D. MILLER & D. J. MAYER. 1977. Evaluation of brain function in severe human head trauma with multimodality evoked potentials. II. Localization of brain dysfunction and correlation with post-traumatic neurological conditions. J. Neurosurg. 47: 163–177.

24. SUTER, C. 1977. Acute seizure problems. MCV Quart. 13(3): 116–122.

25. SCHAEFER, J. & J. J. CARONNA. 1978. Duration of apnea needed to confirm brain death. Neurology 28: 661–666.

APPENDIX I

CRITERIA FOR ESTABLISHMENT OF BRAIN DEATH

Where, from the history and medical record, it is clear that the patient has suffered a sudden and definable episode of brain damage, either from cerebral anoxia, severe head trauma or wounds, or sudden stoppage of respiratory function in the course of illness such as brain tumor, or cerebral hemorrhage, then the following conditions, if they are found six hours or more following such an insult and exist for a period of thirty minutes, shall be considered sufficient criteria for declaring brain death. These criteria shall include the absence of severe hypothermia and the absence of drug overdose; the presence for thirty minutes or more of electrocerebral silence recorded according to the standards set forth by the Ad Hoc Committee of the American EEG Society and interpreted by a duly licensed physician who regularly functions as a specialist in electroencephalography; the absence for a period of thirty minutes of any evidence of cerebral responsivity to any stimuli; the absence of all cranial nerve reflexes; the presence of dilated fixed pupils; evidence that there is no spontaneous respiration. These findings must be confirmed by a consultant in neurology or neurosurgery and be reviewed and concurred in by the attending physician.

In the absence of a clear time of onset of the cerebral insult, then the above conditions must be met for a period of thirty minutes and recorded again six hours later for another period of thirty minutes. If, at this point, the attending physician, the consulting neurologist or neurosurgeon or the electroencephalographer have any doubts that brain death has occurred then other tests (such as tests of cerebral blood flow) should be done and an additional period of time shall be allowed to elapse until the consultants and the attending physician agree that the criteria for brain death have been completely met.

It should be clearly understood by the physicians, nurses and other paramedical personnel as well as by the patient's family that in the presence of brain death, regular cardiac function may remain quite a long time and also that spinal reflexes resulting in the reflex movements of the body below the neck may occur. It should also be understood that these criteria have not yet been established for infants or newborns.

APPENDIX II

CHAPTER 252

An Act to amend the Code of Virginia by adding a section numbered 32-364.3:1 relating to definition of death.

(H 1727)

Approved March 13, 1973

Be it enacted by the General Assembly of Virginia:

1. That the Code of Virginia be amended by adding a section numbered 32-364.3:1 as follows:

§ 32-364.3:1. A person shall be medically and legally dead if, (a) in the opinion of a physician duly authorized to practice medicine in this State, based on the ordinary standards of medical practice, there is the absence of spontaneous respiratory and spontaneous cardiac functions and, because of the disease or condition which directly or indirectly caused these functions to cease, or because of the passage of time since these functions ceased, attempts at resuscitation would not, in the opinion of such physician, be successful in restoring spontaneous life-sustaining functions, and, in such event, death shall be deemed to have occurred at the time these functions ceased; or (b) in the opinion of a consulting physician, who shall be duly licensed and a specialist in the field of neurology, neurosurgery, or electroencephalography, when based on the ordinary standards of medical practice, there is the absence of spontaneous brain functions and spontaneous respiratory functions and, in the opinion of the attending physician and such consulting physician, based on the ordinary standards of medical practice and considering the absence of the aforesaid spontaneous brain functions and spontaneous respiratory functions and the patient's medical record, further attempts at resuscitation or continued supportive maintenance would not be successful in restoring such spontaneous functions, and, in such event, death shall be deemed to have occurred at the time when these conditions first coincide. Death, as defined in subsection (b) hereof, shall be pronounced by the attending physician and recorded in the patient's medical record and attested by the aforesaid consulting physician.

Norwithstanding any statutory or common law to the contrary, either of these alternative definitions of death may be utilized for all purposes in the Commonwealth, including the trial of civil and criminal cases.

_____
President of the Senate

_____
Speaker of the House of Delegates

Approved:

_____
Governor

BRAIN DEATH AND ORGAN TRANSPLANTATION *†

Frank J. Veith

Montefiore Hospital
Bronx, New York 10467; and the
Albert Einstein College of Medicine
Bronx, New York 10461

Brain death is a term commonly used to describe a condition in which the brain is completely destroyed and in which cessation of function of all other organs is imminent and inevitable. The concept of brain death is important to consider since advances in medical technology have resulted in the artificial prolongation of the overall process of dying. In the past, cessation of heartbeat and spontaneous respiration always produced prompt death of the brain, and, similarly, destruction of the brain resulted in prompt cessation of respiration and circulation. In this context it was reasonable that absence of pulse and respiration became the traditional criteria for pronouncement of death. Recently, however, technological advances have made it possible to sustain brain function in the absence of spontaneous respiratory and cardiac function, so that the death of a person can no longer be equated with the loss of these latter two natural vital functions. Furthermore, it is now possible that a person's brain may be completely destroyed even though his circulation and respiration are being artificially maintained by mechanical devices.

It has been argued persuasively that a person whose brain is totally destroyed is in fact dead, and this premise has gained considerable acceptance throughout the world from the public and from professionals in various relevant fields. Accordingly, the pronouncement of death on the basis of irreversible cessation of all brain function has become common. Such brain-death pronouncements are important in organ transplantation because they facilitate the procurement of cadaver organs that are undamaged by ischemic injury or hasty removal. This is the case because, if the brain-death concept is accepted and used, organs can be carefully and deliberately removed without significant ischemic damage from a donor whose circulation is artificially maintained after death has been pronounced on brain-related criteria.

Since physicians associated with transplantation have a vested interest in the acceptance and utilization of brain-related criteria for the pronouncement of death, it is important that they examine the issues related to brain death not from their own or their patients' perspective but from the points of view of others interested in the subject. The present article does this and attempts to

* This work was supported in part by Grants Nos. HL 17417 and HL 16476 from the United States Public Health Service and by the Manning Foundation.

† Many of the concepts expressed herein are based on a pair of articles [1,2] jointly authored by Dr. Veith and Jack M. Fein, M.D., of the Department of Neurosurgery, Albert Einstein College of Medicine; Moses D. Tendler, Ph.D., of the Departments of Biology and Talmudic Law, Yeshiva University; Robert M. Veatch, Ph.D., of the Hastings Institute of Society, Ethics and the Life Sciences; and Marc A. Kleiman, J.D., LL.M., and George Kalkines, J.D., of the New York City Health and Hospitals Corporation.

0077–8923/78/0315–0417 $01.75/0 © 1978, NYAS

establish the scientific, social, philosophical, theological, and legal validity of the brain-death concept and how its use or nonuse will have an impact on society in general.

Any ethical or legal considerations concerning pronouncements of death on a neurologic basis must be founded on the certainty that a person who meets the clinical and laboratory criteria has had actual complete destruction of the brain. In 1968 guidelines were formulated by an Ad Hoc Committee of the Harvard Medical School to permit the determination of irreversible coma.[3] These Harvard criteria require that neurologic examinations disclose unreceptivity, unresponsiveness, absence of spontaneous movements and breathing, absent reflexes, fixed dilated pupils, and persistence of all these findings over a 24-hour period in the absence of intoxicants or hypothermia. A persistently isoelectric electroencephalogram over the same period is also required to confirm the clinical examination. Since 1968 the validity of these widely used criteria has been established in several ways.

These validations include the substantial morphologic evidence that, when the criteria have been fulfilled, there is widespread destruction of the brain. Richardson has found that all the brains of 128 patients meeting the Harvard criteria showed extensive destructive changes.[4] In a larger series of autopsy studies, however, the exact nature and distribution of these fatal morphologic lesions in the brain were also shown to be dependent on the etiology and on the interval between fulfillment of the Harvard criteria and pathologic examination.[5] The latter observation is consistent with the well-known finding in other organs that time must often elapse before morphologic evidence of cellular destruction can be detected.

In addition, patients who fulfill the Harvard criteria have been shown by isotopic techniques to have no significant intracranial blood flow,[6] and absent intracranial blood flow over a 10–15 minute interval is uniformly associated with subsequent necrosis and liquefaction of the brain.[7] The latter finding is based on autopsy studies from several Scandinavian hospitals of more than 120 patients who had nonvisualization of intracranial arteries after cerebral angiography with contrast injections repeated over a 10–15-minute interval. In related studies from several centers, clinical and electroencephalographic evidence of complete brain destruction was almost always associated with angiographic evidence of cessation of intracranial blood flow.[8-11]

Another validation of the Harvard criteria derives from cooperative studies of the value of electroencephalography and neurologic examination in the determination of complete brain destruction.[12, 13] In these studies, members of the American Electroencephalographic Society and of electroencephalographic societies in Europe were questioned. Of the 2,642 cases under study, there was no instance of recovery in a patient who fulfilled the Harvard criteria. Furthermore, since 1970, there have been no adequately documented examples in which the Harvard criteria could be considered invalid.[14] Moreover, many authorities presently consider these criteria too strict in at least two regards.[14-19] First, it has been shown that spinal reflexes, including withdrawal movements, may

‡ This section was written in collaboration with Jack M. Fein.

persist after complete destruction of the brain. Second, it is believed that certain determination that the brain is totally destroyed can be made even when the period of clinical and electroencephalographic evidence of absent brain function is reduced to less than 24 hours.§ The latter is consistent with the opinion that methods for measuring intracranial blood flow will allow a sure determination of complete destruction to be made with periods of observation less than the 24 hours proposed in the original Harvard criteria.[6-11, 17]

Further support for the use of less restrictive criteria is provided by the recently completed Collaborative Study on Cerebral Survival, which was based on an analysis of 503 unresponsive apneic patients. From this experience it was concluded that if all appropriate diagnostic and therapeutic procedures had been performed to exclude reversible conditions, brain destruction was always present if certain criteria were observed for at least 30 minutes, six hours or more after the cerebral insult had occurred. The specified criteria were unresponsivity, apnea, dilated fixed pupils and absent cephalic reflexes, electrocerebral (EEG) silence, and confirmation of absent cerebral blood flow by angiography, isotopic bolus techniques, or echoencephalography.[18, 20, 21] The confirmatory test for absent cerebral blood flow was not deemed necessary in cases where the obvious etiologic factor was known to be a nontreatable condition, such as massive trauma to the brain.

Although some groups have indicated that electroencephalography is not required to determine that brain death has occurred,[16, 22] and although many neurologists and neurosurgeons would agree that brain death can safely be pronounced in the absence of a test for electrocerebral silence in the occasional patient, the recommendation that electroencephalographic criteria be met before brain death is pronounced is probably best for general usage.[17-20, 23] This recommendation appears advisable at present in the light of a report that a patient who ultimately recovered had met the clinical criteria of brain death but never had electrocerebral silence,[24] and in view of the current trend toward increasingly frequent medical malpractice suits.

A final validation of the criteria for measuring total destruction of the brain has been an attempt on the part of the authors to explore purported anecdotal exceptions. In every instance where recovery of brain function was claimed, the criteria had not been fulfilled. Thus, the validity of the criteria must be considered to have been established with as much certainty as is possible in biology or medicine.

PHILOSOPHICAL BASIS FOR USE OF BRAIN-RELATED CRITERIA
FOR PRONOUNCING DEATH ||

The principal reason for deciding that a person is dead should be based on a fundamental understanding of the nature of man. Our present conceptualization of man almost reflexively draws a distinction between a person whose organs are under nervous system influence and the remnant of a person or his

---

§ The immature brain is more resistant to all forms of insult. Therefore, altered, less restrictive criteria for determining total brain destruction in patients under 14 years of age may differ from those in adults. (See the paper by Pampiglione in this volume.)

|| This section was written in collaboration with Robert M. Veatch.

corpse in which residual and nonhomeostatic functions may or may not have completely ceased. Without a brain, the body becomes the convenient medium in which the energy-requiring states of organs run down and the organs decay. These residual activities do not confer an iota of humanity or personality. Thus, in the circumstance of brain death, neither a human being nor a person exists any longer.

Although all members of society will not be able to agree precisely on an acceptable formulation of man's nature, fortunately all that is necessary to establish a public policy is agreement on some widely acceptable, general statements about the nature of man. Almost all segments of society will agree that some capacity to think, to perceive, to respond, and to regulate and integrate bodily functions is essential to human nature. Thus, if none of these brain functions is present and will ever return, it is no longer appropriate to consider the person as a whole as being alive.

If there were no offense, no moral or social costs in treating dead persons as if they were alive, then the safer course would be to continue to do so. Quite clearly, however, this is not the case. In addition to reflecting an inadequate understanding of the nature of man, it is an affront to the individual person or that person's memory to treat a human being who has irreversibly lost all brain function as if he were alive. It confuses the person with his corpse and is morally wrong.

Furthermore, maintenance of a dead person on life-support systems for no reason is an irresponsible squandering of our economic and social resources. Such a practice places an unnecessary financial burden on society and an additional emotional burden on the person's family and is thereby also morally wrong. Thus, even without consideration of the use of the body or its organs for transplantation or other altruistic purposes, there are sound moral and social reasons for treating a body that has lost significant thinking, perceiving, responding, regulating, and integrating capacities as dead. Of course, it is a waste of human resources and a further wrong to continue treating a corpse as if it were alive when such treatment may deprive other living persons of needed organs.

ACCORD OF BRAIN-DEATH CONCEPT WITH ORTHODOX JEWISH LAW ¶

The Orthodox Jewish response to the premise that death may be pronounced on brain-related criteria is, like much of the moral conscience of Western civilization, based on biblical and Talmudic ethical imperatives. According to these, it is axiomatic that human life is of infinite worth. A corollary of this is that a fleeting moment of life is of inestimable worth because a piece of infinity is also infinite. The taking or shortening of a human life is therefore ethically wrong; and premature termination of life or euthanasia is no less murder for the good intentions which were the motivation for the immoral act.

The indices of life are many. Which of them can be viewed, in ethical or religious terms, as the definition or *sine qua non* of the living state rather than a mere confirmation that the patient is still living? It is first important to point out that absent heartbeat or pulse was *not* considered a significant factor in ascertaining death in any early religious sources.[25] Furthermore, the scientific fact that cellular death does not occur at the same time as the death of the

¶ This section was written in collaboration with Moses D. Tendler.

human being is well recognized in the earliest biblical sources. The twitching of a lizard's amputated tail or the death throes of a decapitated man were never considered residual life, but simply manifestations of cellular life that continued after death of the entire organism had occurred.[26] In the situation of decapitation, death can be defined or determined by the decapitated state itself as recognized in the Talmud and the Code of Laws.[26-28] Complete destruction of the brain, which includes loss of all integrative, regulatory and other functions of the brain, can be considered physiologic decapitation and thus a determinant *per se of* death of the person.

Loss of the ability to breathe spontaneously is a crucial criterion for determining whether complete destruction of the brain has occurred. Earliest biblical sources recognized the ability to breathe independently as a prime index of life.[25, 29] The biblical verse in Genesis records: "And the Lord had fashioned man of dust of the earth and instilled in his nostrils the breath of life and man became a living creature." [29] Spontaneous respiration is thus an indicator of the living state. However, it cannot be considered its definition, since a respirator patient whose sole defect is paralysis of the motor neurons to the muscles of respiration due to neurologic disease is surely fully alive despite his inability to breathe spontaneously. Therefore, to define death in biblical terms, loss of respiration must be combined with other more obvious evidence of the nonliving state. Such evidence would be provided by the clinical and laboratory criteria that allow a physician to determine that complete and irreversible destruction of the brain or physiologic decapitation has occurred.

The higher integrative functions of the brain are carried out by portions of the brain other than the brain stem. Irreversible loss of these functions, signifying destruction of corresponding parts of the brain, does not alone constitute a determinant of death in biblical terms. Coincident loss of vegetative functions, represented by loss of spontaneous respiration and indicating destruction of the brain stem, is also a requisite. Thus, destruction of the entire brain, or brain death, and only that, is consonant with biblical pronouncements on what constitutes an acceptable definition of death, i.e., the state in a patient who has all the appearances of lifelessness and who is no longer breathing spontaneously. Patients with irreversible total destruction of the brain fulfill this definition even if heart action and circulation are artificially maintained. This definition is also fulfilled in patients who die with or from irreversible cessation of heart action, because this results in a failure to perfuse the brain, which produces total brain destruction. Thus, cessation of heart action is a cause of death rather than a component of its definition. In the light of these considerations, the Harvard criteria or other neurologic criteria for determining death can be viewed as the scientific expression of those observations which, until recently, were the actual way a patient was known to be dead.

The tumult that has greeted the suggestion that brain death be given legal recognition is partly the reaction of an uninformed public who envision the possibility that a man who can move, feel, and think or who could possibly recover these functions if he had lost them could be erroneously declared dead. The realization that the expression "brain death" is only professional jargon used to describe the state of a patient who exhibits a permanent loss of signs of life, such as spontaneous movement and responsivity, and who has permanently lost the ability to breathe spontaneously, would facilitate society's acceptance of the concept of brain death and would help to gain public support for legislation recognizing that death may be pronounced on the basis of total and irreversible destruction of the brain.

Since the distinction between cellular and organismal death is valid, once the death of the person has occurred and can be determined, there is no biblical obligation to maintain treatment or artificial support of the corpse. Thus, there is no religious imperative to continue to use a respirator to inflate and deflate the lungs, thereby maintaining the cellular viability of other organs in an otherwise dead patient.[30]

Accord of Brain-Death Concept with Roman Catholic Ethics **

Roman Catholic theologians have generally accepted a concept of death based on brain function, although there is no single authoritative pronouncement. The traditional Roman Catholic understanding of the moment of real death has been based on the time of departure of the soul from the body. Since this separation is not an observable phenomenon, it must be related to physically measurable signs for defining apparent death. Because the only certain signs have been the appearance of rigor mortis and the beginning of bodily decomposition, it has been recognized that real death may not coincide with apparent death. Use of such signs as cessation of heartbeat and breathing places the moment of apparent death in greater proximity to the time of true theological death. For practical reasons, theologians have accepted these signs of apparent death as reasonably accurate indicators of irreversible cessation of all vital bodily functions adequate for allowing such processes as embalming and autopsy. When artificial life-support systems are used to maintain heart and lung function and when the brain is irreversibly destroyed, there is also no reasonable hope of restoring vital bodily functions to a person. Accordingly, "It would seem that death is more certain under these conditions than it was at the [time of] cessation of spontaneous heart and lung function. If theologians were willing to accept the latter as signs of apparent death, they should be more willing to accept the irreversible cessation of brain function." [31]

A similar position has been reached by the Catholic theologian, Father Bernard Häring,[32] who after analysis of the theological arguments concludes, "I feel that the arguments for the equation of the total death of the person with brain death are fully valid." In the same vein, the prominent author on Roman Catholic interpretations of medical ethics, Charles J. McFadden, argues that "once the fact of brain death has been established, *the person is dead,* even though heartbeat and respiration are continued by mechanical means." [33] These statements are consistent with the discourse of Pope Pius XII, who, in discussing patients who are terminally unconscious, said "one can refer to the usual concept of separation . . . of the soul from the body; but on the practical level, one needs to be mindful of the connotation of the terms 'body' and 'separation.' . . . As to the pronouncement of death in certain particular cases, the answer cannot be inferred from religious and moral principles, and consequently, it is an aspect lying outside the competence of the Church." [34] We understand the papal point to be that determination of the criteria for deciding the moment of death requires technical measures that can only be established by those with the appropriate medical expertise.

** This section was written in collaboration with Robert M. Veatch.

Accord of Brain-Death Concept with Current Protestant Thought ††

Among Protestant theologians, there are no consistent positions on questions of medical ethics including the definition of death. However, leading spokesmen of widely diverging traditions accept brain-related criteria for pronouncing death.[35-39] The body is an essential element of the person according to Christian theology; but, as many of these authors emphasize, mere cellular and organ system activity alone is not sufficient to treat a human body as if it were alive. Even more conservative thinkers such as Paul Ramsey accept the use of brain-oriented criteria for pronouncement of death. Ramsey recognizes proposals for updating the definition of death as in reality "proposals for updating our procedures for determining that death has occurred, for rebutting the belief that machines or treatments are the patient, for withdrawing the notion that artificially sustained signs of life are in themselves signs of life, for telling when we should stop ventilating and circulating the blood of an unburied corpse because there are no longer any vital functions really alive or recoverable in the patient."[35] Thus, the complete and permanent absence of any brain-related vital bodily function is recognized as death by Jewish, Roman Catholic, and Protestant scholars even if they may disagree among themselves on the precise theoretical foundations of this judgment.

Need for Statutory Recognition that Death May Be Determined by Irreversible Cessation of Brain Function

The fact that physicians can recognize total and irreversible destruction of the brain on the basis of clinical and laboratory criteria is accepted and commonly utilized in many areas of the world. The need to make such pronouncements is based primarily on the requirement of society to respond appropriately to two recent advances in medical technology. The first advance is the hardware that can artificially maintain lung and heart action in the absence of spontaneous respiration and circulation. Although these devices may be life-saving in many situations, their use in maintaining respiration and circulation in a human body that is dead by virtue of total destruction of the brain serves no purpose. In such instances it is reasonable to terminate these artificial support systems.

The second advance which requires pronouncement of death using brain-related criteria is cadaver organ transplantation. Most suitable donor organs come from patients who die from injury or disease of the brain. Only in such patients may the donor's circulation be artificially maintained after death so that needed organs can be removed with minimal ischemic damage. Since destruction of the brain is the cause of the donor's death, there is no reason not to remove these organs before cessation of the donor's artificially maintained circulation. This requires recognition that destruction of the brain is the basis for death of the donor and pronouncement of death on brain-related criteria.

Since the responsibility for pronouncing death resides with physicians, it has been suggested that no statute giving legal recognition to any particular criteria for determining death is necessary or desirable.[40] However, there is a potential dilemma in the absence of legal recognition of the medically accepted

†† This section was written in collaboration with Robert M. Veatch.

practice of pronouncing death on neurologic criteria. Doctors who pronounce death on this basis may be disputed in a judicial proceeding with the contention that death occurs only when spontaneous respiration and heartbeat cease. This contention could be based on the common law definition of death (see below [41]), which is generally held applicable to jurisdictions without specific statutes. Without statutory or case law recognition of the use of brain-related criteria for pronouncing death, it is possible that a valid medical declaration of death could be considered illegal and lead to difficulty in the prosecution of a murderer or criminal or civil liability on the part of a physician or hospital. These possibilities have made many neurologists and neurosurgeons reluctant to pronounce death on brain-related criteria and have given rise to judicial actions in several locales. These cases have been a major factor leading to the passage in many states of statutes recognizing the use of brain-oriented criteria for pronouncing death.

Case law recognition of the legal validity of pronouncing death on brain-related criteria, although helpful, is an inadequate solution to the dilemma that arises from the potential discrepancy between medically accepted practice and legally accepted practice for two important reasons. First, case law is fluid and subject to appeal and change by subsequent judicial action. Second, court decisions to recognize the use of brain-related criteria for pronouncing death may relate to certain special circumstances, such as transplant organ donation. A statute giving general recognition to this concept for all purposes would avoid future inconsistencies under the law and would prevent repeated anguish-producing court cases. Such a law would allow a physician to terminate artificial respiratory support for a patient who is clearly dead by accepted and validated criteria. It would obviate the possibility that the physician, other health professionals, next of kin, guardians, and institutions might be held criminally or civilly liable for actions consistent with standards of current medical practice.

In addition, even if physicians agree that brain-related criteria should be used in death pronouncements, the question is still open as to what the rest of society would choose as its public policy. Public policy can only be determined by some public act such as legislation. Thus, a statutory definition of death would serve as a vehicle to translate a generally accepted medical standard into a form that is accepted by most if not all members of society. As such, it will help to minimize some of the burdens placed on the family and physicians of the dead person by facilitating honest relationships and communication between them in many ways.

Until such public-policy recognition by legislation has occurred, the family confronted with the loss of a relative who is recognized as dead by brain-related criteria is forced to deal with the confusing and misleading assumption, supported by an out-of-date common law, that, while the heart beats, there is life and hope of recovery. Of all the reasons for establishing a statutory definition of death, the simplest and the most important is that it will help the family of the dead patient to appreciate the reality of his death, and to reassure them that the medical determination of death is valid. Such a law will also facilitate relief of the family from financial and emotional pressures and will enable them to confront death with greater dignity and understanding.

In a similar way, the physician's onerous task of conveying to the family in such a situation that the patient is in fact dead would be aided and supported by the passage of an up-to-date statutory definition of death. This would reflect a public policy that recognizes that when the brain is dead, the person as a whole is dead, and there is neither life nor hope despite the mechanically supported respiration and heartbeat. The presence of such a statute will remove from the physician the fear of unjust litigation and thereby allow him to practice medicine in a manner consistent with present scientific knowledge and standards. It will allow him to do this openly after honest discussion with the patient's family, and it will permit him to cooperate in efforts to procure cadaver organs in optimal condition for transplantation into other patients.

A further advantage of having a statutory definition of death is that it would help to guarantee that the highest standards of medical science would be used to make this determination. The recent New Jersey Supreme Court decision [42] in the Karen Quinlan case underscores the need to assure the public that pronouncements of death will be based on standardized and thoroughly validated indices. Even though the criteria of brain death were not fulfilled in Miss Quinlan's case, the court held that her parent, acting as guardian, might authorize cessation of life-sustaining treatment if a physician and a hospital "ethics committee" agreed there was no reasonable possibility of recovery to a cognitive, sapient state. Although this decision and the resulting discontinuation of respiratory support did not alter Miss Quinlan's course because she was able to breathe spontaneously, there has been substantial confusion between the issues in this case and the debate about the definition of death. Such misunderstandings could result in less than optimal nonstandardized determinations of death. These would be prevented by the existence of a statute that mandates use of the best standards of current medical practice to pronounce death.

A statutory definition of death would also have other advantages from a legal point of view. It would provide a clear and precise definition within which legal rights and relationships after death could be determined. It would facilitate the prosecution of murderers and permit the organs of murder victims to be used as transplants without jeopardizing conviction of the murderer. Such a statute would provide for consistency under the law in various jurisdictions, and it would avoid reliance on jury systems to make medical and legal decisions that might be inconsistent with present scientific knowledge.

Many physicians have suggested that the specific criteria for pronouncing brain death should not be placed in a statutory form. This is a reasonable position, since there is always the possibility that the criteria might change. This would mean that the law would have to be changed prior to utilizing any improved criteria. This is obviously a good reason not to legislate *specific* neurologic criteria for pronouncing death. However, it is an inadequate reason for opposing a law which, while leaving the specific criteria flexible, recognizes that death may be pronounced when irreversible cessation of brain function occurs.

LEGAL STATUS OF BRAIN DEATH ‡‡

Until recently, the traditional legal definition of death has been consistent with the prevailing medical concept that death is determined by cessation of the vital functions of respiration and heartbeat. This is reflected in the common law definition of death as stated in *Black's Law Dictionary* [41]: "The cessation of life; the ceasing to exist; defined by physicians as a total stoppage of the circula-

‡‡ This section was written in collaboration with Marc A. Kleiman and George Kalkines.

tion of the blood, and a cessation of the animal and vital functions consequent thereon, such as respiration, pulsation, etc." With the exception of several notable recent decisions, traditional case law has similarly concentrated on the cardiovascular and respiratory functions as prime determinants of the occurrence of death.

In *Smith v. Smith*,[43] the Supreme Court of Arkansas, in a case that turned on the issue of simultaneous death, adopted Black's definition of death verbatim. The court took judicial notice of the fact that "one breathing, though unconscious, is not dead." Similarly, in *Thomas v. Anderson*,[44] a California District Court of Appeals also cited Black's definition and stated that ". . . death occurs precisely when life ceases and does not occur until the heart stops beating and respiration ends. Death is not a continuous event and is an event that takes place at a precise time." Other jurisdictions have also relied on this definition.[45, 46] In addition, other cases have upheld the premise that death has not occurred until cessation of heartbeat and respiration, even in circumstances where the courts have noted complete destruction of the brain.[47-49]

In all the cases cited, the determination of death was dealt with as a question of fact for a jury to decide in connection with the demise of individuals for the purposes of construing and applying "simultaneous death" clauses in testamentary documents. The factual question of the time of death in these cases was judged on the basis of circumstantial evidence relating to the cessation of heartbeat and respiration. This evidence was provided by the testimony of lay persons rather than physicians. These cases, which constitute the leading precedents in this area, predated the landmark report of the Ad Hoc Committee of the Harvard Medical School to Examine the Definition of Brain Death,[3] which is now generally regarded as the first widely recognized index that current medical concepts about the definition of death were changing.

Emerging Case Law

In contrast with these traditional opinions, in several recent cases the issue of death has been considered in the light of expert testimony by physicians concerning the time of irreversible cessation of brain function and such testimony has often been incorporated in jury charges. These cases give explicit or implicit legal recognition to a pronouncement of death based on a determination of irreversible cessation of brain function in accordance with the customary standards of medical practice. These legal actions were relevant because the medical determination of the timing and occurrence of death in these cases was based on brain-related criteria, and legal application of traditional criteria of death would have been inappropriate. Thus, judicial action fortunately kept the law apace of scientific developments.

The first such judicial action occurred in the Oregon case, *State v. Brown*,[50] in which the defendant had been convicted on a charge of second degree murder. On appeal, he contended that the victim's death was caused by termination of life-support systems rather than by the cranial gunshot wound that he had inflicted. The Court held that the defendant's contention was without merit on the basis of expert medical testimony that the gunshot wound with resultant brain damage was the cause of death.

One year later, the impact of current medical thinking on case law was clearly evident in a Virginia case, *Tucker v. Lower*.[51] In a wrongful death action, it was alleged that an individual was not dead at the time his heart and kidneys were removed for purposes of transplantation. The Court rejected a motion for a summary judgment in favor of the defendants on the grounds that the Court was bound by the common law definition of death until it was changed by the State Legislature. However, after considerable debate, the Court instructed the jury that it might properly consider, as a substitute for the traditional criteria for determining the time of death, ". . . the time of complete and irreversible loss of all function of the brain; and, whether or not the aforesaid functions [respiration and circulation] were spontaneous or were being maintained artificially or mechanically." The jury then decided that the transplant surgeons were not guilty of causing a wrongful death. Whether or not this decision was based on the jury's acceptance of the brain-death concept is not known. However, this case has been widely publicized as supporting the use of brain-related criteria for pronouncing death. Furthermore, in commenting on this case, one legal scholar points out that "the jury instructions represent an admission by the courts that the old legal definition of death needs modification in the light of advances in medical science. The new definition—'brain death'—which is gaining recognition, reflects the consensus of informed medical opinion." [52]

Similarly, in a widely publicized California case, *People v. Lyons*,[53] a victim had suffered a gunshot wound of the head and had been declared neurologically dead before a transplant team headed by Dr. Norman Shumway had removed his heart. The defendant pleaded not guilty to a charge of murder, contending that the death of the victim had been caused by the removal of his heart rather than by the gunshot wound inflicted by the defendant. On the basis of expert testimony, the jury was instructed as a matter of law that "the victim was legally dead before removal of the organs from his body." The Court thereby removed from the jury its traditional task of having to determine the exact time of death. The brain-death standard was explicitly accepted.

However, a contrasting ruling was made in the initial phase of another California criminal prosecution, emphasizing the inconsistency that can occur with case law. In this case, the defendant, who had been driving on the wrong side of a freeway while intoxicated, had caused an accident which severely injured a 13-year-old girl. The girl was pronounced dead on brain-related criteria, and her heart was used as a transplant. On the basis of these facts, a Municipal Court Judge at a preliminary hearing did not hold the defendant to answer to a manslaughter charge, apparently determining that the pronouncement of death on neurologic criteria and the subsequent removal of the heart created substantial doubt as to the proximate cause of death. The Court concluded that, ". . . the evidence is not certain as to the cause of death of Colenda Ward, certain enough to charge this defendant with manslaughter." [54] On a subsequent appeal by the District Attorney, the Superior Court authorized the filing of a manslaughter charge and made reference to "unimpeached medical testimony" that conclusively established ". . . that the [victim's] heart could not beat nor could she breathe without artificial support." [55] The defendant was convicted of both manslaughter and felony drunk driving but received a sentence of less than five months. In commenting on this result, the Deputy District Attorney involved observed: "I cannot escape the firm belief that the uncertain state of the case and statutory law on the subject of brain death was a substantial factor in the imposition of such a light sentence." [56]

A rather novel approach to the legal question of when death occurs was taken in 1975 in New York,[57] where a court was requested to set forth, in an action for declaratory judgment, a legal definition of the terms "death" and "time of death" as used in the New York State Anatomical Gifts Act. The Court was asked to include in such definition not only the common law criteria of cardiac and respiratory failure, but also the concept of "brain death." Following extensive uncontroverted testimony concerning brain-death criteria, the Court held that "death" as used in the Anatomical Gifts Act "implies a definition consistent with the generally accepted medical practice of doctors primarily concerned with effectuating the purposes of this statute." Having confined its decision legally recognizing brain-related criteria for pronouncing death to the Anatomical Gifts Act, the Court concluded by urging the State Legislature ". . . to take affirmative action to provide a State-wide remedy for this problem."

These cases have been helpful in resolving particular controversies. However, they have probably had a greater impact by serving to increase public awareness of the need for a statutory definition of death. In all but one instance in which litigation has arisen, legislation that recognizes the validity of brain death as a legally accepted standard for determining death has been enacted shortly thereafter. The single exception is New York, where proposals are currently pending before the State Legislature.

Legislation

At the present time, eighteen states have enacted a statutory definition of death: Kansas, Maryland, Virginia, New Mexico, Alaska, California, Georgia, Michigan, Oregon, Illinois, Oklahoma, West Virginia, Tennessee, Louisiana, Iowa, Idaho, Montana, and North Carolina.[58] §§ All 18 statutes recognize that death may be pronounced on the basis of irreversible cessation of brain function, and none describes in detail the specific criteria for determining brain death. However, the laws vary in certain major and minor ways. In general, they conform to one of three major types or patterns.

The first of these includes laws providing alternative definitions of death. Typical of this pattern is the first statute enacted in 1970 by Kansas:

> A person will be considered medically and legally dead if, in the opinion of a physician, based on ordinary standards of medical practice, there is the absence of spontaneous respiratory and cardiac function and, because of the disease or condition which caused, directly or indirectly, these functions to cease, or because of the passage of time since these functions ceased, attempts at resuscitation are considered hopeless; and, in this event, death will have occurred at the time these functions ceased; or
>
> A person will be considered medically and legally dead if, in the opinion of a physician, based on ordinary standards of medical practice, there is the absence of spontaneous brain function; and if based on ordinary standards of medical practice, during reasonable attempts to either maintain or restore spontaneous circulatory or respiratory function in the absence of aforesaid brain function, it appears that further attempts at resuscitation or supportive maintenance will not succeed, death will have occurred at the time when these conditions first coincide. Death is to be pronounced before artificial

§§ Hawaii has recently enacted a statutory definition of death.

means of supporting respiratory and circulatory function are terminated and before any vital organ is removed for purposes of transplantation.

These alternative definitions of death are to be utilized for all purposes in this state, including the trials of civil and criminal cases, any laws to the contrary notwithstanding.

An identical statute was enacted by Maryland in 1972. In 1973, Virginia passed a similar law, which differed only in that death recognized using brain-related criteria can only be declared by two physicians, one of whom is a specialist in neurology, neurosurgery, or electroencephalography. The Virginia law also mandates that absence of spontaneous respiratory functions accompany "absence of spontaneous brain functions." The New Mexico statute passed in 1973 and the Alaska statute, passed in 1974, are similar to the Kansas law. The Oregon statute enacted in 1975 is the simplest and clearest of the alternative definition type of law:

When a physician licensed to practice medicine acts to determine that a person is dead, he may make such a determination if irreversible cessation of spontaneous respiration and circulatory function or irreversible cessation of spontaneous brain function exists.

All six of these alternative definition-of-death statutes suffer the disadvantage of providing two different definitions of death. The choice of which to use in a specific instance is left to the physician. The major flaw with this type of legislation is that it appears to be based on the misconception that there are two separate types of death. This is particularly unfortunate because it seems to relate to the need to establish a special definition of death for organ transplant donors. These laws could lend support to the fear that a prospective transplant organ donor would be considered dead at an earlier point in the dying process than an identical patient who was not a potential donor. In addition, such laws suffer the legal disadvantage of possibly permitting a physician, either inadvertently or intentionally, to influence the outcome of a will. If, for example, a husband and wife are fatally injured in the same accident, survivorship and consequent inheritance may be determined by the physician's choice of which of the alternative criteria to use in the pronouncements of death.

The second major type of law was suggested by Capron and Kass to remedy this defect and to provide one definition of death that recognizes that death is a single phenomenon that can be determined by brain-related criteria only in situations where artificial support of respiratory and circulatory functions is being maintained [59]:

A person will be considered dead if in the announced opinion of a physician, based on ordinary standards of medical practice, he has experienced an irreversible cessation of spontaneous respiratory and circulatory functions. In the event that artificial means of support preclude a determination that these functions have ceased, a person will be considered dead if in the announced opinion of a physician based on ordinary practice, he has experienced an irreversible cessation of spontaneous brain functions. Death will have occurred at the time when the relevant functions ceased.

This model statute takes cognizance of the fact that the medical standards for pronouncing death may vary with circumstances. However, unlike the previous laws, it does not leave as an arbitrary decision for the physician the choice of which standard to apply, but defines under what circumstances the new or secondary brain-related criteria may be used. This bill avoids establishing a separate kind of death, brain death, and, as pointed out by Capron and Kass, provides "two standards gauged by different functions for measuring different manifestations of the same phenomenon. If cardiac and pulmonary functions have ceased, brain functions cannot continue; if there is no brain activity and respiration has to be maintained artificially, the same state (i.e., death) exists." [59] The Capron-Kass Bill, which clearly appears to be satisfactory if not ideal, was adopted by Michigan and West Virginia in 1975 and by Louisiana in 1976. The latter law specifies that when organs are to be used as a transplant, an additional physician unassociated with the transplant team must also pronounce death. Iowa in 1976 and Montana in 1977 enacted laws based on the Capron-Kass model, with the additional requirement that brain-death pronouncements must be made by two physicians.

The third major type of law follows the suggestion of the American Bar Association, which recognized the need for a standardized statutory definition of death that minimized the risk of confusion from misunderstandings of semantics, medical technology and legal sophistication, and that took into account recent developments in transplantation, supportive therapy, and resuscitation. The suggested law was developed by the Law and Medicine Committee of the American Bar Association in 1974 and approved by the House of Delegates of that organization in 1975 [60]: "For all legal purposes, a human body with irreversible cessation of total brain function, according to usual and customary standards of medical practice, shall be considered dead."

This Committee states that the advantages of its simple direct definition are that it: permits judicial determination of the ultimate fact of death; permits medical determination of the evidentiary fact of death; avoids religious determination of any facts; avoids prescribing the medical criteria; enhances changing medical criteria; enhances local medical practice tests; covers the three known tests ("brain, beat and breath deaths"); covers death as a process (medical preference); covers death as a point in time (legal preference); avoids passive euthanasia; avoids active euthanasia; covers current American and European medical practices; covers both civil and criminal law; covers current American judicial decisions; avoids nonphysical sciences.[60]

Some have objected that this simple model statute fails to recognize the still common practice of pronouncing death on the basis of cessation of heartbeat and respiration. However, in practice, death is only pronounced when the functions of circulation and respiration have ceased long enough to cause destruction of the brain and produce other signs of lifelessness. In these instances, cessations of circulation and respiration represent the specific criteria by which irreversible cessation of brain function or death is determined. Thus, this model statute recognizes traditional as well as brain-related criteria for determining death. It is, therefore, also satisfactory and has formed the basis for the California statute enacted in 1974, the Georgia statute enacted in 1975, and the Idaho statute passed in 1977. All three laws require that deaths pronounced on brain-related criteria be confirmed by a second physician. The Illinois statute enacted in 1975 also resembles the American Bar Association's suggestion in its simplicity. It does not require concurrence of a second physician, although it has the flaw of restricting the use of brain-related criteria to instances involving the Uniform Anatomical Gift Act. It therefore has the disadvantage of implicitly establishing alternative types of death with a special definition to be used for transplant organ donors. The Oklahoma law enacted in 1975 also seems to be based on the American Bar Association model, but is rendered confusing by the addition of a number of qualifying clauses and phrases mandating that it must also appear "that further attempts at resuscitation and supportive maintenance will not succeed." The Tennessee statute enacted in 1976 avoids these flaws and complexities and follows exactly the recommendation of the American Bar Association.

Many factors underlie the variability between the statutes enacted in the different states and account for the difficulty in reaching agreement on what constitutes the wording of a single ideal statutory definition of death. Prominent among these factors is the present climate of public mistrust of the medical profession. This has prompted legislators to enact more complicated laws in an attempt to protect patients from erroneous or premature declarations of death.

It is hoped that this article, by summarizing the overwhelming evidence supporting the validity of the concept of brain death, will help to allay these concerns and facilitate drafting of simple, effective statutes defining death. Furthermore, by showing that pronouncements of death on brain-related criteria are in accord with secular philosophy and with the principles of the three major Western religions, we hope that the present article will help overcome opposition to legislation from those who previously failed to accept the brain-death concept. And lastly, by documenting the compelling reasons to have a statutory definition of death, we hope that this article will help to influence the American Medical Association and others who have felt that legislation defining death is unnecessary to adopt a supportive position, as several of the state medical societies have already done. Such support would greatly facilitate passage of appropriate statutes in the 32 states prevently without them. This, in turn, would make the law in regard to brain death consistent with current medical practice throughout the entire United States.

REFERENCES

1. VEITH, F. J., J. M. FEIN, M. D. TENDLER, R. M. VEATCH, M. A. KLEIMAN & G. KALKINES. 1977. Brain death: I. A status report of medical and ethical considerations. JAMA **238**: 1651.
2. VEITH, F. J., J. M. FEIN, M. D. TENDLER, R. M. VEATCH, M. A. KLEIMAN & G. KALKINES. 1977. Brain death: II. A status report of legal considerations. JAMA **238**: 1744.
3. 1968. A definition of irreversible coma: Report of the Ad Hoc Committee of the Harvard Medical School to examine the definition of brain death. JAMA **205**: 337–340.
4. RICHARDSON, E. 1972. *In* Refinements in Criteria for the Determination of Death: An Appraisal: A report by the Task Force on Death and Dying of the Institute of Society, Ethics and the Life Sciences. JAMA **221**: 48–53; also, personal communication, 1976.
5. WALKER, A. E., E. L. DIAMOND & J. MOSELEY. 1975. The neuropathological findings in irreversible coma: A critique of the "respirator brain." J. Neuropathol. Exp. Neurol. **34**: 295–323.
6. KOREIN, J., P. BRAUNSTEIN & I. KRICHEFF, *et al.* 1975. Radioisotopic bolus technique as a test to detect circulatory deficit associated with cerebral death: 142 studies on 80 patients demonstrating the bedside use of an innocuous IV procedure as an adjunct in the diagnosis of cerebral death. Circulation **51**: 924–939.
7. CRAFOORD, C. 1969. Cerebral death and the transplantation era. Dis. Chest **55**: 141–145.

8. HEISKANEN, O. 1964. Cerebral circulatory arrest caused by acute increase of intracranial pressure: A clinical and roentgenological study of 25 cases. Acta. Neurol. Scand. **40** (Suppl. 7).
9. BERGQUIST, E. & K. BERGSTROM. 1972. Angiography in cerebral death. Acta. Radiol. Diagn. **12:** 283–288.
10. LOFSTEDT, S. & G. VON REIS. 1959. Diminution or obstruction of blood flow in the internal carotid artery. Opuscula Medica **4:** 345–360.
11. GREITZ, T., E. GORDON, G. KOLMODIN & L. WIDEN. 1973. Aortocranial and carotid angiography in determination of brain death. Neuroradiology **5:** 13–19.
12. SILVERMAN, D., M. G. SAUNDERS, R. S. SCHWAB & R. L. MASLAND. 1969. Cerebral death and the electroencephalogram. Report of the Ad Hoc Committee of the American Electroencephalographic Society on EEG criteria for determination of cerebral death. JAMA **209:** 1505–1510.
13. SILVERMAN, D., R. L. MASLAND, M. G. SAUNDERS & R. S. SCHWAB. 1970. Irreversible coma associated with electrocerebral silence. Neurology **20:** 525–533.
14. MASLAND, R. L. 1975. When is a person dead. Resident and Staff Physician April 5 : 49–52.
15. KOREIN, J. & M. MACCARIO. 1971. On the diagnosis of cerebral death: A prospective study on 55 patients to define irreversible coma. Clin. Electroenceph. **2:** 178–199.
16. MOHANDAS, A. & S. N. CHOU. 1971. Brain death: A clinical and pathological study. J. Neurosurg. **35:** 211–218.
17. INGVAR, D. H. & L. WIDEN. 1972. Brain death—A summary of a symposium. Kakartidningen **69:** 3804–3814.
18. WALKER, A. E. 1975. Cerebral death. The Nervous System. Vol. 2: The Clinical Neurosciences. Donald B. Tower, Ed. : 75–87. Raven Press. New York, N.Y.
19. UEKI, K., K. TAKEUCHI & K. KATSURADA. 1973. Clinical study of brain death. Presentation No. 282, Fifth International Congress of Neurologic Surgery, Tokyo, Japan.
20. WALKER, A. E. 1976. The neurosurgeon's responsibility for organ procurement. J. Neurosurg. **44:** 1–2.
21. 1977. An appraisal of the criteria of cerebral death. A summary statement. A collaborative study. JAMA **237:** 982–986.
22. 1976. Diagnosis of Brain Death. (Summary of Conference of Royal Colleges and Faculties of the United Kingdom) Lancet **ii:** 1069–1970.
23. MOLINARI, G. F. Death: The definition, III. Criteria for death. Encyclopedia of Bioethics. In press.
24. BOLTON, C. F., J. D. BROWN, E. CHOLOD & K. WARREN. 1976. EEG and "brain life." Lancet **i:** 535.
25. Bab Talmud Tractate Yoma 85A.
26. Bab Talmud Tractate Chullin 21 A and Mishnah Oholoth **1:** 6.
27. MAIMONIDES: Tumath Meth **1:** 15.
28. Code of Laws: Who is considered as dead although yet living? Yoreh Deah: **370:** 1.
29. Genesis. Chapter **2:** 7.
30. FEINSTEIN, M. On the determination of death in accord with Orthodox Jewish practice. Personal communication, May 5, 1976.
31. CONNERY, J. R. Comment on the proposed act to amend the public health law of the State of New York in relation to the determination of the occurrence of death. (1975–76 Session, dated March 25, 1975).
32. HÄRING, B. 1973. Medical Ethics. Fides Publishers, Inc. Notre Dame, Ind.
33. McFADDEN, C. J. 1976. The Dignity of Life: Moral Values in a Changing Society. : 202. Our Sunday Visitor, Inc. Huntington, Ind.
34. PIUS XII. Acta Apostolicae Sedia 45 : 1027–1033. November 1957.
35. RAMSEY P. 1970. The Patient as Person: Explorations in Medical Ethics. : 101–112. Yale University Press. New Haven, Conn.

36. NELSON, J. 1973. Human Medicine: Ethical Perspectives on New Medical Issues. : 125–130. Augsburg, Minneapolis, Minn.

37. FLETCHER, J. 1969. Our shameful waste of human tissues: An ethical problem for the living and the dead. In *Updating Life and Death: Essays in Ethics and Medicine.* Donald R. Cutler, Ed. : 1–30. Beacon Press. Boston, Mass.; and FLETCHER, J. 1974 New definitions of death. Prism **2:** 13 ff.

38. VAUX, K. 1974. Biomedical Ethics. : 102–110. Harper and Row. New York, N.Y.

39. SMITH, H. 1970. Ethics and the New Medicne. Abington. Nashville, Tenn.

40. 1974. Definition of death. JAMA **227:** 728.

41. 1968. Black's Law Dictionary, 4th ed. : 488. West Publishing Co. St. Paul, Minn.

42. *In the matter of Karen Quinlan,* 355 A.2d 647 (1976).

43. *Smith v. Smith,* 229 Ark. 579, 317 SW2d 275 (1958).

44. *Thomas v. Anderson,* 211 P2d 478 (1950).

45. *United Trust Co. v. Pyke,* 427 P2d 67 (1967).

46. *Schmidt v. Pierce,* 344 SW2d 120 (1961).

47. *Vaegemast v. Hess,* 280 NW 641 (1938).

48. *Gray v. Sawyer,* 247 SW2d 496 (1952).

49. *In re Estate of Schmidt,* 67 Cal. Reptr. 847 (1968).

50. *State v. Brown,* 8 Oreg. App. 72 (1971).

51. *Tucker v. Lower,* No. 2381 (Richmond, Va., L & Eq Ct, May 23, 1972).

52. KENNEDY, I. 1973. The legal definition of death. Medico-Legal Journal **14:** 38.

53. *People v. Lyons,* 15 Crm. L. Rprt. 2240 (Cal. Super. Ct. 1974).

54. *People v. Flores,* Cal. Super. Ct., Sonoma County, 7246-C, p. 1, 1974.

55. *People v. Flores.*[54] p. 2.

56. TUCKER, S. T. (Deputy District Attorney, Sonoma County, Calif.). Personal communication, May 19, 1977.

57. *New York City Health & Hosp. Corp. v. Sulsona,* 81 Misc. 2d 1002 (1975).

58. State Laws: Kan. Stat. Ann. § 77–202 (Supp. 1974); Md. Code Ann. § 32–364.3:1 (Cum. Suppl. 1975); New Mex. Stat. Ann., § 1–2–2.2 (Supp. 1973); Alaska Stat. § 9.65.120 (Supp. 1974); Va. Code Ann. § 32–364.3:1 (Supp. 1975); Cal. Health and Safety Code Ann. § 7180–81 (West Supp. 1975); Ill. Ann. Stat. Ch. 3, § 552, (Smith-Hurd Supp. 1975); Ga. Code Ann. § 88–1715.1 (1975); Mich. Stat. P.A. 158 (Laws 1975); Ore. Rev. Stat. Ch. 565, § 1 (Laws 1975); Ch. 91, Laws 1975, amending Okla. Stat. Ann. tit. 63, § 1–301 (g) (1971); W. Va. Code Ann. § 16–19–1 (Supp. 1975); Tenn. Stat., H.B. No. 1919 Ch. 780 (Laws 1976); La. Acts 1976, No. 233, § 1; Laws of 66th Iowa General Assembly, Ch. 1245, (1976 Senate File 85); Mont. H.B. No. 371, Ch. 228, Laws 1977; 1977 Idaho Session Laws, No. 1197, Ch. 30; Ch. 815, N. Carol. Laws 1977, § 90–322.

59. CAPRON, A. M. & L. R. KASS. 1972. A statutory definition of the standards for determining human death: An appraisal and a proposal. Univ. Penn. Law Rev. **121:** 87–118.

60. DeMERE, M., T. ALEXANDER & A. AUERBACH, et al. Report on definition of death, from Law and Medicine Committee. Adopted by the American Bar Association, February 25, 1975.

DISCUSSION

BERESFORD: Before I direct any comments to Dr. Veith, I would like to stress two aspects of the papers presented in this volume. First, the areas of consensus and the areas of disagreement have been noted. The scientific data base and the degrees of consensus in the areas that remain open, particularly with respect to what technologies are highly useful in determination of loss of brain function, have been discussed. In addition, some of the doctrinal, social, moral and legal issues have been discussed.

Second, aspects of the decision-making process have been evaluated. Many of us have had experience with or have thought very hard about the approach to decisionmaking on these questions. Some have approached these questions in an abstract manner, but few have discussed the point of intersection of the technical, moral, legal and ethical issues in this area.

Let me just make an amendment to Dr. Veith's paper. I think that the Massachusetts highest court has also upheld the brain-death concept and was ruled upon.

VEITH: That is correct in Massachusetts. I wish it were correct in New York, but it is not.

BERESFORD: It is still in the lower court in New York. Dr. Veith has challenged all of you. One certainly cannot accuse him of inertia or misinformation in the face of the challenge that has been posed. Before we comment further, Dr. Milhaud will share with us some of the experience relating to these issues in France.

MILHAUD: I would like to discuss some of the problems relating to the intensive care unit and organ transplantation in France. To take the question from an ethical point of view, in 1963 we || || proposed with M. Cara to remove organs for transplantation from patients with total brain death. Prior to this time, the use of normal living donors was accepted. In France today the use of live donors is very rare (DISCUSSION FIGURE 1), as reported by Jean Dausset.¶¶

Of course, the word "cadavre" as used in DISCUSSION FIGURE 1 could be misleading unless one clearly understands that this represents patients who are totally brain-dead. In France today, numerous cities are participating in this transplantation project (DISCUSSION FIGURE 2).

From a medicolegal point of view, I would like to make three remarks:

1. There must be a definite legal standard of brain death. In France, since the law of December 22, 1976 was passed, every individual is a potential organ donor unless he officially refused during his life. We are now waiting for the full application of this law.

2. Usually, when the victim of a murder or a suicide is diagnosed as being brain-dead, we can remove the kidneys after a telephone call to the "Procureur de la Republique," who is perhaps equivalent to your Attorney General. The same things are true for other organs, including the heart.***

|| || MILHAUD, A. 1964. Quelques questions posées par l'arrêt circulatoire inopiné—Séminaire consacré à l'Enseignement supérieur du secourisme organisé par l'Association des Anesthésiologistes Français, Barbizon, 7 mai 1963. Ann., Anesthesiol., Fr., 5: 639.

¶¶ HORS, J., J. COLOMBANI & J. DAUSSET. 1974. Histocompatibilité HL-A et greffes rénales. Statistiques de France-Transplant. Ann. Anesthesiol. Fr. XV (spécial III): 200–208.

*** CABROL, C. & L. LOYGUE. 1974. Etat actuel de la transplantation cardiaque, transport et conservation des greffons. Ann. Anesthesiol. Fr. XV (spécial III): 233–240.

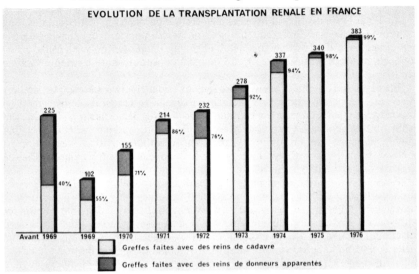

DISCUSSION FIGURE 1. Evalution of renal transplantation in France.

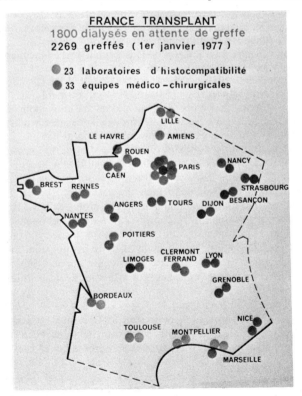

DISCUSSION FIGURE 2.

3. Total brain death and irreversible cerebral damage ††† with coma of long duration are two very different things. The most important diagnostic point is real apnea. We believe that this can be reliably diagnosed only by using a disconnecting test of a duration of more than 15 minutes in pure oxygen and after denitrogenation.

From a logical point of view, some may consider the two states to be similar. However, physicians know very well that irreversible cerebral damage may be deemed to be worse in many ways than brain death. Brain death is, in fact, the death of the person. In a good intensive care unit, patients with irreversible cerebral damage can survive for years with or without artificial ventilation as opposed to patients with total brain death, who cannot survive more than a week despite artificial ventilation and good nursing.

FEIN: I would like to dispute Dr. Tendler's suggestion that legislation for brain death be codified to include specified criteria. This is unwise and very unnecessary. There are many areas in which physicians come into contiguity with socially significant problems, and where diagnoses made by physicians have social significance. To codify the specifics on which each diagnosis should be made would be chaotic. There would be tremendous inertia between developments in diagnostic capabilities and eventually defining these in the form of a codified law.

There are many adequate mechanisms by which the public can seek redress from physicians who are incompetent. The physician is always aware of this, and the public is protected in many ways. The public has recourse to malpractice action should a diagnosis be improper.

BERESFORD: I agree with you, but I wonder if there is somebody who will argue another view?

VEITH: I coauthored an article with Dr. Fein and Dr. Tendler, and so you can appreciate my satisfaction in getting them to agree on anything. In Dr. Tendler's absence and since I have spoken to him about this subject at length, I would like to give his view. Although I disagree with it somewhat, I can see that there are some good reasons for holding to it.

His belief is that in the climate of mistrust that exists in our society with regard to physicians, he would like to have something in writing as a statutory basis for making sure that physicians do not abuse their position. All of us who are physicians know that this is, in fact, the case. Dr. Tendler has on several occasions compromised in the actual wording of proposed law. He has accepted a compromise, for example, in relation to brain-death pronouncements by two physicians who are certified or who are specialists in neurology, neurosurgery and electroencephalography. Accordingly, I think his position, though he states it with great fervor, is not as inflexible as it would appear. His reasons are, as I stated, that there is distrust in society towards the medical profession and that he, as a representative of society, would like to see some guarantee that physicians do not abuse their privileges.

J. ZIMMIT: This comment is addressed to Dr. Suter. Issues concerning a particular member vital to the health care team have not been adequately discussed nor has this member been properly represented at these proceedings.

††† Dr. Milhaud is referring to persistent vegetative or noncognitive state.—*J. K.*

The member I am referring to is the nurse. The nurse is a constant and consistent presence on the floor. He or she works intimately with each patient. In some cases, as in the ICU, the nurse-to-patient ratio is one to one. As a result the nurse is aware of second-to-second, minute-to-minute changes in the patient's status, assesses each situation, utilizes acquired judgment and implements care, interacts with patients and family and observes their behavior, and offers comfort and support.

In this respect it is ironic that a nurse has not been officially represented here. Nurse representatives should be included in these conferences so that nursing views, problems, vantage points and implications could be presented.

BERESFORD: I agree.

SUTER: I must also agree with that. I have, in fact, mentioned the importance of nurses in my paper. It is important in a good intensive care unit that there be a set of rules for the operation of the unit that are devised by the nurses and the doctors. It must be a document that is agreed upon by all members of the team. In decisions relating to use of the ICU, the nursing opinion should have parity with that of other health professionals. If you can determine when the unit is no longer useful for a patient, and it is agreed upon by the nurses and the doctors and documented, then your legal standards are better. Nurses' observations of the patient are as important as those of the physicians.

GRENVIK: In support of Dr. Suter's excellent paper dealing with the problems that we face, the Presbyterian University Hospital in Pittsburgh is a referral center where for many years we have received brain-dead patients as donors of organs for transplantation. There is a great need for strict guidelines at our hospitals, which has been pointed out along with the need for referral of patients to centers that are used for confirming diagnosis of brain death.

A patient (whose name translated into English as "Guest of Horror") was certified as brain-dead at an outlying hospital within a few hours after very severe head injuries, and was then referred to us. However, after donation consents were signed by the parents, we found that he did not fulfill the criteria for brain death and was therefore resuscitated and supportive measures were continued. It only took us two weeks to get him sitting up in a wheelchair, eating, talking, and then after another two months discharged from the hospital with a rather minimal hemiparesis as the only consequence.

BERESFORD: Chilling case.

SUTER: This may be a common occurrence if the determination of brain death is made in a hospital without the proper facilities. One of the problems with the centers is that it has been a little hard to convince our own personnel that when anybody arrives at the facility in that condition they must be admitted to the intensive care unit and not just be evaluated in the emergency room. I refuse to send our patients to the emergency room for any purpose involving transplants, since our ICU is appropriately equipped to make the diagnosis of brain death. The patient must be admitted to the hospital, and then to the ICU, where the determination of brain death will be made. You are quite right; many of these comatose patients are not brain-dead.

BERESFORD: Yes, we have to presuppose that the fact-finding is accurate; otherwise our discussion fails.

VEITH: In our search of the lay literature we have found a number of cases similar to this. We had several cases in our own transplant unit in which patients were sent to us by the referring physician and permission had been granted by the families, but, in fact, when these patients were adequately evaluated, they were found not to be brain-dead. Because of the thoroughness of the evaluation and the aggressive care, these patients, who probably otherwise would have died, recovered. I tell these stories to people like Dr. Tendler to try and reassure him that, in fact, the transplant surgeons are very worried about a mistake being make. Because we, and our neurologists, are so careful about this, I know of no mistake that has been made. I also know a number of anecdotal stories describing patients who have been subjected to this rigorous evaluation and therapy and who have survived when otherwise they probably would have died.

BERESFORD: My impression has always been that physicians involved with organ transplantation have a high degree of visability. Therefore one is very safe in their hands as far as determinations of this nature are concerned. Much publicity has been brought to bear on this subject. Two or three years ago Professor Capron coauthored a book with J. Kass, a Professor of Law and Psychiatry at Yale, called *Catastrophic Diseases—Who Decides What?* in which they laid out a variety of issues relating to organ transplantation, arguably in a somewhat slanted way, but making it very clear that these decisions are being made in the open and that no one conceals the facts related to the organ transplantation. The chances of somebody behaving in a technically inaccurate or unethical way in this particular context are very unlikely.

M. H. GOLDMAN (*Naval Medical Research Institute, Bethesda, Md.*): I would like to add some support to Dr. Veith's statement. The Navy deals with a central location military facility with adequate technical support for diagnosing brain death. There are a number of dispensaries in outlying circumferential areas from which traumatized military personnel arrive, with the clinical and perhaps inadequate diagnosis of brain death. These patients are referred to the U.S. Navy transplant team as potential donors. Under these circumstances, those patients are "medivacced" to the central military facility and admitted not directly to the transplant service, but either to the neurology or the neurosurgery service. I think this is what a number of people have been referring to with respect to civilian facilities. So, if you have a questionably brain-dead person he ought to be referred to the appropriate centrally located facility which is adequately equipped and staffed and has the capability of establishing the diagnosis of brain death.

BACHRACH: I would like to reintroduce the subject of cost-containment. Although I am not an economist, I think we have to come back to some of the economic realities, including tradeoffs, of what we have to do. This is related to the cost-containment policies of government administration. In terms of cost-benefit analysis, it is amazing to me that Dr. Suter has been able to develop and maintain his pavilion without having to obtain a "certificate of need." While it is very commendable to keep a patient in an acute care hospital from Christmas until April, the economic realities we are facing makes such a policy less tenable. The routine use of computerized tomography scans, for example, that has been described may be contrasted to the limit of three to four CT scans for my entire county in Worcester. We should consider the limits imposed upon us by the economic realities as indicated by HEW policy.

BERESFORD: Balanced against the HEW policy, however, is the demand of the public for the highest quality of medical care we are capable of delivering and this may prevent HEW from achieving their stated goals of cost-containment.

SUTER: We feel completely justified, economically and otherwise, in the use and maintenance of our facility. The level of patient care and benefits to the patient speak for themselves.

BERESFORD: I admire your achievement. I think we all envy you your facility.

NESBAKKEN: We have been discussing brain death, persistent vegetative states, euthanasia and other problems, each of which are distinctly separable topics. They should not be confused with one another lest this lead to serious misconceptions that may jeopardize the laymen's acceptance of the entire concept of brain death itself.

BERESFORD: Everyone here at this Conference has been taking great pains to try to distinguish what they mean by total destruction of the brain, i.e., brain death and other states. If anybody here has sat through these discussions and papers and still has a misconception as to the distinction among the various issues, he should carefully read the volume.

VAN TILL: Dr. Veith should not be amazed that there is distrust and ignorance among the public, the legislators, etc. One of the main problems is that the doctors who understand about brain death and its associated problems have not made much effort to inform the medical profession, other health professionals such as nurses, legislators, the news media, and the public in general; this is one of the reasons why newspapermen and T.V. commentators really do not know what it is all about and say absolute nonsense. If one finds contradictory opinions in an attempt to clarify different issues, we become aware of the necessity for deriving a concept such as brain death. The sort of public distrust that followed the first heart transplant can only be dispelled by physicians' educating journalists or the public in general. This also might be accomplished by interdisciplinary statements of doctors, lawyers and other interested parties, first nationally and then on an international level.

VEITH: Although I do not take issue with what you say, in New York State we tried very hard to do just what you are suggesting. However, brain death is not a glamourous issue. Although some of the intelligent journalists have cooperated to a certain extent in our attempt to educate the legislators and the public, our efforts to do this have met with a great deal of frustration. In our efforts to educate, we have found that most physicians do not themselves understand what brain death is. It is not a simple issue and I personally lobbied our State Assembly, probably approaching more than half of 125 Assemblymen. I sat down and explained the issues so that most of them understood it. We had the votes, but we did not get the Bill passed at that session. By the time the session came around again, half of those legislators who had understood and supported the issues were voted out of office. There is a limit to the amount of time and energy that one or two or a group of people can put into this. It is also very difficult to raise money to try to support professional lobbyists and professional educators. Indeed, in our own transplant organization, we have had an incredibly difficult time in raising money to support such an effort. What you say is relevent but in our State the approach was unsuccessful.

KOREIN: I agree with you completely. This matter of education via the news media is one that I was quite interested in and several years ago was quite naive about. It turned out that on T.V. you are usually given up to three minutes to present your issue. I went through about 30 newspaper articles that misquoted me, and one word in four was wrong. The news media are often more interested in obtaining headlines and selling their publications than in informing the public. It is therefore very difficult to transmit information to the public via the media so that they comprehend the difference between a persistent vegetative state and brain death. I will give you one example. I saw an article in a newspaper with an atrocious headline which included the word, "euthanasia." The article itself was literate, but the headline irrelevant. I called up the newspaper and asked the editor how such a misleading headline could be put on the article. Then I found out that the way a newspaper operates, the person who writes the article has nothing to do with the headline. The article is written and then typeset, a space is left over it and there is an individual who makes titles. This person looks through the article, takes out the words that will fit in the space and at the same time will attract the most attention. He then puts the headline in. The headline may have no relationship to the information contained in the article itself. So the use of news media as an educational force must be considered in terms of its limitations.

BERESFORD: The medium is the message.

VEITH: Are the organized societies of neurosurgeons and neurologists behind the efforts to gain passage of a statutory definition of death in the states without it? Is there any effort on the part of those societies to make an impact on the AMA?

R. E. CRANFORD: I have been interested in this area for some time. I am now the new chairman of the ethics committee of the American Academy of Neurology. I made preliminary contact with the AMA, the American Association of Neurological Surgeons and the American Heart Association. What we are going to try to do, and Dr. Beresford is on our committee, is propose through the membership of the Academy a strongly worded resolution on brain death legislation which opposes the position of the American Medical Association. The AMA just recently came out with an opinion from their general counsel. They were strongly against the idea of legislation to legalize brain death criteria. There are two ways to approach this problem. The AMA, the AANS, the AAN and the American Heart Association have formed an interagency committee on Brain death and irreversible coma. This has been a low-profile committee that has tried to draw up uniform brain-death criteria totally apart from the idea of brain-death legislation. These criteria have gone through numerous revisions. They have not been accepted by the member organizations as yet. I think that working through this interagency committee is another way of countering the AMA position. The AMA is now trying to get the ABA to change *their* position. Likewise, the ABA is trying to get the AMA to change their position. I think the AMA is absolutely and totally wrong. It is extremely detrimental to the position of the medical profession. Another approach to the problem is through the state medical associations. We could ask each state medical association to poll their delegates to the AMA convention on this matter. I am also chairman of an ad hoc committee on death of the Minnesota State Medical Association. We have sponsored brain-death legislation in Minnesota.

Another thing that we did at the state level was to draw up uniform brain-death criteria. These criteria have nothing to do with legislation, and have been accepted as official policy of the State Medical Association in Minnesota. This can be used as a basis for an accepted standard of medical practice. This might be done state by state, thereby altering the stance of the AMA. This effort has already begun. Dr. Beresford and I may present a report of our progress at the next AAN meeting and then continue to work with other groups. This may take a year and a half or longer, depending upon the opposition we may face. This summarizes our dual approach to obtaining brain-death legislation.

Index of Contributors

(Italicized page numbers refer to comments made in discussion.)

443

Subject Index

Organ transplantation, 30–31
  anencephalic donors, 141–142
  apallic syndrome and, 210
  ethical issues in, 41–42, 396–397
  "extraordinary care" and, 33
  hypotension and, 64
  legal barriers to, 45–50
  problems of supply, 47
  role of ICUs in, 411–412
  statutes on, 45–49, 423–425
  See also Uniform Anatomical Gift Act
Orthodox Jewish law, *see* Jewish law
Oregon, 1975 statute in, 51, 429
Oxidative metabolism
  of brain, 97–98
  experimental study, 98–103
Oxygen uptake in disconnecting tests, 246

Pancuronium bromide in determining
    ECS, 408
Parental decisions in termination of treat-
    ment, 344–345
Pathology of brain death, 272–279
Patient consent, experimentation and, 360
Patients' rights, 41
  termination of treatment and, 53–56,
    328, 341, 378–379, 382
People v. Flores, 351
People v. Lyons, 370–371, 427
Perioral facial reflex, *see* Snout reflex
Persistent vegetative state
  defined, 8–9, 219–222
  neocortical death and, 8, 21, 27, 160
  proposed statute on, 355–356
  term discussed, 224–225
  See also Quinlan case
Pharyngeal reflex
  cardiac arrest with, 88
  as criteria for brain death, 71, 74, 75,
    80, 83, 85
  in survivors, 80, 93
Physicians
  California Natural Death Act and,
    382–383, 391–393
  euthanasia, 369, 373–374
  needs of terminally ill and, 377
  social attitudes towards, 323–326
  statutory definition of death and, 424–
    425
  termination of treatment and, 341–342,
    344, 345
Pius XII, proclamation of, 28–29
Plantar responses as criteria in brain
    death, 71, 84, 85, 91–92

Posterior fossa
  circulation in, 174, 178, 180–181
  EEG and lesions in, 130
  exclusion of, in bolus technique, 145
  in respirator brain, 276–277
Postmortem autolysis, biochemical changes
    in, 276–277
Primary diagnoses, correlation with EEG,
    113, 114
Privacy, right to, 378
"Prolongation of Life, The" (Pius XII),
    28–29
Protestant thought, accord of brain death
    concept with, 423
"Pseudocoma," 220–222
"Pseudo-isoeletric" EEG, 122–123
Psychological problems, related to coma,
    413
Pulmonary insufficiency, disconnecting
    test with, 263
Pupillary fixation, in comatose patients,
    216–217
Pupillary reflex
  in apallic syndrome, 201
  in cardiac arrest, 88
  in coma, 219–220
  as criteria in brain death, 71, 74, 75,
    82–87
  in presumed brain death, 91–93
Pupil size
  with cardiac arrest, 88, 93
  in presumed brain death, 90–91, 93,
    215
PVO_2, in determining brain death, 238
PVS, apallic syndrome and, 9

Quinlan case, 52, 320–321, 334–341, 425
  termination of treatment and, 346–347

Radial reflexes as criteria of brain
    death, 71, 85
Radioactive tracers
  in evaluating cerebral circulation, 143–
    163
  ^{133}Xe isotope technique, 185, 203, 205
  See also Bolus technique
Radioisotopic bolus technique, 31, 130
  medical ethics and, 395
  See also Bolus technique
Reginia v. Potter, 351
Regional brain glucose metabolism, 106

Religious attitudes
  history of, towards death, 11–14
  toward identification of person with
    brain death, 42–43
REM sleep, 218–219
Research, *see* Human experimentation
Respiration
  in coma, 219
  in survivors, 77, 78, 80
  See also Spontaneous respiration
Respirator brain, 9, 87, 89, 275–278
Respiratory pattern in vegetative state,
  298
Resuscitation
  after cardiac arrest, 281, 284–290
  quality of survival after, 283, 287–288
  stages after, 287–289
Reticular formation lesions, 105–107
Reye's syndrome, 410
Rheoencephalography, 234, 238
RISA, spinal injection of, to determine
  brain death, 236
Roman Catholic ethics, accord of brain
  death concept with, 422–423
Rostral reorganization, 107, 108
Rostral reticular formation lesions, 106

Scavenger cells, in patients with defec-
  tively perfused brains, 270
Seizures, treatment of, 410–411
Simultaneous bilateral reticular formation
  lesions, 106
Skeletal muscle tone, in vegetative state,
  295, 299
Sleep, 218–219
Slow-wave sleep, 218–219
"Small" bolus, 214
Smith v. Smith, 426
Snout reflex
  cardiac arrest with, 88
  as criteria of brain death, 71, 73–75,
    79–80, 82–83, 85, 91
  in normal subjects, 87
Social interaction, loss of capacity for
  as definition of death, 312, 314
Soul, loss of, as definition of death, 309–
  310
Spinal cord
  with absence of bolus, 267
  in respirator brain, 272–273
Spinal reflexes, 10, 85, 86, 418–419
  in apallic syndrome, 201
  defined, 10
  as discrimination indices, 74–76, 84, 91,
    218
  ECS and, 73–74, 115

  in locked-in syndrome, 225–227
  in survivors, 81–83
Spindle activity, in EEG, 408, 410, 411
Spontaneous eye movements, in vegetative
  state, 295, 298
Spontaneous hypothermia, apnea and, 241
Spontaneous movement
  with cardiac arrest, 88
  as criteria in brain death, 71–72, 75,
    84–87, 92
  with ECS, 74, 115
Spontaneous respiration
  in biblical sources, 421
  in comatose patients, 217
  in presumptive brain death, 83, 84,
    215–216
  testing for, 413
State v. Brown, 426
Statutory "conscience clause," 356–357
Statutory definitions of death, 50–52, 363
  American Bar Association (1975), 51,
    356, 365–366
  California (1974), 354
  Capron-Kass model statute (1972), 51,
    349, 354, 361
  degree of specificity in, 352
  euthanasia and, 354
  Georgia (1976), 51, 354
  Idaho (1977), 354
  Kansas (1970), 50, 51, 349, 353, 354
  Maryland (1972), 349
  medical opposition to, 350, 353
  North Carolina (1977), 357
  Oklahoma, 51
  Oregon (1975), 51
  scientific basis for, 353
  uniformity in, 352–353, 357
  See also Case law
Steady potentials, in diagnosing brain
  death, 235–236
Stroke, ICUs and, 401, 403, 404
Subcortical activity, ECS and, 126–127
Succinylcholine, 406–408
Suicide
  euthanasia as, 369
  rejection of treatment and, 370
Suppression burst pattern, in EEG, 123
Survival, quality of, 287–289
Survivors, of presumptive brain death,
  76–83
Swallow reflex
  as criteria of brain death, 71, 74, 75,
    84, 85
  in survivors of presumptive brain death,
    80, 81, 93
Swedish criteria of brain death, 64, 66–67
Systemic death, defined, 6, 21